Suzanne Fisher

CRANIOSPINAL TRAUMA

TRAUMA MANAGEMENT
Volume V

Series Editors

F. William Blaisdell, M.D.
Professor and Chairman
Department of Surgery
University of California, Davis
Sacramento, California

Donald D. Trunkey, M.D.
Professor and Chairman
Department of Surgery
The Oregon Health Sciences University
Portland, Oregon

CRANIOSPINAL TRAUMA

Lawrence H. Pitts, M.D.
Professor and Vice-Chairman
Department of Neurosurgery
University of California, San Francisco
San Francisco, California

Franklin C. Wagner, Jr., M.D.
Professor and Chair
Department of Neurological Surgery
University of California, Davis
Sacramento, California

Joint Section on Neurotrauma and Critical Care
American Association of Neurological Surgeons
and the Congress of Neurological Surgeons

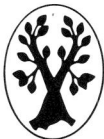

1990
Thieme Medical Publishers, Inc., NEW YORK
Georg Thieme Verlag, STUTTGART • NEW YORK

Thieme Medical Publishers, Inc.
381 Park Avenue South
New York, New York 10016

CRANIOSPINAL TRAUMA
Lawrence H. Pitts, Franklin C. Wagner, Jr.

Library of Congress Cataloging-in-Publication Data

Craniospinal trauma / [edited by] Lawrence H. Pitts, Franklin C.
 Wagner, Jr.
      p.   cm. — (Trauma management : v. 5)
    "Joint Section on Neurotrauma and Critical Care, American Association
 of Neurological Surgeons and the Congress of Neurological Surgeons."
    ISBN 0-86577-322-X
    1. Head—Wounds and injuries. 2. Spine—Wounds and injuries
 I. Pitts, Lawrence H. II. Wagner, Franklin C. III. Joint Section
 for Neurotrauma and Critical Care. IV. Series.
    [DNLM: 1. Brain Injuries 2. Spinal Cord Injuries. WO 700 T776
 1982 v. 5]
  RD529.C75   1990
  617.5'1044—dc20
  DNLM/DLC
  for Library of Congress   89-5239
                                            CIP

Important note: Medicine is an ever-changing science. Research and clinical experience are continually broadening our knowledge, in particular our knowledge of proper treatment and drug therapy. Insofar as this book mentions any dosage or applications, readers may rest assured that the authors, editors, and publishers have made every effort to ensure that such references are strictly in accordance with the state of knowledge at the time of production of the book. Nevertheless, every user is requested to carefully examine the manufacturers' leaflets accompanying each drug to check on his own responsibility whether the dosage schedules recommended therein or the contraindications stated by the manufacturers differ from the statements made in the present book. Such examination is particularly important with drugs that are either rarely used or have been newly released on the market.

Some of the product names, patents, and registered designs referred to in this book are in fact registered trademarks or proprietary names even though specific reference to this fact is not always made in the text. Therefore, the appearance of a name without designation as proprietary is not to be construed as a representation by the publisher that it is in the public domain.

Printed in the United States of America.

5   4   3   2   1

TMP ISBN 0-86577-322-X
GTV ISBN 3-13-741601-9

Contents

Continued

v

Contributors

E. Francois Aldrich, M.D.
Assistant Professor
Division of Neurosurgery
The University of Texas Medical Branch
Galveston, Texas

Brian T. Andrews, M.D.
Assistant Chief
Neurological Surgery Service
San Francisco General Hospital
San Francisco, California

Nicholas M. Barbaro, M.D.
Assistant Professor
Department of Neurosurgery
University of California, San Francisco
San Francisco, California

Sheldon Berrol, M.D.
Associate Professor
Physical Medicine and Rehabilitation
  Services
San Francisco General Hospital, and
University of California, San Francisco
San Francisco, California

Rebecca P. Brightman, M.D.
Division of Neurosurgery
The Ohio State University
Columbus, Ohio

Ralph G. Dacey, M.D.
Professor
Division of Neurosurgery
University of North Carolina at Chapel Hill
Chapel Hill, North Carolina

Paul J. Donald, M.D., F.R.C.S. (C)
Professor
Department of Otolaryngology/Head & Neck
  Surgery
University of California, Davis
Sacramento, California

Howard M. Eisenberg, M.D.
Professor
Division of Neurosurgery
The University of Texas Medical Branch
Galveston, Texas

Thomas A. Gennarelli, M.D.
Associate Professor
Division of Neurosurgery
University of Pennsylvania
Philadelphia, Pennsylvania

Steven L. Giannotta, M.D.
Associate Professor
University of Southern California School of
  Medicine
Department of Neurosurgery
Los Angeles, California

Mark N. Hadley, M.D.
Department of Neurological Surgery
Barrow Neurological Institute
Phoenix, Arizona

Bryan Jennett, M.D., F.R.C.S.
Institute of Neurological Sciences
University of Glasgow
Glasgow, Scotland, and
King's Fund Institute
London, England

Sanford J. Larson, M.D., Ph.D.
Professor and Chairman
Department of Neurosurgery
Medical College of Wisconsin, and V.A.
  Medical Center
Milwaukee, Wisconsin

Lawrence F. Marshall, M.D.
Professor of Surgery/Neurosurgery
Division of Neurological Surgery
University of California Medical Center
San Diego, California

Carole A. Miller, M.D.
Associate Professor
Division of Neurosurgery
The Ohio State University
Columbus, Ohio

Raj K. Narayan, M.D.
Associate Professor
Department of Neurosurgery
Baylor College of Medicine
Houston, Texas

Lawrence H. Pitts, M.D.
Professor and Vice-Chairman
Department of Neurosurgery
University of California, San Francisco, and
Chief of Neurosurgery
San Francisco General Hospital
San Francisco, California

Jeffrey Robinson, M.D.
Assistant Professor
University of Duneeden Medical School
South Island, New Zealand

Michael J. Rosner, M.D.
Professor
Division of Neurosurgery
University of Alabama at Birmingham
Birmingham, Alabama

Michael C. Rowbotham, M.D.
Clinical Instructor of Neurology
Department of Neurology
University of California, San Francisco
San Francisco, California

Thomas G. Saul, M.D.
Mayfield Neurological Institute
Director of the Neurological Intensive Care
    Unit
Good Samaritan Hospital
Associate Professor of Clinical Neurosurgery
Unversity of Cincinnati Medical Center
Cincinnati, Ohio

Richard K. Simpson, Jr., M.D., Ph.D.
Professor
Department of Neurosurgery
Baylor College of Medicine
Houston, Texas

Donald S. Soloniuk, M.D.
Assistant Professor
Department of Neurosurgery
State University of New York at Buffalo
Buffalo, New York

Volker K.H. Sonntag, M.D.
Department of Neurological Surgery
Barrow Neurological Institute
Phoenix, Arizona

George W. Sypert, M.D.
Professor
Department of Neurosurgery
University of Florida Health Center
Gainesville, Florida

Benjamin H. Venger, M.D.
Professor
Department of Neurosurgery
Baylor College of Medicine
Houston, Texas

Dennis G. Vollmer, M.D.
Assistant Professor
Division of Neurosurgery
University of North Carolina at Chapel Hill
Chapel Hill, North Carolina

Franklin C. Wagner, Jr., M.D.
Professor and Chair
Department of Neurological Surgery
University of California, Davis
Sacramento, California

John D. Ward, M.D.
Professor
Division of Neurosurgery
Department of Surgery
Medical College of Virginia
Virginia Commonwealth University
Richmond, Virginia

Chi-Shing Zee, M.D.
Associate Professor
University of Southern California School of
    Medicine
Department of Radiology
Los Angeles, California

Foreword

Although its importance has long been appreciated by neurosurgeons, neurotrauma has recently become more widely recognized by trauma surgeons as the most important single factor in the outcome of the injured patient. Head injury, in particular, is now recognized as the single largest cause of death and persistent disability after injury. Therefore, Drs. Pitts and Wagner, in conjunction with the Joint Section on Neurotrauma and Critical Care of the American Association of Neurological Surgeons and the Congress of Neurological Surgeons, provide in this volume a comprehensive review of the state of the art of neurotrauma care. Because a head injury occurs every 7 seconds in the United States, surgeons who deal with trauma will be confronted with neurotrauma almost every day. The principles outlined in this volume can be used by neurosurgeons and non-neurosurgeons to develop a system for the rapid and efficient evaluation and management of the neurotrauma patient. Hopefully, these principles will be integrated into the overall trauma care systems that are crucial to the outcome of all injured patients. The authors and the editors of this volume have provided a major service to the injured patient and are due congratulations from the trauma care community.

Thomas A. Gennarelli, M.D.

Preface

We are very proud of the material put together by Drs. Pitts and Wagner regarding *Craniospinal Trauma*. As trauma care progresses with the organization of trauma systems ensuring prompt delivery of critically-injured patients to those centers best capable of managing them, more and more patients survive. It is apparent that as our ability to control life-threatening torso trama and internal and external hemorrhage increases, we are still left with unsolved problems related to central nervous system trauma.

Head injury alone now accounts for the majority of deaths in any trauma program. Central nervous system trauma, whether it be head injury or spinal cord injury, constitutes far and away the commonest cause of late morbidity and permanent disability.

The prompt application of principles outlined in this book should result in significant improvement on this mortality and morbidity. Nonetheless, we still have a long way to go. We congratulate the authors on a job well done.

F. William Blaisdell, M.D.
Donald D. Trunkey, M.D.

Acknowledgments

The editors wish to express their gratitude to the many individuals who have helped make this volume a reality. We appreciate the permission of the Board of Directors of the American Association of Neurological Surgeons and the Executive Committee of the Congress of Neurological Surgeons to allow the Joint Section on Neurotrauma and Critical Care to present this work. We understand that there are a number of acceptable techniques and management schemes in caring for patients with craniospinal trauma. We are most grateful for the able assistance of an Editorial Board who reviewed the individual chapters and made suggestions to ensure the broadest possible acceptance of this material. We would like to thank Drs. Brian Andrews, Raj Narayan, Ralph Wicker and Harold Wilkinson for their help. We also would like to thank Ms. Shirley Hamilton, Ms. Sue Stevenson, and Ms. Cheri Albericci for their help in processing the manuscripts, and Ms. Jennifer Pitts for manuscript editing. We also appreciate the considerable help of the editorial and production staff of Thieme Medical Publishers, who have been invaluable in seeing this book to completion. Finally, we are most grateful to the many authors who have given their time and their ideas to the treatment of craniospinal trauma to help neurosurgeons and trauma surgeons optimally manage nervous system injury.

Lawrence H. Pitts, M.D.
Franklin C. Wagner, Jr., M.D.

Historical Development of Head Injury Care

BRYAN JENNETT

Neurosurgery began with the treatment of head injuries. Compound depressed fractures due to arrows have been preserved from the Chinese dynasties, and trephine openings to evacuate traumatic clots with evidence of healing and therefore of survival have been found in many remains from the Incas onward. Hippocrates classified head injuries and recommended trephining for some; he coined the aphorism that no head injury is too trivial to ignore nor too serious to despair of. More than a millennium later, Macewen of Glasgow was pioneering elective intracranial surgery based on deductions from recent knowledge of cerebral localization.[12] This was in the 1870s, years before x-rays were discovered and when Harvey Cushing was still a schoolboy. Macewen worked for a time as casualty surgeon to the Central Police Division in Glasgow, one of the roughest of Victorian cities. One article from this period discussed the distinction between traumatic and alcoholic pupillary abnormalities. Another reported how the observation of focal epilepsy led to the detection and localization of complications at a distance from the site of trauma to the head; he described first an abscess and then a subdural hematoma—the latter successfully removed. A link between his era and ours is a patient who more than half a century after being operated on by Macewen came to our clinic at the Institute in Glasgow where a computed tomography (CT) scan showed the bone defect resulting from Macewen's surgery.

LESSONS FROM 20TH CENTURY WARS

War provides an opportunity for surgeons to learn about trauma. When Cushing came to Europe for World War I, he found that no less than 60% of deaths after dural penetration were due to sepsis. He maintained that many were avoidable if delay in debridement could be reduced, and by the end of that conflict he had reduced mortality from 54 to 29%.[6] Neurosurgical services for the British army in World War II were organized by Cairns, who had been a resident with Cushing. In order to minimize the delay that Cushing had warned about, Cairns set up mobile neurosurgical units, each staffed by a neurosurgeon, a neurologist, and an anesthetist.[4] He was fortunate to have the opportunity of making the first tests with penicillin, which marked the beginning of a new era in the treatment of war wounds. Many soldier-surgeons later became academics, but Cairns was already Professor of Surgery at Oxford before he became a Brigadier. He imposed on his medical officers the academic discipline of careful note-taking from the time of first medical contact in the field. This provided data not only for accurate correlation of the severity and type of injury with the immediate outcome, but also for research on the sequelae of head injury that continued for 20 years or more. The base hospital that he set up in Oxford admitted injured men a few days after their surgery near the front, thanks to the development of air evacuation. This hospital remained until the mid-1950s and several of us who were too young for the war served our National Service there and the experience led to our having a lifelong interest in head injuries.

The Korean conflict saw the further development of Mobile Army Surgical Hospitals (MASH) near the front with early helicopter evacuation to base hospitals. Yet the lesson that delay leads to high infection rates, even when antibiotics have been given prophylactically, had to be learned yet again. Early in that campaign the infection rate was 41%, but it had fallen to 1% by the end.[31] Vietnam saw even more rapid evacuation of casualties to surgical facilities, which were often reached within an hour or less, and almost always within 6 hours. One consequence was that the mortality rate increased as casualties who in previous wars would have died on the battlefield now reached a hospital. However, most of the cases were irrecoverable and triage determined that many of these died without surgery. Such deaths accounted for 20% of admissions, whereas of 1455 who were operated on only 9% died in the hospital, the rate for those who were not in coma being only 3%.[11] Several of these lessons of war have had to be learned over again by surgeons dealing with head injuries in civilian life—in particular the importance of organization to minimize delay before injured patients reach a specialist, and the importance of triage.

THE LAST 30 YEARS IN CIVILIAN LIFE

Since World War II, there have been two major developments in the management of head injuries. In 1958 a neurosurgeon, an otolaryngologist, and an anesthetist from Newcastle in England reported improved survival after severe injuries as a result of what later came to be known as intensive care. Their regimen involved frequent use of tracheostomy and they also recommended drugs that reduced spasticity and facilitated the control of increased body temperature.[27] Since then, there has been a mushrooming of intensive care units, from almost zero to 50,000 in the United States between 1960 and 1980. The main impetus was that mechanical ventilators became available in more and more hospitals, and this brought anesthetists on the scene as major actors in the management of severe head injuries. They have developed regimens of intensive medical therapy for severe head injuries in collaboration with neurosurgeons. It became clear that only a small minority of patients with head injuries ever need surgery, whether they are mild or severe. Consequently most head injuries, especially the less severe injuries, are now looked after by disciplines other than neurosurgery. In the United States, however, where there are a large number of neurosurgeons, most head trauma is managed by them.

The other dramatic advance has been CT scanning. When this became available in the mid 1970s, it did away with amateur angiograms in the middle of the night and it put an end to the woodpecker surgery of exploratory burr holes for patients suspected of harboring a life-threatening hematoma (see Editors' note). As scanning became more widely used, it was realized that significant hematomas could be detected in patients who had not yet developed the clinical features of cerebral compression, and earlier intervention became possible. Scanning has also taught us much about the nature of the lesions that are associated with less severe injuries that seldom come to autopsy—on which we had previously relied for data about pathologic aspects of head injury. Magnetic resonance imaging is extending that knowledge still further by revealing lesions that were not shown on CT scans—in particular demonstrating how extensive brain damage can be in patients who by clinical standards have been only mildly injured.

The wide availability of CT scanning in the United States changed attitudes to the investigation and management of head injuries, both severe and mild. This has led to interest in the organization of care for head-injured patients in the hospital system as a whole, as distinct from what goes on in neurosurgical and intensive care units. This has brought actors onto the scene, in particular radiologists, trauma surgeons, and emergency room doctors. The demand for scanners to deal with head injuries in the acute stage was one factor that created a need for information about the scale of occurrence of these injuries, and epidemiologists on both sides of the Atlantic then came to recognize that head injury presents a major public health problem. At the same time, there has been an unprecedented period of interest on the part of a small group of pathologists and neurosurgeons in exploring human lesions at autopsy and in developing experimental models for head injury.

PATHOLOGY, HUMAN AND EXPERIMENTAL

The autopsy has traditionally been the source of knowledge about the damage sustained by the brain during and after head injury. Although new imaging techniques have given fresh insights, the interpretation of some of the radiologic findings has depended on recognizing during life lesions that had hitherto been known only after death. For many years, however, the literature on the pathologic aspects of head injury had been dominated by forensic pathologists whose accounts included much data based on the injured who had died at the scene of the accident. These account for only about half of all head injury deaths and the lesions found after such overwhelming injuries are often different in kind from those in patients who survive even 24 to 48 hours. However, attempts to undertake detailed neuropathologic examination of the brain after death in the hospital have been frustrated for years by the belief that the demand for an immediate report for legal purposes necessitated the slicing of the unfixed brain. Special arrangements with the legal authorities in Glasgow several years ago have allowed academic neuropathologists to receive uncut brains for prolonged fixation—an essential condition for carrying out detailed dissection and quantitative histologic examination. This has now been carried out on more than 600 brains by Adams et al.[1] who have mapped out the pattern of primary and secondary damage.

These studies have shown that obvious cortical contusions are a much less important form of primary damage than is diffuse axonal injury in the white matter, a lesion seldom detected without microscopy. It also became evident that the brainstem was not the main, and never the only, site of damage, although clinicians had for years been referring to comatose patients with extensor responses as having "brainstem injury." These studies also showed how frequent was secondary brain damage. Widespread hypoxic or ischemic lesions were found in 80 to 90% of hospital deaths with evidence of increased intracranial pressure (ICP) in 70% or more. The cause of the hypoxic brain damage was considered to be intracranial hypertension combined with arterial hypotension or reduced oxygen content of the blood. These systemic abnormalities commonly result from blood loss and respiratory insufficiency, usually a consequence of major extracranial injuries that are found in about a third of patients with severe head injuries. Another contribution of these clinicopathologic studies in Glasgow has been to identify how frequently patients "talk and die."[39] With this came the concept of avoidable factors contributing to death after head injury, the most common reason being delayed evacuation of an intracranial hematoma.[40]

Experimental primate studies by Gennarelli et al.[9] over the last 20 years have confirmed and extended the work of Russell and Denny-Brown at Oxford in the first years of World War II, who showed that brain damage was more extensive when the head of a monkey was free to move when struck.[7] Their findings also confirmed the predictions of the Oxford physicist Holbourn who in the 1940s experimented with gelatin models of the brain and simulated the shearing lesions of white matter that we now call diffuse axonal injury. From collaborative research by teams in Philadelphia and Glasgow, it appears that all the lesions found in man can be reproduced experimentally by varying the degree, duration, and direction of applied acceleration and deceleration forces.[9] There now seems no doubt that shearing forces acting on nerve fibers and blood vessels are the main mechanism for producing impact or primary damage. These experiments also show that axonal damage in continuity can occur; whether or not this progresses to a permanent lesion may depend on factors that might be influenced by pharmacologic interventions. This alters the philosophy of impact brain damage, which has hitherto been based on the assumption that damage is maximal at onset and is irreversible.

CLINICAL RESPONSE TO PATHOLOGIC DATA

The finding that many patients who died had hypoxic or ischemic brain damage and increased ICP seemed to explain the benefit claimed from intensive respiratory care and other medical measures. There followed several years of efforts to control ICP by steroid drugs, osmotic agents, and hyperventilation[3] to reduce the brain's metabolic rate by inducing general body hypothermia and by the use of depressant drugs.[28A] At the same time, there was an abundance of experimental work on intracranial pressure and cerebral blood flow using a number of models that were one step removed from trauma, lesions usually induced by ischemia or cold. Means of measuring ICP and cerebral blood flow were also used in intensive care units in academic centers.[28] Much of the data was confusing, however, with no consistent correlation between pressure, blood flow, and clinical outcome, except at the extremes of normality and abnormality.

It also came to be appreciated that most monitoring and therapeutic interventions involved some hazards and that it was uncertain whether the trade-offs in improved outcome justified some of the components of modern intensive care (often labeled "aggressive management"). It was tempting to assume that most severely injured patients who survived after such treatment would have died without it. In 1978, Langfitt[25] concluded that there was little evidence of a large decrease in head injury mortality over the previous 50 years. The validity of comparisons between series was, however, limited by the lack of an accepted measure of the severity of injury. It had long been recognized that deeper and more long-lasting coma, and injury in older patients, each produced higher mortality rates. Yet the course followed by individual patients often seemed capricious, with some patients who initially looked hopeless not only surviving but sometimes even making a reasonable recovery, whereas others whose impact injury had been less serious sometimes deteriorated and died.

It was this dilemma, in the context of the limited availability of expensive intensive care, that led the Glasgow neurosurgeons in 1968 to begin prospective data collection in severely injured patients. The specific intention was to develop prognostic criteria that might help with decision-making in the acute stage. This led to the development of the Glasgow Coma Scale, a simple descriptive and numerical means of classifying the responsiveness of patients with impaired consciousness,[43] and also of the Glasgow Outcome Scale.[16] Data collection was later extended to include two centers in the Netherlands and one in Los Angeles. This international trauma data bank defined "coma" as no eye opening, not obeying commands, and not uttering any understandable words. It also defined a head injury as "severe" only if coma lasted for at least 6 hours. Analysis of the first 700 severely head-injured patients revealed that the details of intensive therapy had differed considerably in the three countries (for example, the use of steroids, osmotics, controlled ventilation, and of tracheostomy). Despite this, the mortality and degree of recovery in survivors was strikingly similar in the three countries.[22] The mortality was about 50%, similar to that found in Langfitt's review of previously published series, albeit that severity was less well defined in these. It seemed that in many cases the outcome depended more on the degree of brain damage and the patient's age than on the details of treatment, and in 1976 we reported that a confident prediction of outcome at 6 months could be made within a few days of injury in about half the patients.[20]

These conclusions were confirmed by analysis of 1250 cases from the data bank[21] and again by comparison of more than 700 more recent cases from Glasgow with more than 400 from San Francisco.[13,36] Several reports from other places challenged these findings and claimed that by the use of various intensive therapeutic regimens the results could be improved.[3,28A,28,33] A recent critique of these conflicting reports has drawn attention to the pitfalls inherent in the evaluation of therapy for a life-threatening conditions such as severe head injuries.[35] Most variations in outcome can be explained by differing selection criteria for entry, often reflecting local features in the organization of care and methods of triage for severe injuries. When age and severity of injury are carefully accounted for, it proves possible to predict with considerable accuracy what the outcome will be.[13,20,21,36,37] The same was later found by Knaus for patients in general intensive care units in different parts of the United States,[23] and when patients in the United States were compared with those in France, where fewer interventions were undertaken.[24] The message of the international head injury study was sometimes misrepresented as indicating that treatment was of no value. In fact, all the cases in that study had been nursed in specialist intensive care units and had had the benefit of first class neurosurgical care, in particular the early detection and removal of intracranial hematomas.

MANAGEMENT OF INTRACRANIAL HEMATOMA

None of these activities in the last 30 years has altered the importance of ensuring that acute intracranial hematomas are detected and dealt with expeditiously. Policies directed to this end should mean that fewer patients would develop secondary brain damage that leads to death or permanent disability.[29] Such policies seem likely to make more impact on reducing mortality and morbidity from head injuries in patients who reach the hospital than other measures. Hopes ran high that the CT scanner would do much to this end—so effective was it in detecting hematomas. However, three neurosurgical centers in Britain reported no improvement in the outcome of head injury during the first 3 to 4 years after scanning became available. It became clear from the Glasgow study that the potential for benefit depended on organizational changes that would ensure that more patients at high risk of this complication, or suspected of already having developed it, were transferred early to centers able to provide not only scanning but skilled surgical intervention. Once transfer policies were changed, there were more patients scanned per year, more hematomas detected, and fewer patients in coma by the time of surgery; both mortality and morbidity from operated intracranial hematoma improved.[42]

Both CT scanners and neurosurgeons are much scarcer in Europe than in the United States, and they are largely located in regional units, making the issue of triage for scanning and for neurosurgical consultation more important than in the United States. Intracranial hematoma is an infrequent complication (1 in 6000 attenders at emergency departments and 1 in 900 of those admitted in Britain). It is therefore vital to identify as soon as possible which patients are at risk of developing this complication, particularly among those who are awake and talking because they might not be suspected of being at risk and therefore in need of further observation and investigation. Study of several thousand such patients in accident departments and general surgical wards in Scotland has shown that a fracture of the skull is a much more powerful predictor of hematoma than is altered consciousness, and patients who had recovered from briefly impaired consciousness and had no fracture were extremely unlikely to develop a clot.[32] On this basis, guidelines were agreed on nationally by neurosurgeons in Britain—for x-raying the skull in accident departments, for admission for further observation, and for CT scanning and neurosurgical consultation.[10] Where these have been applied, there has been a reduced admission rate for mild injuries at low risk, whereas the detection rate for hematomas has increased. The wide availability of CT scanners in the United States has reduced the use of plain radiographs of the skull, particularly when a CT scan seems indicated,[30,44] but that is not the case in Europe.[15]

RECOVERY AFTER HEAD INJURY: REHABILITATION

When the Newcastle team reported improved survival rates after severe head injuries in 1958, they stated that most survivors made a good physical and mental recovery and predicted that most would be fit to return to productive work.[27] Ten years later, reports were appearing that showed that several years after injury less than half such patients were working at all; many of those working were doing jobs of lower status than before the injury.

An English orthopedic surgeon reported in 1967 that 40% of 230 patients he treated were left disabled, and he coined the term "lamebrain."[26] An editorial questioned whether survival might not sometimes be more tragic than death and stressed the paucity of prognostic criteria to inform decision-making in the acute stage.[2] Noting the tendency to use overoptimistic terms to describe recovery associated with disability (satisfactory, practical, useful, worthwhile) Jennett and Bond[16] introduced the simple Glasgow Outcome Scale. This scale showed that 6 months after severe head injury only 40% of survivors had made a good recovery, 30% were moderate, 25% severely disabled, and 5% were vegetative.[22] Since the average age of disabled survivors is about 27 years, many of these patients face some 40 years of disability. The features of this disability have been extensively studied in the last decade and it is clear that the physical or neurologic sequelae are much less disabling than the mental, which include disorders of memory, behavior, cognitive function, and emotional control.[18] Relatives report serious personality change in most injured survivors and the burden of caring commonly results in family disruption. Psychologists have studied the nature of those deficits that can be measured by their tests and have been prominent in setting up numerous rehabilitation facilities, especially in the United States. There is some confusion between interventional treatment and the provision of continuing support, and there remains considerable controversy about the impact that different forms of therapy have on either the rate of recovery, the achieved level of function.[41] Most patients reach their final category on the Glasgow scale within 6 to 12 months.[18]

EPIDEMIOLOGY, PREVENTION, AND ORGANIZATION OF CARE

Accidents are now the leading cause of death under the age of 45 years in Western countries. Head injuries account for 70% of accidental deaths and for most of the persisting disability after trauma, being 10 to 40 times more common than spinal cord injury. Routinely collected statistics provide limited data that are most reliable about deaths. However, the last decade has seen large-scale surveys of patients in Scotland, in several areas of the United States, and in two Australian states.[8,17,45] Death rates from head injury per 100,000 vary from 9 for Britain to 25 for the United States to 28 for Australia. Ten times as many patients are admitted as die in the United States, but in Britain the ratio is 30 to 1; attenders at accident departments outnumber admissions by 5 to 1 in Britain, where they account for 10% of all patients coming to such departments.[17] Add to this the accumulation of disabled survivors with their long expectation of life, and the much larger number of patients having symptoms for a few weeks after mild injuries, and the scale and scope of the problem posed by head injuries becomes obvious. Less than 10% of patients admitted to the hospital have serious impairment of consciousness, yet about half of all the patients who eventually need neurosurgery and half of those who stay in the hospital for more than a month come from the large number whose initial injuries were mild or moderate.[34] This fact, together with recognition that paying so much attention to the most severe injuries has yielded only modest gains, is leading to increasing interest in milder injuries.

In regard to causation and prevention it is possible to overstate the importance of road accidents and the risk to vehicle occupants. Although road accidents are the most common single cause of severe and fatal injuries, they account for only 50 to 60% of these, and for a much smaller proportion of milder injuries.[19] Many accidents occur with pedestrians, especially in the young and the elderly, in whom falls are also common. Alcohol is an important element not only in road accidents (including pedestrians), but also in assaults and in falls. Preventive measures include control of drinking, improvements in vehicle and road engineering, and the use of seat belts and protective helmets.

Perhaps the main challenge for the health care system is to organize the management of the large numbers of mild head injuries that come to the hospital in such a way that the minority who are at risk from complications are identified and are appropriately dealt with.

In Britain many of these mild injuries are managed both in the emergency room and in the ward of first admission by doctors without training in neurosurgery. In the United States most patients hospitalized after head injury are cared for by neurosurgeons or surgeons with some trauma training. A variety of disciplines are involved in the care of head-injured patients according to local arrangements, including emergency physicians, general, orthopedic, or trauma surgeons, pediatricians, neurologists, and radiologists. The role of the neurosurgeon may be different in the United States than in Europe because of the large differences in the availability not only of neurosurgeons but of specialized diagnostic and therapeutic facilities.[15] These differentials have been estimated at seven times for neurosurgeons and ten times both for CT scanners and for intensive care beds. Although neurosurgeons outside the United States deal with only a small minority of the head-injured patients who are admitted to the hospital, they need to provide national and local leadership in devising policies of collaboration with other disciplines for the management of milder injuries.[14,19] These guidelines should include clear indications for investigations, for admission to the hospital, and for referral to specialist units such as those developed in Britain.[10] In the United States there is a strong trend toward more regional organization of facilities for trauma in general as well as for head injuries.[5,38] Services provided for head injuries in a community should be monitored by audits that record the number of cases attending, admitted, investigated, and treated in various ways, with the catchment population as the denominator. The number of patients who talk and die and the number of hematomas detected per year, together with the proportion of survivors who make a resonable recovery, can provide useful indicators of the quality of that service. Trauma registries, including these data, are mandated in trauma systems now being designed in the United States.

The specialty of neurosurgery can expect to prosper in the competitive field of health care only if it is seen to deal effectively with the major problems of the community within its area of expertise.[14] Neurosurgery seems likely therefore to need head injuries for its future welfare as much as head-injured patients need neurosurgeons for their best chance of survival and recovery.

EDITORS' NOTE: Although the vast majority of patients requiring operations for traumatic hematomas have CT scans before surgery, some surgeons have advocated diagnostic burr holes before CT scanning in patients who have signs of transtentorial herniation (Andrews) or who deteriorate abruptly and have signs of herniation (Rockswold) after head injury.

REFERENCES

1. Adams JH, Graham DI: An Introduction to Neuropathology. Edinburgh: Churchill Livingstone, 1988.
2. Anon: Severe head injuries. Lancet 1:514, 1968.
3. Becker DP, Miller JD, Ward JD, et al.: The outcome from severe head injury with early diagnosis and intensive management. J Neurosurg 47:491, 1977.
4. Cairns H: Neurosurgery in British Army 1939–1945. Br J Surg [War Surg Suppl] 1:9–26, 1947
5. California Association of Neurological Surgeons' Emergency Services Committee Report: Guidelines for Establishment of Trauma Centers. J Neurosurg 65:569, 1986.
6. Cushing H: A study of a series of wounds involving the brain and its enveloping structures. Br J Surg 5:558, 1918.

7. Denny-Brown D, Russell WR: Experimental cerebral concussion. Brain 64:93, 1941.
8. Frankowski RF, Annegers JF, Whitman S: The descriptive epidemiology of head trauma in US. In Becker DP, Povlishock JT (eds): Central Nervous System Status Report. Bethesda, MD: National Institutes of Health, 1985
9. Gennarelli TA, Thiebault LE, Adams JH, et al.: Diffuse axonal injury and traumatic coma in the primate. Ann Neurol 12:564, 1982.
10. Guidelines for initial management after head injury in adults. Br Med J 288:983, 1984.
11. Hammon WM: Analysis of 2187 consecutive penetrating wounds of the brain from Vietnam. J Neurosurg 34:127, 1971.
12. Jennett B: Sir William Macewen 1848–1924: Pioneer Scottish neurosurgeon. Surg Neurol 6:57, 1976.
13. Jennett B: Outcome of intensive therapy for severe head injuries: An inter-center comparison. In: Parillo JE, Ayres SM (eds): Major Issues in Critical Care Medicine. Baltimore: Williams & Wilkins, 1984.
14. Jennett B: The future role of neurosurgery in the care of head injuries. Neurosurg Rev 9:129, 1986.
15. Jennett B: Skull x-rays after mild head injuries. Arch Emerg Med 4:133, 1987.
16. Jennett B, Bond M: Assessment of outcome after severe brain damage. A practical scale. Lancet 1:480, 1975.
17. Jennett B, MacMillan R: Epidemiology of head injury. Br Med J 282:101, 1981.
18. Jennett B, Snoek J, Bond MR et al: Disability after severe head injury. J Neurol Neurosurg Psychiatry 44:285, 1981.
19. Jennett B, Teasdale G: Management of Head Injuries. Philadelphia: FA Davis, 1981.
20. Jennett B, Teasdale G, Braakman R, et al.: Predicting outcome in individual patients after severe head injury. Lancet 1:1031, 1976.
21. Jennett B, Teasdale G, Fry J, et al.: Treatment for severe head injury. J Neurol Neurosurg Psychiatry 43:289, 1980.
22. Jennett B, Teasdale G, Galbraith S, et al.: Severe head injuries in three countries. J Neurol Neurosurg Psychiatry 40:291, 1977.
23. Knaus WA, Draper EA, Wagner DP, et al.: Evaluation outcome from intensive care: A preliminary multihospital comparison. Crit Care Med 10:491, 1982.
24. Knaus WA. Wagner DP, Loirat P, et al.: A comparison of intensive care in the USA and France. Lancet 2:642, 1982.
25. Langfitt TW: Measuring the outcome from head injuries. J Neurosurg 48:673, 1978.
26. London PS: Some observations on the course of events after severe injury of the head. Ann R Coll Surg Engl 41:460, 1967.
27. MacIver IN, Frew JC, Matheson JG: The role of respiratory insufficiency in the mortality of severe head injuries. Lancet 1:390, 1958.
28. Marshall LF, Smith RW, Shapiro HM: The outcome with aggressive treatment in severe head injuries. Part I: The significance of intracranial pressure monitoring. Neurosurgery 50:20–25, 1979.
28A. Marshall LF, Smith RW, Shapiro HM: The outcome with aggressive treatment in severe head injuries. Part II: Acute and chronic barbiturate administration in the management of head injury. Neurosurgery 50:26–30, 1979.
29. Marshall LF, Toole BM, Bowers SA: The National Traumatic Coma Data Bank. Part 2: Patients who talk and deteriorate: Implications for treatment. J Neurosurg 59:285, 1983.
30. Masters SJ, McClean PM, Arcarese JS, et al.: Skull x-ray examinations after head trauma: Recommendations by a multidisciplinary panel and validation study. N Engl J Med 316:84, 1987.
31. Meirowsky AM: Neurological surgery of trauma. Washington, DC: US Government Printing Office, 1965.
32. Mendelow AD, Teasdale G, Jennett B, et al.: Risks of intracranial haematoma in head injured adults. Br Med J 287:1173 1983.
33. Miller JD, Butterworth JF, Gudeman SK, et al.: Further experience in the management of severe head injury. J Neurosurg 54:289, 1981.
34. Miller JD, Jones PA: The work of a regional head injury service. Lancet 1:1141, 1985.
35. Miller JD, Teasdale GM: Clinical trials for assessing treatment for severe head injury. In Becker DP, Povlishock JT (eds): Central Nervous System Status Report. Bethesda, MD: National Institutes of Health, 1985.
36. Murray GD: Use of an international data bank to compare outcome following severe head injury in different centres. Stat Med 5:103, 1986.
37. Murray GD, Murray LS, Barlow P, et al.: Assessing the performance and clinical impact of a computerised prognostic system in severe head injury. Stat Med 6:403, 1986.
38. Planning neurotrauma care. Appendix I to the Hospital Resources Document. Bull Am Coll Surg 71:22, 1986.
39. Reilly PL, Graham DI, Adams H, et al.: Patients with head injury who talk and die. Lancet 2:375, 1975.
40. Rose J, Valtonen S, Jennett B: Avoidable factors contributing to death after head injury. Br Med J 2:615, 1977.
41. Rosenthal M, Griffiths ER, Bond MR, et al.: Rehabilitation of the Head Injured Adult. Philadelphia: FA Davis, 1983.

42. Teasdale G, Galbraith S, Murray L, et al.: Management of traumatic intracranial haematoma. Br Med J 285:1695, 1982.

43. Teasdale G, Jennett B: Assessment of coma and impaired consciousness. A practical scale. Lancet 2:81, 1974.

44. Thornbury JR, Masters SJ, Campbell JA: Imaging recommendations for head trauma: A new comprehensive strategy. AJR 149:781, 1987.

45. Trauma Subcommittee of the Neurosurgical Society of Australasia: Neurotrauma in Australia (Report on Surveys), Aust N Z J Surg Suppl 1986.

2

Initial Assessment and Management of Head Injury

THOMAS A. GENNARELLI

Because a head injury occurs every 7 seconds, and a patient dies of a head injury every 5 minutes, a neurosurgeon who deals with trauma is confronted with a head-injured patient almost every day. Approximately 60% of all trauma deaths are associated with head injury, and more than 70% of vehicular trauma deaths are due to head injury. Because of the immense importance of neurotrauma,[1] it is necessary that the neurosurgeon develop an assessment plan that will yield the most useful information about the severity of injury, the potential for deterioration, the necessity for acute surgical intervention, and the prognosis. Most neurosurgeons are well aware of the basic principles of the initial assessment and management of the head-injured patient. However, since almost all head-injured patients will be seen first by physicians with little expertise in brain injury, it is crucial that the neurosurgeon educate these physicians so that they know what to look for and what to convey to the neurosurgeon. The purpose of this chapter is to provide one assessment plan that the neurosurgeon may use himself or use to educate non-neurosurgeons who deal with head-injured patients. In addition, this chapter is consistent with the American College of Surgeons Advanced Trauma Life Support (ATLS) course. More than 75,000 physicians have taken the ATLS course, so it is important that the neurosurgeon who has not been exposed to ATLS become familiar with its methods, as they relate to brain injury.

TYPES OF HEAD INJURY

After resuscitation of the trauma patient, the emergency management of the patient with a head injury is aimed at: (1) determining the severity of the brain injury; (2) establishing a specific anatomic diagnosis of the head injury; (3) assuring the metabolic needs of the brain; and (4) preventing secondary brain damage from treatable causes of cerebral injury. The non-neurosurgeon must develop a working understanding of the types of brain injury and their relative importance because, as he and the neurosurgeon begin to evaluate the patient, their first priority is to identify those patients who require potentially lifesaving surgical procedures. To do so, a rudimentary knowledge of the types of head injury is needed.[3]

Head injuries include: skull fractures, diffuse brain injuries, and focal injuries. The latter two are often called closed head injuries to distinguish them from open head injuries caused by impalement and missile injuries. The pathophysiology, severity, need for urgent treatment, and outcome is different in each group. A review of these head injuries will aid and help simplify the initial diagnosis.

Skull Fractures

Skull fractures are common, but do not, by themselves, cause neurologic disability. Many severe brain injuries occur without skull fracture, and many skull fractures are not associated with severe brain injury. Although identifying a skull fracture is important, diagnosing a brain injury does not depend on it. Searching for a skull fracture should never delay patient management. Attention should be directed to the brain injury. The significance of a skull fracture is that it identifies the patient with a higher probability of having or developing an intracranial hematoma. For this reason, all patients with skull fractures should be admitted for observation. All patients with skull fractures require neurosurgical consultation.

Vault Fractures

Fractures of the cranial vault can be linear or stellate, but they require no particular treatment. Instead, management is directed toward any underlying brain injury. Fractures across vascular arterial grooves or suture lines should raise suspicion of the possibility of epidural hemorrhage. It is important that the non-neurosurgeon understand that not all depressed skull fractures are neurosurgical emergencies. To reduce the risk of possible sequelae, such as a seizure disorder, any fragment depressed more than the thickness of the skull may require operative elevation of the bony fragment.

By definition, open skull fractures have a direct communication between a scalp laceration and the cerebral substance, because the dura is torn. This condition can be diagnosed if brain is visible or if cerebrospinal fluid (CSF) is leaking from the wound. Open fractures require early operative intervention, with elevation or removal of the fragments and closure of the dura. Compound fractures differ because the dura is intact. These fractures may require early operative intervention with elevation or removal of the fragments and exploration for tears of the dura.

Basal Skull Fractures

These fractures are often not apparent on skull films. They can be diagnosed indirectly by the presence of intracranial air or an opaque sphenoid sinus. The diagnosis is more often based on physical findings, such as CSF otorrhea or rhinorrhea. When CSF is mixed with blood, it may be difficult to detect. An aid is the "ring sign," detected by allowing a drop of the fluid to fall onto a piece of filter paper. If CSF is present, blood remains in the center, and one or more concentric rings of clearer fluid develop.

Hemotympanum or ecchymosis in the mastoid region (Battle's sign), or both, also indicate a basal skull fracture. Cribriform plate and orbital roof fractures are often associated with periorbital ecchymosis (raccoon eyes). These signs may take several hours to appear and may be absent immediately after injury. Whenever a frontal basal skull fracture is present, there is danger of passing a nasogastric tube into the brain and thus emergency room personnel should be discouraged from using the nasal route in such patients.

Diffuse Brain Injuries

Diffuse brain injuries are produced when rapid head motions (acceleration or deceleration) cause widespread interruption of brain function in most areas of the brain. Often, as with concussion, the disturbance of neural function is temporary. With more severe injuries (diffuse axonal injury [DAI]), microscopic structural damage throughout the brain may cause permanent deficits. It is important to try to distinguish these injuries from focal injuries, because diffuse brain injuries do not have mass lesions requiring emergency surgery.

Concussion

Concussion is brain injury accompanied by brief loss of neurologic function. In its more mild form, it may cause only confusion and amnesia. More commonly, concussion causes temporary loss of consciousness. The period of unconsciousness is usually short, but more severe forms exist. Many neurologic abnormalities may be described in the first few minutes after concussion, but these disappear quickly, usually before the patient gets to a medical facility. Therefore neurologic abnormality seen when the patient arrives at the hospital generally should not be attributed to a concussion.

Most patients with a concussion will be awake or awakening when seen in the emergency department, even though some mental confusion may persist. After the confusion clears, they may be able to describe portions of the accident, but do not remember the actual impact. They may complain of headaches, dizziness, or nausea, but the minineurologic examination will not show localizing signs. These patients should be observed in the hospital and then at home only if their mental state clears completely. Patients sustaining a severe concussion should be admitted for observation, because of the potential for associated serious brain injuries. The decision to admit the patient should be based on the length of unconsciousness and the reliability of the persons with whom the patient resides. A rule of thumb is that if a patient has been unconscious for 5 to 15 minutes, he should be observed in the hospital. The duration of amnesia or retrograde amnesia also must be considered. If the patient is under the age of 12 years, it is best to admit for observation. Any patient whose confusion does not clear completely must be admitted.

Diffuse Axonal Injury

DAI—often called brainstem contusion, closed head injury, or diffuse injury—is similar to severe concussion but is characterized by prolonged coma, often lasting days to weeks. DAI is a frequent injury, occurring in 40% of coma-producing head injuries. Overall mortality is 33% and, in its most severe form, DAI has a 50% mortality.[4] DAI results primarily in microscopic damage that is scattered widely throughout the brain and does not benefit from surgery. Although the length of coma cannot be determined in the emergency department, recognition of DAI is important because it may mimic other injuries that do require emergency surgery. The diagnosis is justified when an emergency computed tomography

(CT) scan shows no mass lesion in a patient who remains deeply comatose, often with extensor (decerebrate) or flexor (decorticate) posturing. Brain swelling, as part of DAI or due to superimposed hypoxia or ischemia, may also be present. Autonomic dysfunction producing high fever, hypertension, and sweating is common but may not occur acutely. It may be necessary or beneficial to transfer the patient to a facility equipped to care for long-term coma patients.

Focal Injuries

Focal injuries are those in which macroscopic damage occurs in a relatively local area. They consist of contusion, hemorrhages, and hematomas and may require emergency surgery because of their mass effects. Diagnosis during the early postinjury period is important because they are treatable and frequently require emergency operative intervention.

Contusion

Cerebral contusions can be single or multiple, small or large, and the patient may present in several ways. Most commonly, contusions are associated with serious concussions characterized by longer periods of coma and mental confusion or obtundation. Contusions can occur beneath an area of impact (coup contusions) or in areas remote from impact (contre-coup contusions); the tips of the frontal and temporal lobes are especially common sites. The contusion itself may produce a focal neurological deficit if it occurs near the sensory or motor areas of the brain, but a focal deficit may not be apparent if the contusion is elsewhere. If the contusion is large or associated with pericontusional edema, the mass effect may cause herniation and brainstem compression, resulting in secondary or delayed neurological deterioration.

Before the era of CT, contusions were diagnosed clinically in patients who were unconscious for long periods. Predictably, this practice resulted in many incorrect diagnoses. Today, a CT scan of the head will determine with certainty the presence, location, and size of contusions.

Patients sustaining cerebral contusion should be admitted to the hospital for observation because delayed edema or swelling around the contusion may cause neurologic deterioration. Contusions require surgery only if they cause substantial mass effect, but careful observation is necessary to detect patients with delayed bleeding into the contusion. This factor is especially important for patients with measurable blood ethanol levels, because acute or chronic alcohol abuse seems to produce a high incidence of delayed bleeding.

Intracranial Hemorrhages

Due to great variation in location, size, and rapidity of bleeding, there is no typical picture for intracranial hemorrhages. CT has made the diagnosis and localization very precise. It must be stressed that epidural hematoma and temporal lobe intracerebral hematoma can mimic each other, because the symptoms and the clinical findings are usually that of tentorial herniation.

Acute Epidural Hemorrhage.   Epidural bleeding almost always occurs from a tear in a dural artery, usually the middle meningeal artery. A small percentage may occur from a tear in a dural sinus. Although epidural hemorrhage is relatively rare (0.5% in unselected head injuries and 9% of coma-producing head injuries), it must always be considered because it may be rapidly fatal. Arterial tears are usually associated with linear skull fractures over the parietal or temporal areas that cross the grooves of the middle meningeal artery; however, fracture is not an absolute requirement for the diagnosis.

A typical course for an epidural hematoma is loss of consciousness (concussion) followed by an intervening lucid interval (the lucid period may not be a return to full consciousness) usually associated with a severe local headache. Secondary depression of consciousness follows and there generally is contralateral hemiparesis and ipsilateral pupillary dilation due to brainstem compression. Less frequently, the dilated, fixed pupil may be on the side opposite the hematoma or the hemiparesis may be on the same side as the hematoma.[9]

This injury requires immediate surgical intervention. If treated early, prognosis is usually excellent because the underlying brain injury is often not serious. Outcome is directly related to the status of the patient before surgery. For patients not in coma, the mortality from epidural hematoma approximates zero. For obtunded patients, mortality is 9%, and for patients in deep coma, it is 20%. Secondary brain injury will occur rapidly if the hematoma is not quickly evacuated.

Acute Subdural Hematoma.   Subdural hematomas are also life threatening and are much more common (30% of severe head injuries) than epidural hematomas. They most frequently occur from rupture of bridging veins between the cerebral cortex and dura, but also can be seen with lacerations of the brain or cortical arteries. A skull fracture may or may not be present. In addition to the problems caused by the mass of the subdural blood, underlying primary brain injury is often severe. The prognosis is often dismal, and the mortality remains 60%. However, recent studies demonstrate improved outcome if the hematoma is evacuated very early.[10]

Intracerebral Hematomas.   Hemorrhages within the brain substance can occur in any location. CT provides a precise diagnosis. Many small, deep intracerebral hemorrhages are associated with other brain injuries, especially severe DAI. Symptoms vary with the region or regions involved, the size of the hemorrhage, and whether or not bleeding continues.

Open Head Injuries

Impalement Injuries

Emergency room personnel should be instructed not to remove foreign bodies protruding from the skull. They should be left in place until they can be removed by a neurosurgeon in the operating room. Roentgenograms of the skull are required to determine the object's angle and depth of penetration.

Bullet Wounds

The larger the caliber and the higher the velocity of the bullet, the more likely death will occur. Through-and-through and side-to-side injuries, and those lower in the brain tend to be ominous. The outcome is related to the patient's condition. Patients in coma have a very high mortality. Skull films and a CT scan help plan the surgical approach when operation is deemed necessary. Entrance and exit wounds should be covered with antiseptic-soaked dressings until definitive neurosurgical care is provided. A bullet that does not penetrate the skull may still result in intracranial injury and such patients require a CT scan.

ASSESSMENT OF THE HEAD-INJURED PATIENT

Once the physician has a knowledge of the types of head injuries, he is in a position to collect the information that will be useful in making emergency management decisions.

History

It is important to determine the mechanism of injury, since many types of head injury are common or are rare in any given circumstance. The overall cause of injury is usually obvious, but knowing the mechanism is very useful. For example, simply knowing that the patient was injured in a fall instead of a vehicular crash quadruples that patient's risk of having an intracranial hematoma. Similarly, the incidence of severe diffuse brain injury is low in falls and assaults. More detailed information can often be helpful. For instance, belted and unbelted vehicle occupants and helmeted and unhelmeted motorcyclists are prone to develop very different head injuries.

Prehospital personnel should be instructed to record the circumstances of the traumatic events and to observe the neurologic status at the scene immediately after their arrival. Information obtained by ambulance personnel should be documented in writing and provided when the patient is delivered to the emergency department. It must be emphasized that the importance of initial assessment is that it provides the baseline for sequential reassessment, which is the critical basis for many subsequent decisions in management of the patient.

Because many factors influence the neurologic evaluation, documentation of the cardiorespiratory status must accompany the neurologic examination. Emergency resuscitation—airway, breathing, and circulatory control and management—takes priority. Systolic blood pressure less than 60 mmHg or systemic hypoxemia can alter cerebral function. Similarly, a drug screen for alcohol and other nervous system depressants should be obtained so that toxic factors that may influence head injury assessment are taken into account. The initial neurologic examination must consider these metabolic abnormalities.

Assessment of Vital Signs

Although brain injury may alter the vital signs, it is very difficult to be sure that changes in the vital signs are due to head injury and not to other factors. Some useful clinical rules include:

1. Never presume that brain injury is the cause of hypotension. Although bleeding from scalp lacerations can cause hemorrhagic shock, intracranial bleeding cannot produce shock, except in infants. Hypotension arising from brain injury is a terminal event, resulting from failure of the medullary center.
2. The combination of progressive hypertension associated with bradycardia and diminished respiratory rate (Cushing response) is a specific response to an acute and potentially lethal increase in intracranial pressure. In head injury, the cause is usually a lesion demanding immediate operative intervention.

Minineurologic Examination

A minineurologic examination is directed toward a rapid determination of the presence and severity of gross neurologic deficits, especially those that may require urgent operation. The American College of Surgeons ATLS course teaches the AVPU method of defining the global neurological state, which describes the patient's level of consciousness:

> A: Alert
> V: Responds to vocal stimuli
> P: Response to painful stimuli
> U: Unresponsive

The AVPU system is too crude for accurate sequential assessment, so a minineurologic examination should be taught to emergency department personnel and used by them repeatedly in any patient with a head injury. The examination assesses: level of consciousness, pupillary function, and lateralized extremity weakness. Generally, patients with abnormalities of all three components will have a mass lesion that may require surgery.

Level of Consciousness

The Glasglow Coma Scale (GCS) provides a quantitative measure of the patient's level of consciousness. The GCS is the sum of eye opening, verbal response, and best motor response. Each is graded separately and the total sum (3 to 15) is recorded.

Coma is defined as having no eye opening (eye score of 1), and not following commands (motor score less than 6), and no word verbalization (verbal score of 1 or 2). This means that all patients with a GCS less than 8 and most of those with a GCS of 8 are in coma. Patients with a GCS more than 8 are not in coma.

Assessment of Pupillary Function

The pupils are evaluated for their size, equality, and response to bright light. A difference in pupil diameters of more than 1 mm is abnormal. Even though eye injury may be present, intracranial injury must be excluded. Light reactivity must be evaluated for the briskness of response; a more sluggish response may be indicative of intracranial injury.

Lateralized Extremity Weakness

Spontaneous movements are observed for equality. If spontaneous motion is minimal, the response to a verbal or painful stimulus is assessed. A delay in onset of movement, less movement, or need for more stimulus on one side is significant. Often, the motor component of the GCS can be used to score the best and the worst extremity movement. A clearly lateralized weakness or asymmetric posturing suggests an intracranial mass lesion.

Purposes of Neurologic Examination

The minineurologic examination can help to determine the severity of the brain injury, and its sequential use will detect neurologic deterioration. The GCS has been used to categorize injuries as mild (13 to 15), moderate (GCS 9 to 12), and severe (3 to 8). In addition, irrespective of the GCS, a patient is considered to have a serious head injury if the patient exhibits any of the following:

1. Unequal pupils
2. Unequal motor examination
3. An open head injury with leaking cerebrospinal fluid or exposed brain tissue.
4. Neurologic deterioration
5. Depressed skull fracture

A reduction in the GCS score of 2 or more points clearly means the patient has deteriorated. A decrease of 3 or more points is a catastrophic deterioration that demands immediate treatment if the cause if remediable. However, these changes are rather gross and are often preceded by more subtle signs of deterioration. Neurologic deterioration includes any of the following:

1. Increase in severity of a headache or an extraordinarily severe headache
2. An increase in the size of one pupil
3. Development of weakness on one side
4. Increasing confusion or worsening level of consciousness

It cannot be overemphasized that the initial neurologic examination is only the beginning. The initial findings are only the reference with which to compare results of repeated neurologic examinations to determine whether a patient is deteriorating or improving. All previous efforts are wasted if signs of neurologic deterioration are not appreciated. The brain cannot withstand unrelieved compression for very long before brain damage is irreversible. The neurologic assessment is designed to detect this secondary brain damage so that timely treatment can be initiated.

Special Assessment

Skull Roentgenograms

Skull roentgenograms are of little value in the early management of patients with obvious head injuries, except in cases of penetrating injuries. The unconscious patient should have skull roentgenograms only if precise care of the cardiorespiratory system and continuing reassessment can be assured. Physical examination is usually more valuable than skull roentgenograms. For example, when there is a scalp laceration, a skull fracture can often be diagnosed by visual inspection or careful palpation with a gloved finger. Clinical signs of basal fractures are more useful than radiographs of the skull base in diagnosing fracture. For a patient with a minor head injury, skull roentgenograms may be recommended before considering the discharge of a patient from the emergency department.

Computed Tomography

The CT scan has revolutionized diagnosis in patients with head injuries and is the diagnostic procedure of choice for patients who have or are suspected of having a serious head injury. Although not perfect, the CT scan is capable of showing the exact location and size of most mass lesions. Specific diagnosis allows more precise planning of definitive care, including operation. The CT scan has supplanted less specific and more invasive tests, such as cerebral angiography.

Except for patients with trivial head injuries, all head-injured patients will require CT scanning at some time. The more serious the injury, the earlier and more emergent is the need for the scan. Consequently, injured patients seen first at facilities without CT capability may require transfer to a hospital with a scanner.

Once initial resuscitation has been undertaken and the need for a CT scan determined, care must be taken to maintain adequate resuscitation during the scan and assure the best possible quality of the scan. The patient must be attended constantly in the CT suite to monitor closely his vital signs and initiate immediate treatment should his status deteriorate.

Movement of the patient results in artifacts and a poor quality scan. This artifact may mask significant intracranial lesions requiring urgent surgical intervention. Movement artifact can be eliminated by sedating restless or uncooperative patients. However, extreme caution must be exercised to avoid sedating patients whose restlessness or "lack of cooperation" is a clinical manifestation of hypoxia. Often endotracheal intubation for controlled ventilation becomes necessary if the scan is considered mandatory and the patient can be rendered motionless only with paralyzing drugs.

Other Tests

Lumbar puncture, electroencephalogram, and isotope scanning have no role in the acute management of head trauma.

Brainstem reflexes can indicate the integrity of portions of several brainstem neural pathways. Although these may permit more specific diagnosis in some instances, their use can be hazardous, their interpretation difficult, and they add little to the emergency management of the patient. They are not recommended for the non-neurosurgeon.

The emergency room physician should complete these initial assessments and relay the following information to the neurosurgeon, who, in turn, must verify it and detect any changes that have occurred:

1. Age of patient and mechanism of injury
2. Respiratory and cardiovascular status
3. Results of the neurologic examination, especially the level of consciousness, the pupillary reactions, and the presence of lateralized extremity weakness
4. Presence and type of noncerebral injuries
5. The results of diagnostic studies, if obtained

EMERGENCY MANAGEMENT OF HEAD INJURIES

Establishing a Specific Diagnosis

The immediate purpose of a specific diagnosis is to determine which patients need an emergency or urgent neurosurgic operation.[5,7] Patients requiring emergency surgery are those with massive depressed or open skull fractures and those with a large focal mass lesion. The former category is usually obvious, but the latter must be distinguished from diffuse brain injuries where no mass lesion exists.

Rules of Thumb in Assessing the Need for Surgery

Injuries requiring surgery are likely to occur in different circumstances than injuries not requiring surgery. Therefore a gross estimate of a patient's potential need for surgery can be based on knowledge concerning three factors: whether the patient is comatose, whether the trauma was vehicular or nonvehicular, and whether there is a lateralized motor deficit (Table 2–1).

Thus, irrespective of the patient's clinical status, head injuries resulting from nonvehicular accidents are much more likely to require emergency surgery than vehicle occupants or pedestrians. Patients with injuries from falls and assaults develop focal mass lesions more frequently; vehicular injuries tend to produce greater numbers of diffuse brain injuries that do not require surgery. If all one knows is that the patient is comatose, has unequal movements, and was not a vehicle occupant or a pedestrian, the odds are at least four to one that he needs surgery. Although these guidelines cannot govern management of specific patients, they are extremely useful to remember.

Diagnostic Triage System

Based on the minineurologic examination, a practical and systematic approach can be established for diagnosing patients with head injuries. It must be understood that this scheme is only a guideline (Fig. 2–1). Because of the complexity and multiplicity of brain injuries, this system is not and cannot be either foolproof or all-inclusive. However, this system, offers one approach to determine not only the initial diagnosis, but also the severity of injury, so that emergency treatment decisions can be made.

The first priority is determining the level of consciousness, based on the GCS. If a patient has a score of less than 9, the physician must immediately determine whether the pupils are unequal or whether there is a lateralized motor deficit. If either of these exist, a large focal lesion (epidural, subdural, or intracerebral hematoma, or large contusion) must be presumed present. Preparation must be made for emergency operation to evacuate the lesion. Simultaneously, efforts must be taken to decrease the intracranial pressure (ICP). Presumptive evidence of a progressive lesion capable of producing lethal brain herniation (usually an epidural hematoma) is one of the few neurosurgical emergencies that may require operative intervention within minutes. The deterioration may be so rapid or the situation so desperate that burr hole decompression may be required before a CT scan is obtained.[2]

Table 2–1 Approximate Percent of Patients Potentially Requiring Surgery*

	MOTOR/PUPILS (%)			
	NOT IN COMA		COMATOSE	
	Equal	*Unequal*	*Equal*	*Unequal*
Vehicular	20	40[†]	20	30
Nonvehicular	40	70	60	80

*These percentages are, of course, very rough and exclude all patients with very minor injuries.
[†]Very few patients in this group.

LEVEL OF CONSCIOUSNESS
GCS · 9

HEAD INJURY
TRIAGE SCHEME

YES — PUPILS UNEQUAL OR LATERALIZED DEFICIT
NO — PUPILS UNEQUAL OR LATERALIZED DEFICIT

YES   NO   YES   NO

OPEN INJURY ?
YES   NO

NEUROLOGICALLY NORMAL ?
NO   YES

NO LOC, LOC·15MIN OR LOW RISK?
NO   YES

BEST DX:

LARGE MASS	DIFFUSE AXONAL INJURY	POSSIBLE MASS	BASILAR FX PENETRATING INJURY	CONTUSION SMALL MASS POST-CONCUSS	CONCUSSION FRACTURE	MINOR INJURY

ACTION:

ADMIT INTUBATE HV MANNITOL STAT CT OPERATE	ADMIT INTUBATE HV STAT CT ICU MONITOR	ADMIT URGENT CT ICU OBSERVE	ADMIT URGENT CT OBSERVE OR OPERATE	ADMIT ELECTIVE CT OBSERVE	ADMIT ELECTIVE CT OBSERVE	DISCHARGE WITH INSTRUCTION

NS:

STAT	STAT	URGENT	URGENT	URGENT	SELECTIVE	SELECTIVE

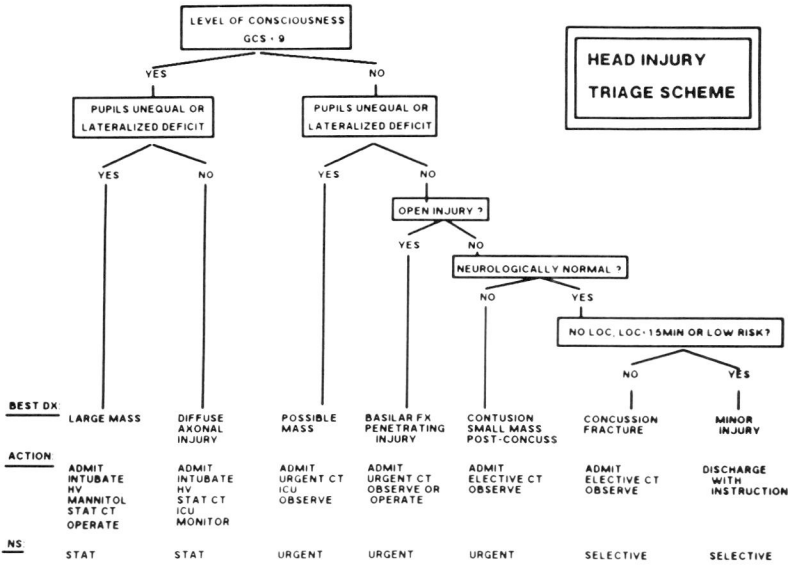

Figure 2–1. A diagnostic triage system for head injuries. CONCUSS: concussion; DX: diagnosis; FX: fracture; HV: hyperventilation; ICU: intensive care unit; LOC: loss of consciousness; NS: neurosurgery.

A comatose patient with equal pupils and motor responses may still have a surgical mass lesion but is more likely to have DAI, acute brain swelling, or cerebral ischemia. After immediate measures have been taken to reduce ICP, an emergency CT is needed to exclude a mass lesion.

A patient who is not comatose that is, (GCS more than 8) still may harbor an injury requiring operation. If pupillary asymmetry or lateralized weakness is present, the patient must be suspected of having a focal lesion that is not (yet) of sufficient size to compress the brainstem and cause coma. A CT scan is urgently required.

If the pupils and movements are equal, the presence or absence of an open head injury must be determined by searching for CSF leaking from the nose, ears, or a scalp wound. If there is no open injury (in the noncomatose patient who has equal pupils and movements), a complete neurologic examination must be performed. If the examination is not normal, a focal lesion must be excluded by CT scan. If the examination is normal, and the patient has been unconscious only briefly and is in the low-risk group[8] for an intracranial lesion (Table 2–2), discharge may be considered after appropriate instructions are given to the patient. If any of these conditions are not met, the patient should be admitted for postconcussion observation. A normal neurologic examination includes a normal mental status examination. No patient with signs of head injury should be discharged because he is intact "except for being intoxicated." Do not presume that altered mental status is due to alcohol. The patient should be observed until his mental status is completely normal, or he should be admitted for observation.

Table 2–2   Relative Risk of Intracranial Lesion

LOW RISK GROUP	MODERATE RISK GROUP	HIGH RISK GROUP
Asymptomatic	Change of consciousness	Depressed consciousness
Headache	Progressive headache	Focal signs
Dizziness	Alcohol or drug intoxication	Decreasing consciousness
Scalp hematoma	Unreliable history	Penetrating injury
Scalp laceration	Age > 2 years	Palpable, depressed fracture
Scalp contusion	Post-traumatic seizure	
Scalp abrasion	Vomiting	
Absence of moderate or high-risk criteria	Post-traumatic amnesia	
	Multiple trauma	
	Serious facial injury	
	Signs of basilar fracture	
	Possible skull penetration	
	Possible depressed fracture	
	Suspected child abuse	

Emergency Treatment

Once a working diagnosis is established, treatment must be commenced; urgency of treatment depends on the nature and severity of injury. Emergency treatment of the seriously injured patient is aimed at protecting the brain from further (secondary) insults by maintaining adequate cerebral perfusion and metabolism and preventing and treating intracranial hypertension.

Maintenance of Cerebral Metabolic Needs

Cerebral ischemia or hypoxia result in insufficient subtrate delivery to the injured brain. These conditions are present in more than 90% of patients who die from head trauma, are associated with poor outcome in survivors, and are the most important preventable complications of head injury.

The principal metabolic requirements of the brain are oxygen and glucose, which are normally used at extremely high rates. The injured brain usually has a lowered cerebral metabolism and therefore requires less oxygen and glucose. However, the damaged brain is more susceptible to the lack of these substrates, and thus temporary severe or prolonged moderate deprivation causes worse damage than in the uninjured brain. Therefore emergency management of head injury includes maintenance of adequate cerebral metabolic fuels.

The physician must assure delivery of adequate levels of glucose and oxygen to the brain. Delivery of these substrates depends on their arterial concentrations and the blood flow to the brain. Blood glucose concentration is not a common problem in trauma, but if it is, correction with supplemental intravenous glucose is needed.

Oxygen content depends on arterial hemoglobin and oxygen concentrations. Arterial oxygen concentration can be assessed with blood gases and supplemental oxygen delivered to maintain the arterial partial oxygen tension (PO_2) greater than 80 mmHg. Blood transfusion may be necessary to provide sufficient hemoglobin to maintain normal oxygen-carrying capacity. Cerebral blood flow is dependent on systemic arterial pressure and arterial partial carbon dioxide tension (PCO_2), especially shortly after head trauma. Normalization of blood pressure and maintenace of PCO_2 at greater than 25 mmHg is sufficient to maintain adequate cerebral blood flow under most circumstances.

Preventing or Treating Intracranial Hypertension

Induced Hypocapnia.   Arterial carbon dioxide concentration profoundly affects cerebral circulation. When abnormally elevated, cerebrovasodilation occurs, increasing intracranial blood volume and ICP. Conversely, reduction of PCO_2 reduces intracranial blood volume and, secondarily, ICP. Additionally, hyperventilation tends to reduce intracerebral acidosis and increase cerebral metabolism, both of which are beneficial. Therefore, hyperventilation is recommended to reduce arterial PCO_2, maintaining it at 26 to 28 torr. This procedure usually requires endotracheal intubation, controlled ventilation, and intermittent iatrogenic paralysis. Intubation should be performed early for the comatose patient.[6] Care must be taken to assure that injudicious intubation does not cause further intracranial problems due to increased ICP elevations from coughing or gagging during intubation. Hypocapnia can reduce cerebral circulation to the point where cerebral ischemia occurs; therefore blood gases must be monitored closely.

Fluid Control.   Intravenous fluids should be administered judiciously to prevent overhydration, which augments cerebral edema. Similarly, intravenous fluid used for maintenance must not be hypo-osmolar.

Diuretics.   Diuretics such as mannitol, which produce diuresis by increasing intravascular volume and osmolality, are widely used for severe brain injury. Mannitol can be very effective in shrinking the brain and lowering ICP. It is recommended for all patients who develop unilateral pupillary dilation, decorticate or decerebrate posturing, or if the GCS decreases by 2 points. For the average adult patient, 1 gm/kg is used. The neurosurgeon may also recommend loop diuretics, such as furosemide (40 to 80 mg intravenously for adults). These medications act by medically decompressing the brain and may reduce ICP for several hours.

Steroids.   The use of steroids for patients with head injury, although very common in the recent past, has become increasingly controversial. Many neurosurgeons no longer routinely use steroids in the management of head injury.

SUMMARY

The basic principles for the initial assessment and early management of the head-injured patient have been known to neurosurgeons for years. After stabilizing the airway, breathing, and circulation, a minineurologic examination should be used to evaluate the level of consciousness, pupillary reactivity, and lateralized motor signs. This examination, with a few simple steps, can be used effectively to triage most head-injured patients into diagnostically meaningful categories within a few minutes so that emergency management can be instituted promptly. The challenge to the neurosurgeon is to convey these principles of initial assessment and triage to those non-neurosurgeons who are the first to encounter the head-injured patient so that the patient receives the most appropriate care at the earliest possible time.

REFERENCES

1. Anderson DW, McLaurin RL: The National Head and Spinal Cord Injury Survey. J Neurosurg 53:S1–543, 1980.
2. Andrews BT, Pitts LH, Lovely MP, et al.: Is computed tomographic scanning necessary in patients with tentorial herniation? Results of immediate surgical exploration without compared tomography in 100 patients. Neurosurgery 19:408–414, 1986.
3. Cooper PR (ed): Head Injury, 2nd ed. Baltimore: Williams & Wilkins, 1987.
4. Gennarelli TA, Spielman GS, Langfitt TW, et al.: Influence of the type of intracranial lesion on outcome from severe head injury: A multicenter study using a new classification system. J Neurosurg 56:26–32, 1982.
5. Gennarelli TA: Emergency department management of head injuries. Emerg Med Clin North Am 2:749–760, 1984.
6. Gildenberg PL, Makela M: Effect of early intubation and ventilation on outcome following head injury. In Dacey RG (ed): Trauma of the Nervous System. Raven Press: New York, 1985, pp 79–90.
7. Jennett B, Teasdale G: Management of Head Injuries. Philadelphia: FA Davis, 1981.
8. Masters SJ, McClean PM, Arcarese JS, et al.: Skull x-ray examinations after head trauma: Recommendations by a multidisciplinary panel and validation study. N Engl J Med 316:84–91, 1987.
9. Pitts LH: Neurological evaluation of the head injury patient. Clin Neurosurg 29:203–224, 1982
10. Seelig JM, Becker DP, Miller JD, et al.: Traumatic acute subdural hematoma: Major mortality reduction in comatose patients treated within four hours. N Engl J Med 304:1511–1518, 1981.

3

Imaging in Acute Head Injury

STEVEN L. GIANNOTTA AND CHI-SHING ZEE

Since its introduction into clinical medicine in the early 1970s, computed tomography (CT) scanning has become the primary imaging modality in the evaluation of head-injured patients. Among the advantages of CT over previously utilized imaging techniques, such as plain skull radiographs, cerebral angiography, radionuclide brain scanning, and ventriculography, are improved resolution, safety, and economy of time.

In the following discussion we will emphasize the CT presentation of the more common cranial and intracranial traumatic lesions. The role of angiography and magnetic resonance imaging (MRI) in complementing and supplementing information gained from CT will be presented in terms of current (1989) clinical practice.

COMPUTED AXIAL TOMOGRAPHY

Standard transaxial CT is performed with conventional angulation of slices relative to the orbitomeatal line. In certain circumstances with cooperative patients, coronal plane images can be obtained. In general, computerized reformatting following the initial acquisition of CT data will allow examination of alternative orientations.

Patient motion can significantly degrade the image. However, later generation scanners require only a few seconds or less to record each slice. In conjunction with appropriate head positioning and immobilization, supplemented with judicious use of sedatives or even muscle relaxants with assisted respiration, a highly acceptable examination can be accomplished in a relatively short time.

Accuracy of CT assessment depends on completeness of the examination. Contiguous slices should be obtained from the upper reaches of the cervical spine to the vertex. Any slice badly degraded by motion artifacts should be repeated.

The majority of acute traumatic intracranial lesions can be adequately assessed without the use of intravenous iodinated contrast agents. However, in certain circumstances, the use of contrast enhancement may prove beneficial. The decision to use contrast agents is dictated by a number of factors, not the least of which is the patient's condition, since this procedure substantially increases the length of the examination. The indications for the use of intravenous contrast will be discussed in conjunction with specific lesions.

CRANIAL LESIONS

Skull Fracture

In most instances CT is superior to skull roentgenography in the detection of skull fractures. Close scrutiny of a comprehensive CT evaluation will detect most calvarial and base fractures, thereby eliminating the need for further time-consuming studies. Evaluation of depressed fractures can be especially gratifying. Axial planes can frequently delineate the extent and depth of fracture fragments. CT does have its limitations in this regard. Vertex or horizontally oriented fractures may not be seen on axial slices. The scout or localizer view may suggest evidence of a vertex injury, which can then be better targeted with repositioning or coronal plane reconstruction.[14]

Skull base fractures can be effectively delineated using thin (5 mm or less) or overlapping slices (Fig. 3–1). Indirect evidence of skull base injury may also be identified. An air-fluid level may be demonstrated in one of the paranasal sinuses, indicating the presence of blood or cerebrospinal fluid (CSF). Persistence of an air-fluid level or clinical evidence of rhinorrhea would favor the CSF origin. Although most leaks will resolve spontaneously, the use of intrathecal water-soluble contrast agents can be valuable in the evaluation of chronic post-traumatic CSF leaks before their surgical treatment.[1]

Of critical importance in the examination of head trauma using CT is the added information afforded by altering window width.[9,14] Without the use of bone window settings, fractures can easily be missed, and depressed fragments may mimic other lesions, such as epidural hematomas. Overlying metallic foreign bodies may cast artifacts that can be minimized by judicious use of window settings, allowing for accurate identification of facial injuries, including lamina papyracea fractures, blowout injuries of the orbit, and fractures of the petrous bone.

Intracranial Mass Lesions

Before the advent of CT scanning, cerebral angiography was used to determine the presence of a surgically treatable intracranial traumatic lesion. Although displacement of arteriographically defined landmarks can signal the size and approximate location of a mass lesion, differentiation between hematomas and other space-occupying lesions is unreliable. The ability of CT to differentiate between various attenuation values aids in defining the nature of most mass lesions. Edema, for example, can be easily distinguished from acute hematoma. Whole blood with a hematocrit of 45% has an attenuation value of 56 Houndsfield units, much greater than that of brain.[3,4,16] Attenuation values of blood are due largely to the protein fraction of hemoglobin, with a linear relationship linking the two factors.

Subdural Hematoma

Acute subdural clots on CT appear as high-density, homogenous, crescent-shaped masses that parallel the margin of the bony calvarium, expanding in an anteroposterior direction. They also can present subfrontally, subtemporally, or near the vertex, in which case they are more difficult to image in the standard axial plane.

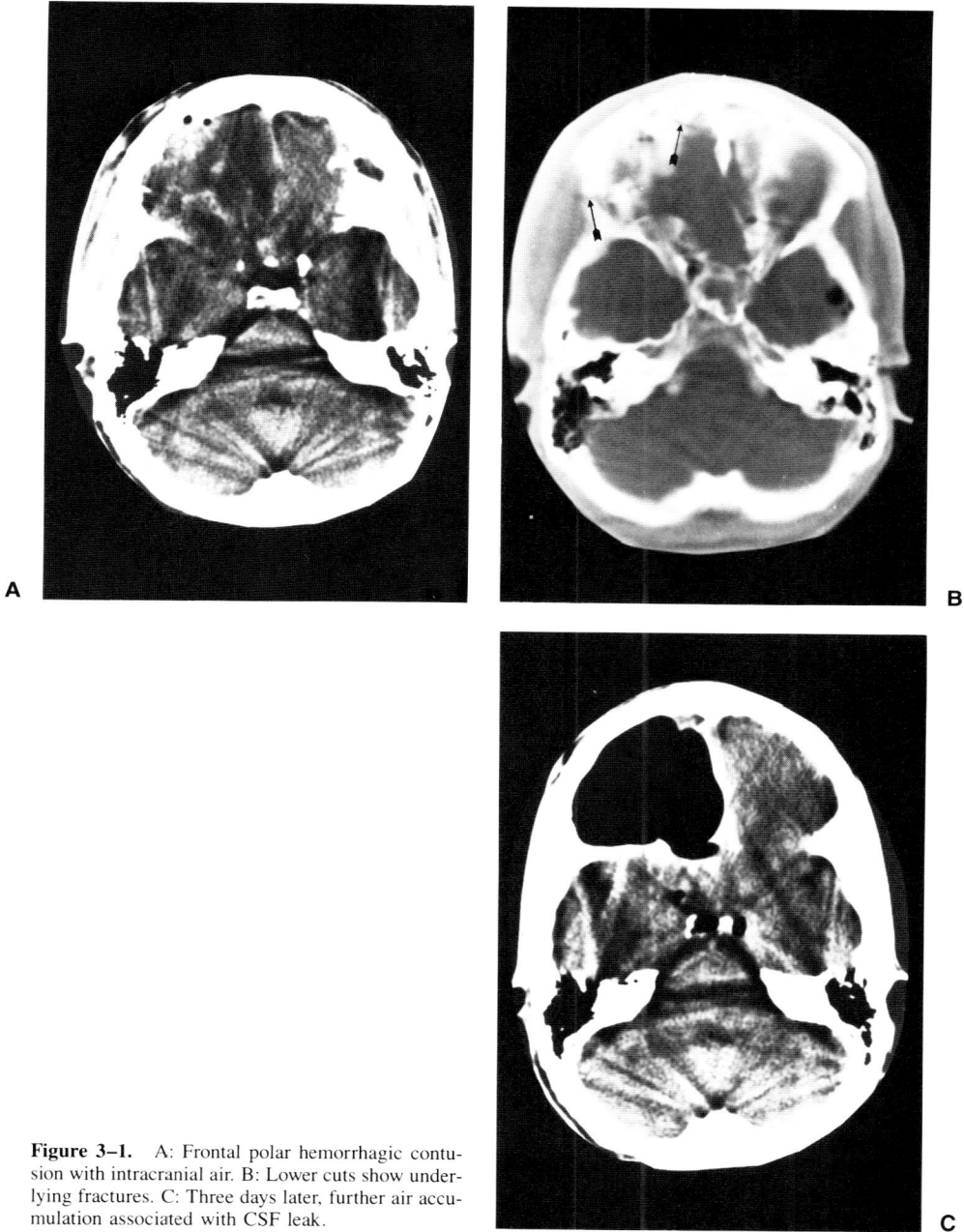

Figure 3–1. A: Frontal polar hemorrhagic contusion with intracranial air. B: Lower cuts show underlying fractures. C: Three days later, further air accumulation associated with CSF leak.

Since attenuation is related to hemoglobin content, it is not surprising that up to 10% of acute subdural hematomas may be isodense with brain, owing presumably to the trauma patient's preexisting anemia.[16,19] If not removed, a high-density clot will become isodense with adjacent brain between 1 and 12 weeks. Unless rebleeding occurs, most are hypodense with brain by 2 months.[4]

Associated lesions such as edema or contusion can be identified with CT. Frequently, the shift of midline structures is out of proportion to the mass of the clot, due to the presence of these and other coexisting factors.

Interhemispheric subdural hematomas were difficult to define prior to CT. They appear as high-density lesions compressing the ipsilateral lateral ventricle and are frequently associated with adjacent parenchymal injury.[15] They usually resolve without surgery and are considered one of the hallmarks of the battered child syndrome.

Chronic subdural hematomas present as crescent-shaped masses with CT densities less than those of the adjacent brain. Mass effect is proportional to the size of the clot. Rebleeding may cause differing densities within the clot cavity; occasionally loculations will form.

Isodense clots present a special challenge; often indirect evidence of their presence is all that is available. Ventricular distortion, sulcal compression, or adjacent white matter buckling are signatures of an overlying isodense lesion.[12] Bilateral isodense subdurals may be detected by the presence of bilateral loss of sulcal pattern and unusually small ventricles. Intravenous contrast enhancement can be helpful because it may delineate the subdural membrane, demonstrate the displacement of cortical vessels away from the inner table of the calvarium, or actually increase the density of the clot contents above the attenuation values of the overlying brain after a 4- to 6-hour delay[9] (Fig. 3–2).

Extradural Hematoma

Much of the foregoing discussion on the CT characteristics of subdural hematomas applies to epidural hematomas. However, extradural clots are distinguished by their biconcave shape and restriction to a region under the calvarium limited by the cranial sutures. Associated skull fracture is common, but associated brain lesions are less common than with subdural hematomas. Occasionally, an intracerebral lucency due to vascular compression produced directly or indirectly by the clot will be present. High-convexity hematomas may be easily overlooked if vertex slices are not obtained or carefully scrutinized. Chronic epidural hematomas may be enhanced with contrast administration.[17]

Intracerebral Hematoma

Acute traumatic intracerebral hematomas (ICHs) appear as areas of increased attenuation within the brain. They tend to be fluffy, irregular, and poorly marginated compared with spontaneous hemorrhages. Multiplicity and a more peripheral location in the brain further distinguish traumatic ICH from spontaneous hematomas. Traumatic ICH may be surrounded by a zone of decreased density attributable to an associated contusion or edema.

Attenuation values will naturally decrease as hemoglobin decreases.[9] After about 12 weeks, the density appears less than that of normal brain and ultimately will heal as a low-density slit with associated atrophy. In the subacute and chronic aftermath, contrast administration may demonstrate a ringlike enhancement of the lesion due to a combination of loss of integrity of the blood-brain barrier and the presence of neovascularity in the clot periphery.[25] This may be confused with an intrinsic brain tumor.

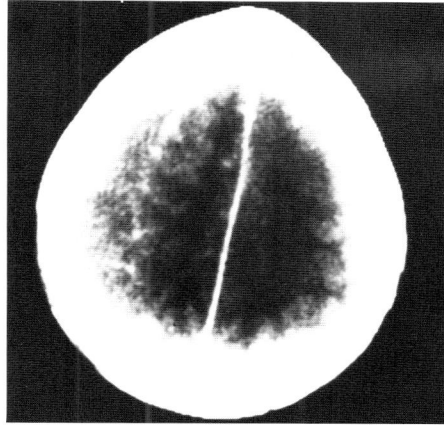

Figure 3–2. Chronic isodense hematoma on CT demonstrated by displacement of contrast-enhanced cortical vessels away from calvarium.

Cerebral Contusion

Contusions appear on CT initially as heterogenous areas of high and low density within the cerebral parenchyma.[24] The density of a given contusion may overlap that of ICH, depending on the relative volumes of hemorrhage, edema, and necrosis. Unless further hemorrhage into the contusion occurs (an entity known as delayed traumatic intracerebral hematoma), the density will decrease with time, although the mass effect may increase due to edema or infarction.[14] At 12 to 14 days, contusions may enhance, making them more easily discernable during their isodense stage. With healing, a slitlike cavity may remain, producing little further structural change after 1 year.

Contusions tend to be located at the polar regions of the cerebrum (Fig. 3–1A). Frontal, temporal, and occipital polar contusions are common and may occur opposite the side of the direct blow due to the contrecoup impaction of brain against the opposite calvarial surface.

Cerebral Edema and Cerebral Swelling

Cerebral edema is increased brain water resulting from loss of vascular integrity and extravasation of fluid and plasma protein into the extracellular space or, in the case of cytotoxic edema, an increase in intracellular water. Cerebral edema appears on CT as an area of homogeneously decreased attenuation, with blurring of gray and white matter distinction. There is usually associated mass effect that, if severe enough, can result in obliteration of basilar cisterns and subarachnoid space. Edema is most intense 1 to 3 days after the initial trauma and is most commonly found in association with hematomas, contusions, or infarctions.

Cerebral swelling, as a distinct clinical entity, usually occurs in children after head injury, and is believed to be due to cerebral vasodilation and a resulting increase in cerebral blood volume.[6] CT characteristics of cerebral swelling include small or absent cerebral ventricles with compression of perimesencephalic, quadrigeminal, and suprasellar cisterns.[23] Cerebral tissue may have an increased attenuation value in contradistinction to that produced by edema. Cerebral swelling can be detected as early as 30 minutes after the traumatic incident and is generally seen in patients under the age of 17 years.

Cerebral Herniation

Intracranial shifts of cerebral structures may be readily identified on CT. The earliest sign of transtentorial herniation is encroachment of the uncus on the lateral aspect of the suprasellar cistern.[18] This is followed by widening of the ipsilateral crural and ambient cisterns. With more severe herniation, obliteration of the cisternal space at the tentorial level is seen; the suprasellar cistern may be difficult to identify. Hydrocephalus of part of the ventricular system not directly exposed to the traumatic lesion may occur, probably from obstruction of the aqueduct or foramen of Monroe. Infarction in the posterior cerebral artery distribution may occur from vascular kinking and compression at the tentorial edge.

Diffuse Cerebral Injury

Especially in the case of high-velocity deceleration trauma, the poor neurologic condition of the patient may be out of proportion to CT scan findings. Careful scrutiny of the images may show elements of cerebral swelling in conjunction with eccentric corpus callosum hemorrhages or brainstem contusions. Small hemorrhages at the gray-white matter junction also may be produced by the shearing forces thought to be responsible for diffuse axonal injuries. Serial examinations often demonstrate delayed diffuse ventricular enlargement.[9]

Subarachnoid hemorrhage usually accompanies diffuse injury, appearing as areas of increased density in the basilar cisterns and adjacent to the falx. These usually resolve within 1 week.

Penetrating Injuries

CT scanning can provide invaluable information about penetrating brain injuries if the physician takes care when performing the examination. One can distinguish entrance and exit wounds by altering window level and width, and metallic fragments causing streak artifacts can be tracked.[14] Pneumocephalus is an important finding, especially if cranial penetration is unsuspected. CT is exquisitely sensitive in dipicting intracranial air because of its extremely low attenuation value. Air is absorbed in time. If pneumocephalus persists, a CSF leak should be suspected.

CT Imaging of Vascular Lesions

There are clear advantages of using CT in place of cerebral angiography in the radiologic evaluation of head trauma. Occasionally, however, CT scanning will not demonstrate certain vascular complications of head trauma. If there is any reason to suspect a traumatic vascular lesion, angiography should be done after CT.

Indirect evidence of vascular abnormalities may be present on CT. Low-density areas in a typical vascular distribution may herald traumatic arterial occlusion either intra- or extracranially. Dural venous sinus occlusion may present with hemorrhagic infarctions adjacent to the sinus affected.[7] Delayed deposition of blood into the subarachnoid space or cerebral substance can be due to the presence of a traumatically induced aneurysm.[21]

Direct imaging of vascular lesions can occur with the use of intravenous contrast agents. Carotid-cavernous fistula and traumatic aneurysms are examples. Occasionally, preexisting vascular lesions may cause the traumatic event. Contrast enhancement of CT images assumes more importance if the diagnosis or mechanism of injury remains in question.

CEREBRAL ANGIOGRAPHY

Despite advances made in noninvasive imaging for brain trauma, angiography remains the most precise method of identifying traumatic vascular lesions or the nature of vascular events that may have led to trauma.[13] Some indications for cerebral angiography after head injury include: focal neurologic deficits unexplained by CT, transient ischemic attacks following trauma, delayed neurologic deterioration, unexplained cranial nerve palsies, and severe epistaxis, cranial bruits, or proptosis.

EXTRACRANIAL VASCULAR INJURIES

Traumatic carotid artery occlusion after head injury usually presents as an abrupt blockage of flow within the internal carotid artery 1 to 3 cm above the bifurcation[22] (Fig. 3–3). Although arterial injury may have occurred at a higher level (usually near the tubercle of C1 or at the skull base), an entire segment is usually occluded by the time the study is performed.[5] Upper cervical, petrous, or cavernous segments may be reconstituted collateral sources. If intracranial branches can be imaged, emboli may be seen causing branch occlusions in some cases.

Traumatic dissection of the carotid artery appears as an irregular narrowing over several centimeters, usually beginning near the C1-C2 vertebral segments. Normal caliber is frequently resumed as the vessel traverses the carotid canal.[20]

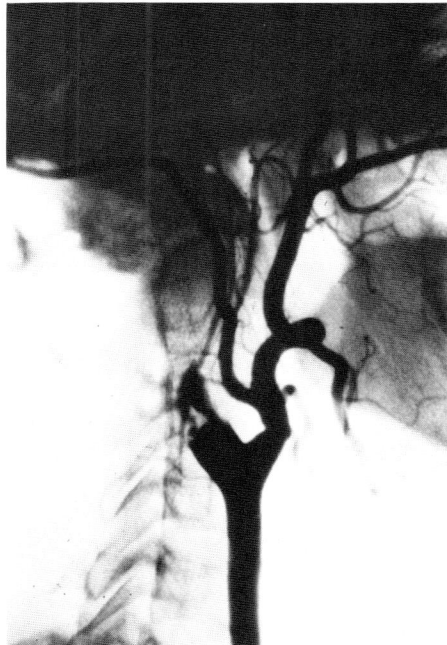

Figure 3–3. Total occlusion of the internal carotid artery in association with blunt head trauma.

Carotid disruption can result in aneurysm formation (Fig. 3–4). Generally, this presents as an irregular enlargement or outpouching of the dye column in association with segmental narrowing. As time progresses, these lesions tend to look more saccular, although many are false aneurysms with walls formed by organized clot. Irregularity of the lumen in this case is likely due to the presence of mural thrombus.

INTRACRANIAL VASCULAR INJURIES

Traumatically induced intracranial vascular injuries occur in less than 3% of head injuries.[8] Cerebral arterial occlusions are probably the most common entity, followed by fistulas and aneurysms.

The intracranial carotid artery is the most common cerebral vessel to be traumatically occluded. This appears as an abrupt, usually smooth stenosis. Distal emboli causing branch occlusion often occur. Cortical arteries may be occluded also, usually in association with overlying calvarial fractures. A sharp angulation in the affected vessel or "Z-sign" is caused by tethering of the artery between the fracture fragments. Occasionally, the middle cerebral artery may be occluded at its origin, presumably due to impact against the sphenoid ridge. Basilar artery occlusion is rare and usually is associated with fracture of the clivus. Midline or occipital fractures can cause major venous sinus occlusion or injury (Fig. 3–5).

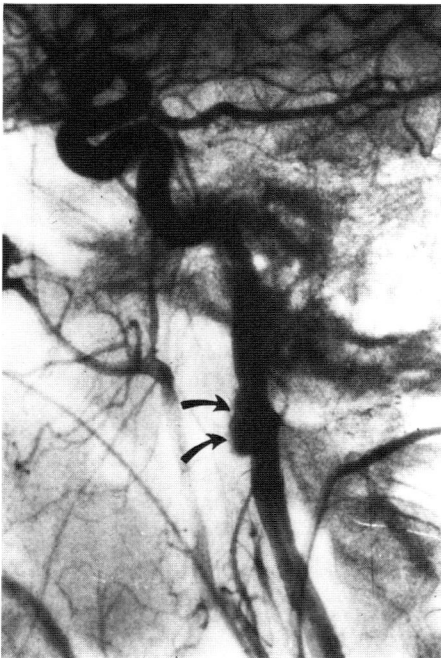

Figure 3–4. Cervical internal carotid artery aneurysm associated with blunt head trauma.

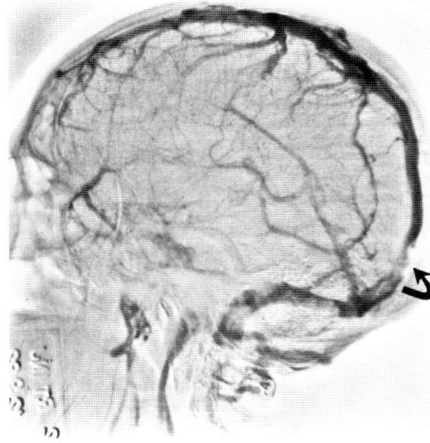

Figure 3–5.   Injury to sagittal sinus from overlying calvarium fracture.

Traumatic Aneurysms

Despite their relative rarity, more than 50 cases of traumatic cerebral artery aneurysms have been identified at Los Angeles County-USC Medical Center since 1968.[21] The majority of these cases came to light before the introduction of CT as the primary imaging modality for trauma. Those cases that were not identified incidentally presented with subarachnoid hemorrhage following head trauma, delayed onset of neurologic deterioration, epistaxis, delayed cranial nerve palsy, and extracerebral hematomas after trivial trauma. Angiographic hallmarks of traumatic aneurysms include delayed filling and emptying, irregular contour, absence of a neck, and peripheral location usually not at a branching point (Fig. 3–6).

Arteriovenous Fistula

Traumatically induced arteriovenous fistulas are an unusual but well-recognized concomitant of head trauma. The most dramatic example of this genre of lesions is the carotid-cavernous sinus fistula (CCF) (Fig. 3–7). CCFs have been categorized according to their vessels of origin and the velocity of the shunt; however, it is the type A cases that are most often associated with a traumatic etiology.[2] The type A CCF is a direct communication between the internal carotid siphon and the cavernous sinus through a single tear in the arterial wall. The clinical features of proptosis, chemosis, orbital bruits, and cranial nerve palsies are easily recognized. Angiographically, the cavernous sinus opacifies almost simultaneously with the carotid artery. Venous drainage typically involves the superior ophthalmic vein, but the contralateral cavernous sinus, pterygoid and petrosal veins, and inferior ophthalmic veins also may drain the cavernous sinus. Treatment regimens by interventional radiologic techniques, such as using detachable balloons, depend on correct identification of the exact site of the abnormal communication. Therefore high-speed multiplanar serial angiographic studies are mandatory.

Blunt head injury may produce scalp arteriovenous fistulas or aneurysms of the

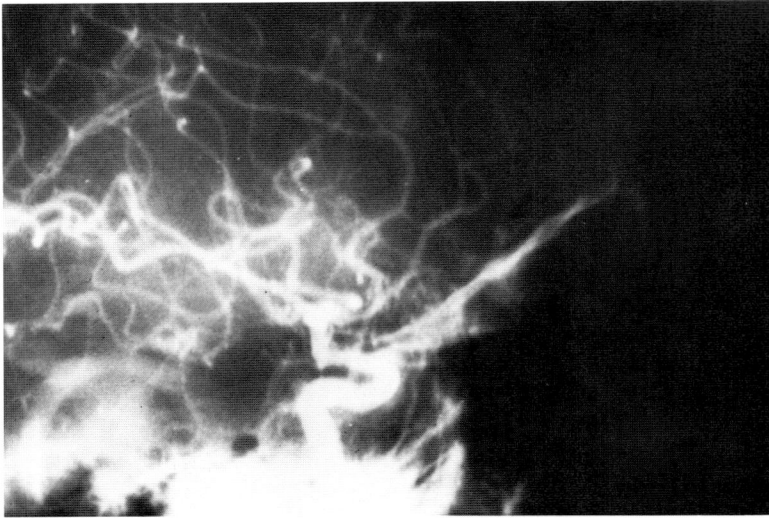

Figure 3–6.   Traumatic aneurysm (arrow) off branch of anterior cerebral artery.

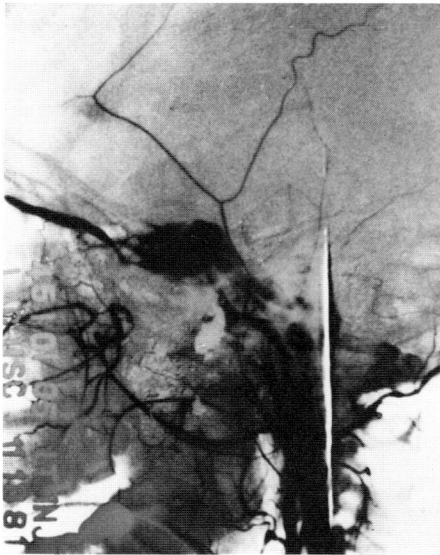

Figure 3–7.   Traumatically induced carotid-cavernous sinus fistula.

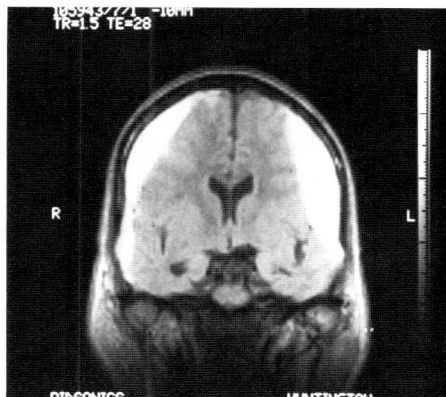

Figure 3–8. Bilateral chronic subdural hematomas detected by MRI.

superficial temporal artery.[10] A traumatic middle meningeal fistula may be formed with simultaneous opacification of both middle meningeal artery and veins causing the so-called "railroad track" or "tram track" sign.

MAGNETIC RESONANCE IMAGING

Magnetic resonance has some distinct advantages over CT in imaging certain intracranial conditions. However, in the setting of acute head injury, these advantages are largely theoretical. Practical concerns limit the use of the MRI in the acute trauma patient; studies require more time to complete than those of conventional CT, with longer patient immobilization and delays of other therapeutic and diagnostic procedures. Life-supporting devices containing metallic components cannot be used in the vicinity of the MRI unit.

MRI depicts intracranial hemorrhage differently than does CT. Acute intraparenchymal clot is isointense or slightly hypointense to gray matter on T_1 weighted images and may remain so for up to 1 week. On T_2 weighted images, the signal intensity of the hematoma center is low. In the subacute stage, hematomas exhibit high-signal intensity on T_1. This hyperintensity persists for up to 1 year. Thus, MRI is more sensitive in defining subacute or chronic blood intracranially than CT. Conversely, acute hematomas are better seen on CT scans.

Subacute and chronic extracerebral hematomas are hyperintense on MRI, making this modality much more sensitive than CT in delineating these lesions (Fig. 3–8). Small petechial hemorrhages not detected by CT are readily seen with MRI, as are small shear injuries at the gray-white matter junction.

At present, practical problems related to patient handling limit MRI applicability in acute head trauma. The value of MRI lies in its ability to identify many of the more subtle structural alterations from trauma, allowing perhaps more accurate assessment of prognosis and timely intervention for some of the delayed but no less surgically important sequelae of acute head trauma.[11]

REFERENCES

1. Ahmadi J, Weiss MH, Segall HD, Schultz DH, Zee C, Giannotta SL: Evaluation of cerebrospinal fluid rhinorrhea by metrizamide computed tomographic cisternography. Neurosurgery 16:54–60, 1985.
2. Barrow DL, Spector RH, Braun IF, Landman J, Tindall SC, Tindall GT: Classification and treatment of spontaneous carotid cavernous fistulas. J Neurosurg 62:248–256, 1985.
3. Bergstrom M, Ericson K, Levander B, et al.: Variations with time of attenuation values of intracranial hematomas. J Comput Assist Tomogr 1:57–63, 1977.
4. Bergstrom M, Ericson K, Levander B, et al.: Computed tomography of cranial subdural and epidural hematomas: Variations of attenuation related to time and clinical events such as rebleeding. J Comput Assist Tomogr 1:449–455, 1977.
5. Boldrey E, Maas L, Miller E: The role of atlantoid compression in the etiology of internal carotid thrombosis. J Neurosurg 13:127–139, 1956.
6. Bruce DA: Diffuse cerebral swelling following head injuries in children: The syndrome of "malignant brain edema." J Neurosurg 54:170–178, 1981.
7. Buonanno FS, Moody DM, Ball MR: Computed cranial tomographic findings in cerebral sinovenous occlusion. J Comput Assist Tomogr 2:281–290, 1978.
8. Caveness WF: Incidence of craniocerebral trauma in the United States in 1976 with trend from 1970 to 1975. Adv Neurol 22:1–3, 1979.
9. Dolinskas CA: Intracranial trauma. In Gonzalez CF, Grossman CB, Masdeu, JC (eds): Head and Spine Imaging. New York: John Wiley & Sons, 1985, pp 357–396.
10. Feldman RA, Hieshima G, Giannotta SL, Gade GF: Traumatic dural arteriovenous fistula supplied by scalp, meningeal, and cortical arteries. Case report. Neurosurgery 6:670–674, 1980.
11. Gentry LR, Godersky JC, Thompson B, Dunn VD: Prospective comparative study of intermediate field MR and CT in the evaluation of closed head trauma. AJNR 9:91–100, 1988.
12. George AE, Russell EJ, Kricheff II: White matter buckling: CT sign of extra-axial intracranial mass. AJR 135:1031–1036, 1980.
13. Giannotta SL, Ahmadi J: Vascular lesions in head injury. In Wilkins RH, Rengachary SS (eds): Neurosurgery. New York: McGraw-Hill, 1984.
14. Giannotta SL, Weiss MH: Pitfalls in the diagnosis of head injury. Clin Neurosurg 29:288–299, 1982.
15. Ho SU, Spehlmenn R, Ho HT: CT scan in interhemispheric subdural hematomas: Clinical and pathological correlation. Neurology (Minneapolis) 27: 1097–1098, 1977.
16. New PFJ, Aronow S: Attenuation measurements of whole blood and blood fractions in computed tomography. Radiology 121:635–640, 1976.
17. Omar MM, Binet E: Peripheral contrast enhancement in chronic epidural hematomas. J Comput Assist Tomogr 2:332–335, 1978.
18. Osborn AG: Diagnosis of descending transtentorial herniation by cranial computed tomography. Radiology 123:93–96, 1977.
19. Smith WP, Batnitzky S, Rengachary SS: Acute isodense subdural hematomas: A problem in anemic patients. AJR 136:543–546, 1981.
20. Stringer WL, Kelly DL Jr: Traumatic dissection of the extracranial internal carotid artery. Neurosurgery 6: 123–130, 1980.
21. von Hanwehr RJ, Giannotta SL, Weiss MH: The impact of traumatic cerebral aneurysms and their sequelae on selective morbidity following head trauma. In: Kikuchi H, Fukushima T, Watanabe K (eds): Intracranial Aneurysms, Surgical Timing & Techniques. Niigata, Japan: Nishimura, 1986, pp 96–104. Proceedings from the 1st International Workshop on Intracranial Aneurysms held April 2–4, 1986 in Tokyo, Japan.
22. Yamada S, Kindt GW, Youmans JR: Carotid artery occlusion due to nonpenetrating injury. J Trauma 7:333–342, 1967.
23. Zimmerman RA, Bilaniuk LT, Dolinskas C, Obrist W, Kuhl D: Computed tomography of pediatric head trauma: Acute general swelling. Radiology 126:403–408, 1978.
24. Zimmerman RA, Bilaniuk LT, Dolinskas C, et al.: Computed tomography of acute intracerebral hemorrhagic contusion. J Comput Assist Tomogr 1:271–279, 1977.
25. Zimmerman RD, Leeds NE, Naidich TP: Ring blush associated with intracerebral hematoma. Radiology 122:707–711, 1977.

4

Surgical Treatment of Extracerebral Lesions in Head Injury

LAWRENCE F. MARSHALL

Surgical therapy for extracerebral brain lesions of the brain is one of the oldest surgical techniques known. One can trace the history of trephination for thousands of years, beginning before the time of Christ and continuing on, not only in modern societies, but also in societies with little or no contact with Western medicine. The efficacy of surgical therapy has dramatically improved since the advent of computed tomographic (CT) scanning in 1973. Although much has been written, both pro and con, about the proliferation of CT scanners, clearly there is lower mortality from extra-axial mass lesions as a result of widespread use of CT. In fact, a relatively recent report from Glasgow noted a reduction in mortality from such lesions of greater than 25%.[7] Thus, the accurate and rapid noninvasive diagnosis of extracerebral masses has changed the prognosis during the acute phase and the outcome on a long-term basis. Although criteria for the evacuation of such lesions have been discussed in detail in general texts as well as in more focally directed texts of neurosurgery, it is appropriate to review the generally established criteria presently used in head injury centers with considerable experience.

EXTRADURAL HEMATOMA

An extradural hematoma (EDH) represents a potentially lethal lesion, which, in the absence of other major structural injury, should almost never cause a fatal or vegetative outcome. Bricolo and Paasut[3] demonstrated a mortality of less than 5% in patients with EDH, and this seems an appropriate standard. Although most EDHs require surgical treatment, some physicians have advocated a more conservative approach. This is appropriate only for the smallest lesions, that is, those that do not produce shift of the midline structures or compression of the mesencephalic cisterns. Given the extremely low mortality and morbidity of surgical intervention for an extradural hematoma, it is inappropriate, in my view, to maintain a patient on pharmacologic therapy for intracranial hypertension when a simple surgical removal will usually resolve the problem completely.

The type of craniotomy needed to evacuate such lesions depends on other structural pathologic conditions demonstrated on the CT scan. If a patient with an EDH is neurologically normal, or nearly so, the flap can be placed directly over the EDH. However, if multiple basilar or other fractures are present, then a flap that allows adequate exploration of the likely source of hemorrhage is mandatory (Fig. 4–1). For a posteriorly located EDH, particularly those likely to involve the transverse sinus, it is important that the exposure allows direct repair of the venous tear or, at least, direct compression.

What is initially done during the craniotomy and craniectomy should directly reflect the patient's clinical state. If a patient is deteriorating rapidly, or has evidence of brainstem compression, then the first limb of the flap should be turned directly at the site where a burr hole can be made to allow initial evacuation of the clot (Fig. 4–2). Although not all of the hematoma can be removed through a burr hole, a substantial amount often can be, and this will alleviate some of the pressure on the brainstem. A full craniotomy can then be done and an appropriate exploration carried out.

In general, there is no need to open the dura when an EDH is removed. Exceptions are when a large contusion is seen on CT or an inappropriate degree of brain swelling occurs after evacuation. The emphasis is on "inappropriate," and this should be more clearly defined. In patients in whom the EDH has been present for a considerable period of time, either because the lesion was missed or because the patient's transfer to a neurosurgical center was delayed, postoperative brain swelling is extremely common. However, if the clot is removed within 2 to 4 hours of its occurrence, such brain swelling is rare. If it does occur, then the possibility should be considered that the fullness of the brain is due to a second lesion that has developed since the evacuation or because of a contusion directly underneath the hematoma. We have seen three instances of tandem lesions, not noted on the initial CT scan, which were found at the time of surgical exploration and which undoubtedly devel-

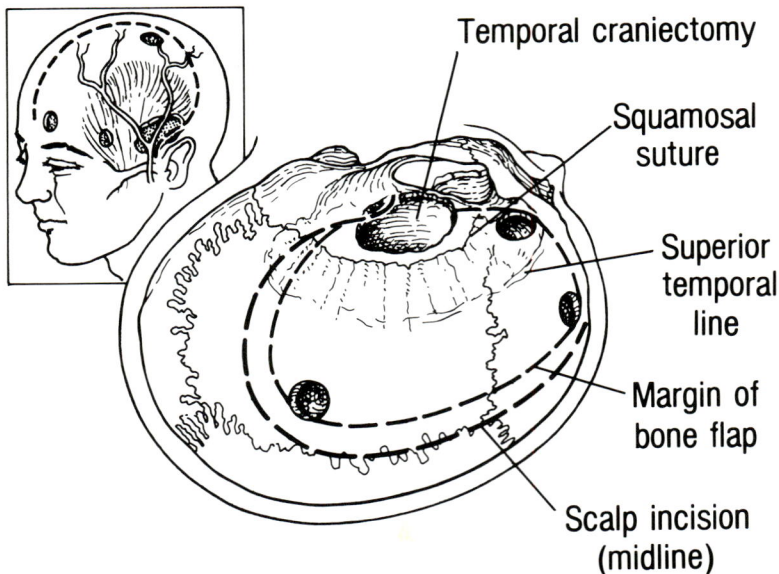

Figure 4–1.   A standard flap utilized in most operations for acute extradural and subdural hematomas. (From Youmans.[8] Reprinted with permission.)

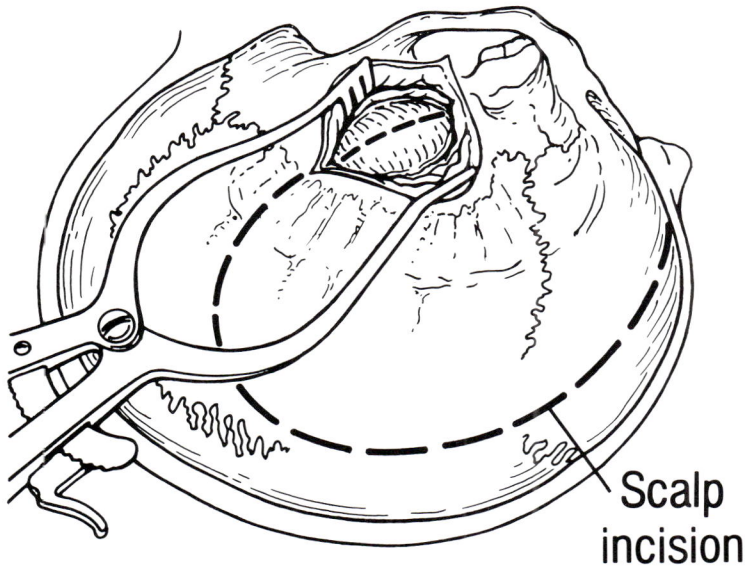

Figure 4–2. Initial approach in the deteriorating patient. Note the incorporation of the small craniectomy site into the craniotomy flap. (From Youmans.[8] Reprinted with permission.)

oped as a result of brain decompression. We also have seen two patients in whom a contralateral subdural hematoma of significant size developed immediately after an extra-dural exploration. When such brain swelling is noted after wound closure, the patient should be taken from the operating theater directly to the scanner and a scan obtained.

Once the hematoma is evacuated, a meticulous closure is required to ensure hemostasis. The dura should be tacked up to prevent reaccumulation of the extradural collection and the bone flap should be secured in place. The muscle, galea, and skin are closed separately. If brain swelling has been demonstrated on the CT scan or is seen during the operation, the surgeon might dress only the suture line to allow access to the fullness of the flap as an indication of intracranial hypertension.

We routinely place an intracranial pressure (ICP) monitor in all patients who are unconscious at the time of hematoma evacuation. Almost 50% of patients in the National Institute of Neurological and Communicative Disorders and Stroke Traumatic Coma Data Bank (TCDB) who had any type of hematoma evacuated had postoperative intracranial hypertension that required therapy. In patients who are not in coma at the time of hematoma removal, the degree of tightness or slackness of the brain serves as an index as to whether or not ICP monitoring is advisable.

ACUTE SUBDURAL HEMATOMA

In contrast to EDH, which is not associated with severe structural injury in the majority of patients, acute subdural hematoma (SDH), in many cases, is a marker of diffuse injury upon which a major mass lesion is superimposed. Acute SDH represents the most frequent traumatic lesion in the seriously injured requiring surgical therapy.

The outcome from SDH is related almost entirely to two factors: the rapidity with which the clot can be removed in the declining patient and the degree of associated brain damage. Although the surgeon has little control over the latter, he has substantial control over the former. The worldwide experience shows that mortality rates of more than 50% are common. In a survey of the mortality from intracranial mass lesions carried out in New South Wales, Australia, a mortality rate of almost 90% was noted for acute SDH.[6] Results of a preliminary analysis of the TCDB show a 50% mortality rate (Table 4–1). This outcome from SDH represents a modest improvement over the results reported by others. Whether this mortality can be reduced further by more stringent adherence to a systematic approach to such patients is unknown. There will always be significant mortality and morbidity because of the structural injuries that occur at the time of impact.

Patients with acute SDH can deteriorate as precipitously as those with extradural collections. In fact, a classic presentation is the awake patient with an uncontrollable headache followed by rapid decline. If a patient with such a headache presents, the possibility of an acute SDH or EDH must be uppermost in the surgeon's mind.

In patients with traumatic injuries, most acute SDH occur from one of several mechanisms. The sylvian or cortical veins on the brain surface may be torn, in which case pressure on the brain is due primarily to the acute SDH. Bleeding may also occur at the site of a brain laceration, or be adjacent to or contiguous to an area of brain contusion or intracerebral hemorrhage, usually of the frontal or temporal lobes. In the temporal lobe, this has been termed a "pulped" or "burst" temporal lobe. The underlying parenchymal injury and the SDH combine to produce the mass effect. Occasionally, arterial bleeding into the subdural space can occur from lacerations or tears of cortical arteries, usually at sites where the brain had become adherent to the dura. Deterioration in such patients is so rapid that unless arrival at the hospital is within minutes, the patient usually dies.

Surgical Management

Surgical management of patients with acute SDH is predicated on the same basic principles as those cited previously for extradural lesions. If, for some reason, a scan cannot be

Table 4–1   Traumatic Coma Data Bank
Outcome after Evacuation of Subdural Hematomas

	PATIENT AGE (YR)		
GLASGOW OUTCOME SCALE	*40 or Less*	*More than 40*	*Total*
Good	4	0	4
Moderate	12	4	16
Severe	21	9	30
Vegetative	7	3	10
Dead	30	30	60
Total	74	46	120

obtained immediately, then emergency trephination should be considered if the patient is declining precipitously. In general, exploratory burr holes or diagnostic trephination should be reserved only for specific circumstances in which the likelihood of finding an extracranial mass is high. These include: (1) patients who have had a precipitous downhill course with mydriasis; and (2) patients in whom the cause of the head injury is such that a hematoma is common, such as falls or assaults.[1]

Trephination should occur on the side of the enlarged pupil, since pupillary localization will be false in only 5% of patients.[5] If the patient is deteriorating but mydriasis has not yet occurred, then the first exploratory burr hole should be placed on the side of the skull fracture or external scalp injury, or contralateral to the side of the worst motor deficit. It should be located in the temporal region 2 cm anterior to the tragus and 2 cm above the zygomatic arch (Fig. 4–2).

Acute SDH or EDH are contralateral to the motor deficit about 75% of the time, and subjacent to a fracture about 80% of the time. Under circumstances in which the first burr hole is negative, we use air ventriculography, as described by Becker and associates,[2] placing approximately 5 cc of air after evacuating 5 cc of cerebrospinal fluid (CSF) to determine whether or not there is significant shift of the midline structures. If the shift exceeds 5 mm and CT scanning is not available following initial trephination, then we perform a large trauma flap incorporating exposure of the frontal, temporal, and parietal area as the next step.

In the management of patients with acute SDH, one must consider the frequently associated brain contusion as a single entity. The purpose of surgical therapy therefore is twofold: to remove the acute hematoma and to debride areas of brain contusion or intra-parenchymal hemorrhage. Support for this philosophy comes most recently from evidence produced in laboratory models. The deleterious effect of blood products, per se, on brain function and blood flow has been demonstrated when blood is present within the brain for long periods. Although the primary goal of operation is to reduce ICP and decompress the brainstem, the secondary objective of cleansing the subdural space should not be neglected. The use of the large craniotomy trauma flap has several major advantages. Patients with acute SDH often have frontal and temporal contusions that require debridement. Additionally, the source of the hemorrhage causing the hematoma may be cortical veins, which often are not reachable if a small flap is turned directly over the central portion of the SDH. If adequate exposure for medial torn veins is not obtained when the clot is removed, substantial intraoperative hemorrhage can occur because the tamponade is lost. It may be appropriate to limit the flap's upward extent if the hemorrhage is primarily temporal and subtemporal, but if there is any possibility of bleeding from bridging veins, then the flap should be extended almost to the midline, as shown in Figure 4–1. Meticulous handling of tissues, both soft tissue and brain, is mandatory.

If the patient has deteriorated immediately before operation or is in a state of extremis, the initial incision should be the same as that recommended in the management of acute EDH (Fig. 4–2). This incision can be carried quickly through the temporalis muscle, and then a burr hole and craniectomy accomplished in a short time by the experienced neurosurgeon. A lifesaving reduction of ICP can be achieved by immediately decompressing the brain through the removal of even a small portion of the clot.

Once this burr hole has been placed, we perform the craniotomy using a free bone flap. This type of flap can be turned more rapidly and reduces the possibility of hemorrhage from an osteoplastic flap, a particular risk in patients with clotting disturbances. The physician should take advantage of fracture lines if they are present, but also may choose, if possible, to incorporate the entire fracture within the craniotomy flap.

Opening the Dura

The dural opening should begin in the temporal region (Fig. 4–3). The advantage of this is that if herniation of the brain occurs it will be from a relatively silent region rather than from more important areas of symbolic language or reasoning. If brain swelling occurs during opening of the dura, cooperative effort with the anesthesiologist is essential. Hyperventilation and adequate doses of osmotic agents, such as mannitol, are important treatments if brain swelling occurs. Short-acting barbiturates and modest hypotension may also be helpful in reversing brain swelling.

   Adequate exposure of the frontal lobes to the frontal tip and of the entire temporal lobe is essential. The flap should be carried low enough along the base so that bleeding from the skull base can be controlled. Although most of the hematoma often can be taken out easily with general suction and irrigation, occasionally cup forceps may be required. Great care should be taken in removing a clot from areas in which adequate exposure has not been achieved. If bipolar coagulation cannot control a bleeding vessel, a small bit of Surgicel or Gelfoam can be used. Pressure tamponade should be maintained for several minutes, so that absolute hemostasis is achieved.

   Once the SDH has been removed, the surgeon can systematically investigate the brain

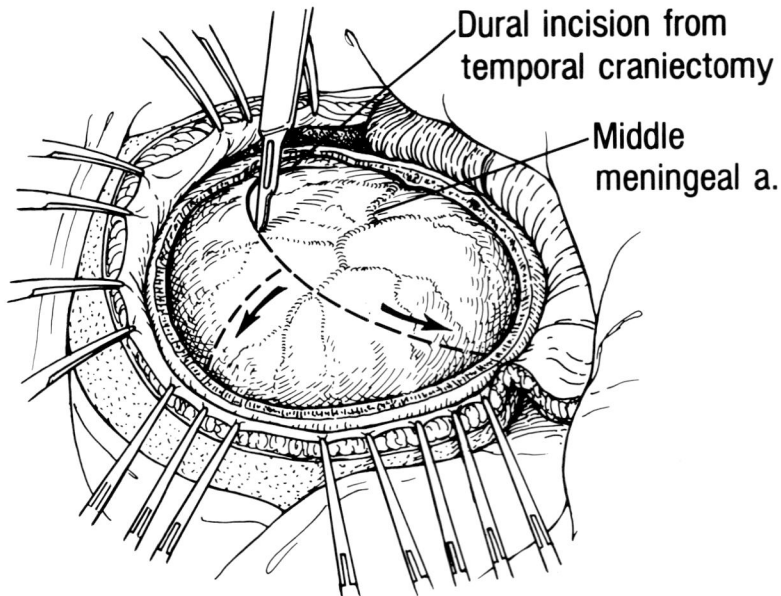

Dural incision from temporal craniectomy

Middle meningeal a.

Figure 4–3.   Dural opening for evacuation and exploration of the patient with an acute subdural hematoma. (From Youmans,[8] Reprinted with permission.)

regions most likely to harbor areas of contusion and hemorrhagic necrosis. They are most frequently found on the inferior surface of the frontal lobe, particularly at the junction of the frontal and temporal lobes at the sphenoid wing. Areas of hemorrhagic tissue should be carefully removed. The preservation of all normal tissue is the primary goal, and the use of small sucker tips and magnification can facilitate this. Whenever possible, we try to achieve a watertight dural closure. If brain swelling has occurred, we attempt to close the dura after the swelling has been reversed. Infrequently, the dura may be left open and the bone flap left out. Brain swelling that cannot be controlled with barbiturates and by reducing mean arterial pressure is uncommon. If it occurs, the anesthesiologist should confirm adequate oxygenation and gas exchange.

Occasionally, a dural graft, usually temporalis fascia, is used. Trauma patients frequently have external injuries, and infection is always a possibility. Management of such infections is easier if the dura is closed. In addition, a CSF fluid leak is less likely after dural closure. The possibility of a contralateral extra-axial collection as a result of brain decompression should also be considered.

The concept that a decompressive craniectomy is useful requires careful reanalysis. Brain frequently herniates through areas of bony decompression and undoubtedly dies. Figure 4–4 illustrates the CT scan done 3 hours after injury in a patient with an acute SDH. It shows a massive area of edema. Once surgical mass lesions have been removed, brain swelling is best managed by a systematic approach to elevated ICP. It is my view that leaving the bone flap out only makes management more difficult.

Once the wound is adequately closed, a systematic management protocol should be followed in such patients. ICP monitoring is mandatory after the evacuation of an acute SDH in a patient whose consciousness has been impaired, since approximately one half of these patients will have postoperative brain swelling.

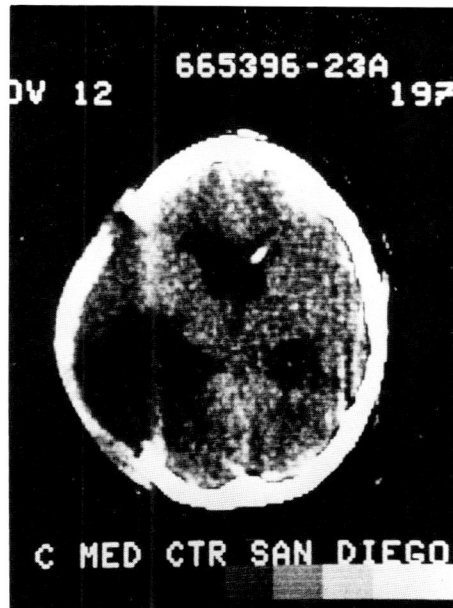

Figure 4–4. Massive edema following removal of bone flap to control ICP in a patient with a subdural hematoma.

SUBACUTE SUBDURAL HEMATOMA

Confusion reigns with regard to the definition of subacute SDH. An arbitrary but pragmatic definition might be: those hematomas that occur within 48 hours to 7 days of injury and are not usually associated with an abrupt decline in the condition of the patient. Patients with a subacute SDH are often older and less ill than those with acute SDH and usually have had a recent fall or blunt injury. Acceleration or deceleration injuries of the type associated with motor vehicle accidents are less common. Headache is frequent, as is focal neurologic deficit, but neurologic decline usually will be slower than that associated with acute SDH. Subacute SDHs can be easily identified on CT scan and usually are not associated with significant other areas of primary brain injury.

Surgical Management

The treatment of subacute SDH is predicated on the assumption that the patient's neurologic deficit is due solely to brain compression from the overlying hemorrhage and that the source of the hemorrhage will be less easily identified than it is in patients with acute SDH. Therefore in patients with subacute SDH we place the craniotomy over the hematoma in contrast to acute SDH where a large craniotomy flap is strongly recommended. An illustration of such a flap is shown in Figure 4–5. In elderly patients, a smaller and more focused flap and a shorter operation are desirable. If a patient has deteriorated, we give mannitol before surgery to protect the patient from the potentially deleterious effects of anesthesia and intubation and from the continuing effects of the hematoma until it can be removed. As in the treatment of the acute SDH, once the clot is removed the underlying

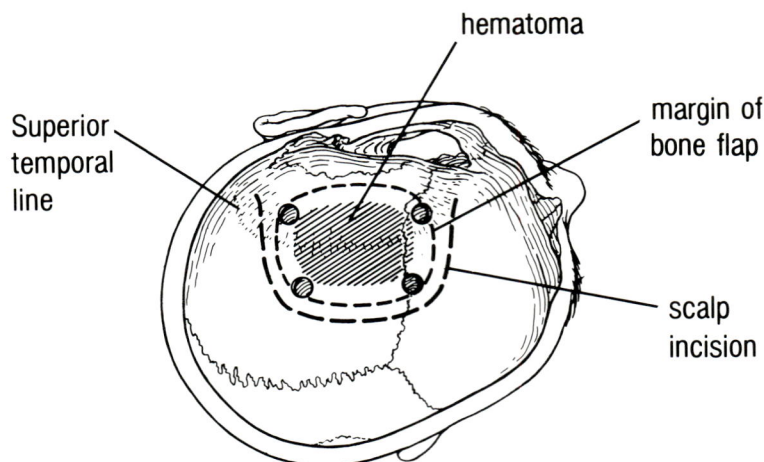

Figure 4–5.   Flap for evacuation of a subacute subdural hematoma. The flap is limited to the area of the hematoma.

brain should be carefully inspected and the dura meticulously closed. It is rare that the bone flap cannot be replaced in such patients. ICP monitoring is usually not necessary because postoperative brain swelling is uncommon. However, if the patient has declined to a point where function is seriously compromised, then ICP monitoring is appropriate.

CHRONIC SUBDURAL HEMATOMAS

Chronic SDH represents an entirely different entity than acute or subacute hemorrhages in terms of their manifestations, time course, and likely outcome. Chronic SDHs become symptomatic later than 1 week after injury. It is uncommon, even in the CT era, for a chronic SDH to be associated with significant underlying parenchymal injury. The accumulation or development of membranes about a subdural hematoma is the most important indication of the chronic nature of the lesion.[4] This lesion is uncommon in patients younger than 40 years in the absence of brain atrophy, which usually is secondary to alcoholism or chronic substance abuse. In approximately 10% of the patients, the lesions are bilateral; this number increases with increasing age of the patient.

Most patients with chronic SDH develop symptoms between 2 and 8 weeks after the initiating event, if the cause can be identified. Patients often have mild symptoms. Aside from headache, a slowing of cognitive processing is the most frequently recognized finding. Disturbances of memory and mild to moderate focal signs, such as a hemiparesis, may be seen. Some patients will present with no focal deficit, but with a picture typical of senile dementia. Thus, chronic subdural collections should be excluded before an untreatable dementia is diagnosed in such patients. Given the ease of establishing the diagnosis with CT scanning, this is now a reasonable requirement. As the lesion increases in size, usually because of recurrent hemorrhages from the sinusoidal capillary channels found in the outer layer of the membrane, more significant disturbances of brain dysfunction may develop, including diplopia, pupillary abnormalities, and papilledema.

A chronic subdural collection may be discovered that is not responsible for the patient's symptoms. As longevity in western society increases, such collections are found increasingly, for example, in patients with chronic renal failure on hemodialysis or in other disorders. The surgeon must decide whether or not the collection is significant in producing the patient's symptoms. If there is a shift of the midline structures, then the subdural collection probably is responsible for the patient's neurologic symptoms. If, however, the midline structures are not shifted, the ventricles are not compressed, and there is evidence of significant brain atrophy, then one must be extremely cautious in draining such collections because the complications of such treatment, particularly in the elderly, infirm patient can be substantial.

In the typical elderly patient with a subdural collection, one should do the least that will likely produce a favorable result, that is, evacuation of the hematoma. Thus, craniotomies usually are not required for the removal of such hematomas. Either twist drill drainage with the placement of a small drain, or evacuation of the hematoma through one or two burr holes, usually two, one placed in the frontal and one placed in the parietal regions, are favored. We usually use twist drill evacuation in the operating room with an anesthesiologist in attendance. In patients who can cooperate with the procedure, a twist drill hole may be placed while the patient is in an appropriate intensive or intermediate care unit, where nursing personnel can assist and where the patient can be carefully observed after the procedure.

Technique of Evacuation

The patient is placed in the supine position with the head slightly elevated. Skull fixation is not used in older patients because it produces substantial discomfort and is not required for such a brief procedure. The head is turned slightly to the opposite side. The skin is infiltrated with 1% lidocaine with 1:1000 epinephrine, and then a small skin incision, approximately 2 cm in length, is placed approximately 6 to 8 cm lateral to the midline over the thickest part of the collection, which is usually in the right frontal region.

A twist drill hole, approximately 3/16 inch in diameter, is placed and the dura penetrated with a size 14 gauge needle. A small amount of fluid is allowed to escape, following which a larger dural opening is made, either with an 11 blade or by repeat perforation of the dura with a needle. A small catheter (8 to 10 F) is placed in the subdural space, gently and carefully, to avoid rupturing fragile bridging cortical veins or those of the cortex. Hematoma drainage need not be complete but sufficient enough to reverse neurologic events and prevent further hematoma formation. The drain is then sutured in place and the wound closed. The drain is attached to a collection device. In our unit we tie a sterile glove tightly to the drain. Fluid can be emptied every 24 hours by tying off and excising a finger of the glove.

Sometimes burr holes are placed to drain chronic SDHs because of the location and size of the clot, e.g., larger and more medial. The first burr hole is placed in the frontal region, over the collection, approximately 4 to 5 cm lateral to the midline. A self-retaining retractor is used for exposure, and the dura is carefully incised and opened. Usually, the dura will appear blue in these patients because of the outer membrane, which must be incised. We open the subdural membrane carefully and allow slow drainage. Once a substantial amount of fluid has drained, a second burr hole is placed, usually in the temporal region directly anterior to the auditory meatus and approximately 4 cm above it. A small red rubber drain is placed over the hemisphere using direct vision and warm saline solution irrigated between the two burr holes. When the hematoma has been adequately drained, and if the brain reexpands, we remove the drain and close both skin incisions with inverted galeal sutures and appropriate skin sutures. If brain reexpansion does not occur, a drain is left in place, similar to the technique used for twist drill evacuation.

In many elderly patients, reexpansion of the hemisphere will be slow, if it occurs at all. Failure of the brain to reexpand is not necessarily associated with lack of improvement. If the patient deteriorates or does not improve, we obtain a CT scan. Trapping of subdural air, or tension pneumocephalus, is a significant and serious complication. This occurs as air replaces the chronic SDH after it is drained and the brain does not expand to fill the cavity. After closure with a drain, the air pressure increases as the brain expands. If the air is under pressure, tapping the subdural space with a needle will allow most of the air to exit.

Illustrations of the potential complications that occur after evacuation of a chronic SDH are shown in Figures 4–6 and 4–7. Note the development, first, of a collection of air, and then, following its evacuation, of an acute SDH that resulted in the patient's abrupt deterioration. In this instance, the passage of the catheter appears to have caused a cortical laceration.

If the policies described here are followed, a very low mortality and morbidity are achievable. Some patients will not improve because the subdural collection is not responsible for the patient's symptoms. In some, the hematoma will have been present too long before evacuation to reverse a significant dementing illness. Although the great majority of patients do improve after evacuation of such lesions, should the patient improve initially and

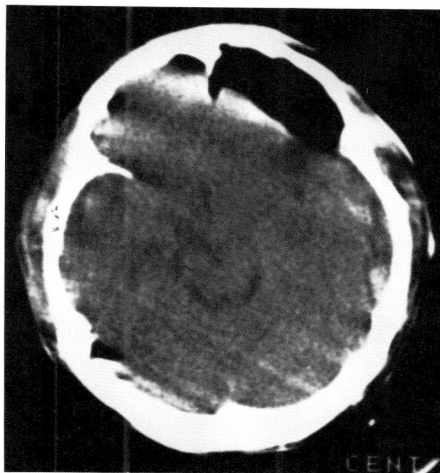

Figure 4–6.   Air entrapped in a patient after evacuation of a chronic subdural hematoma. The patient deteriorated after the initial procedure.

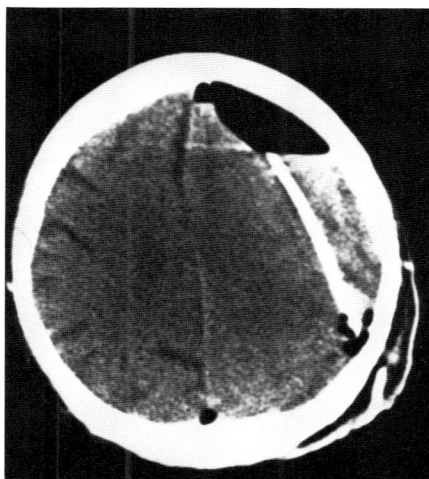

Figure 4–7.   Same patient as in Figure 4–6. Evacuation of the air resulted in the further accumulation of an acute subdural hematoma.

then deteriorate with reaccumulation of the hematoma, the surgeon should attempt to evacuate it again.

SUMMARY

The surgical treatment of extra-axial hematomas is one of the oldest surgical endeavors known to man. Modern technology, coupled with meticulous technique, offers the opportunity to improve substantially the outcome for patients with these lesions. It is incumbent on the neurosurgeon to treat the traumatically injured brain with the same care and respect he does the tissue surrounding an intracranial aneurysm or a benign tumor. Attention to meticulous technique and a systematic and logical approach to each patient are mandatory if the optimal result is to be realized.

REFERENCES

1. Andrews BT, Pitts LH, Lovely MP, Bartkowski HR: Is computed tomographic scanning necessary in patients with tentorial herniation? Results of immediate surgical exploration without computed tomography in 100 patients. Neurosurgery 19:408–414, 1986.
2. Becker DP, Miller JD, Ward JD, Greenberg RP, Young HF, Sakalas R: The outcome from severe head injury with early diagnosis and intensive management. J Neurosurg 47:491–502, 1977.
3. Bricolo AP, Paasut LM: Extradural hematoma: Toward zero mortality. A prospective study. Neurosurgery 14: 8–12, 1984.
4. Brihaye J: Chronic subdural hematoma. In Vigoroux RP, McLaurin RL (eds): Advances in Neurotraumatology: Extracerebral Collections. Vienna: Springer-Verlag, 1986, pp 101–145.
5. Pitts LH: Neurological evaluation of the head injury patient. Clin Neurosurg 29:203–224, 1981.
6. Stening WA, Berry G, Dan NG, Kwok B, Mandryk JA, Ring I, Sewell M, Simpson DA: Experience with acute subdural haematomas in New South Wales. Aust N Z J Surg 56:549–556, 1986.
7. Teasdale G, Galbraith S, Murray L, Ward P, Geuttanna D, McKath M: Management of traumatic intracranial hematomas. Br Med J 285:1695–1697, 1982.
8. Youmans JR: Neurological Surgery, vol 4. Philadelphia: WB Saunders, 1982

5

Traumatic Intracerebral Hematomas

DONALD S. SOLONIUK, E. FRANCOIS ALDRICH, AND HOWARD M. EISENBERG

In the management of patients with post-traumatic intracerebral hematomas (ICH) the decision to evacuate the hematoma surgically can often be simple. This is true in those hematomas that are large, causing mass effect, in relatively silent areas of the brain. The decision for conservative management can be relatively easy in small hematomas in vital areas with little mass effect. Frequently, however, in the management of the patient with a post-traumatic ICH, the neurosurgeon is faced with a difficult dilemma. In hematomas in which size and location do not force the decision to treat conservatively or to evacuate, factors such as overall condition of the patient and the potential for deterioration must be taken into account. Optimum timing of surgery must also be considered.[41]

It is the purpose of this chapter to elucidate the problems that must be dealt with in the management of patients with ICH following trauma and to develop guidelines that may be useful in making management decisions.

DEFINITIONS

In evaluating computed tomography (CT) scans of the head injured, the differentiation between a large contusion and a hematoma is often arbitrary. For our purposes, we define a contusion as a heterogenous area of brain necrosis, hemorrhage, and infarction, which is demonstrated on CT scan as mixed density changes. An ICH is defined as a homogenous coalescent area of high attenuation measuring 2 cm or greater with or without surrounding brain contusion or edema. These hematomas can occur in continuity with the surface of the brain. The so-called burst lobe is an ICH in continuity with a subdural hematoma.

CLINICAL MANIFESTATIONS

Post-traumatic intracerebral hematomas have been identified often since CT scanning became routinely available. The incidence of intracerebral hemorrhage is dependent on the type of injury sustained by the patient. Recent series report an overall incidence of between 4 and 12% in patients with severe cranial trauma,[27,88] although an incidence as high as 30% has been reported.[61] The highest hematoma incidence is in patients aged 21 to 40 years,[32] and men are involved more frequently than women.[32,58,59,70] Motor vehicle accidents are the most common cause of ICH;[32] falls either from the standing position or from a height are next in frequency, followed by assaults.

In their series, Jamieson and Yelland[32] found that location of hematoma was related to site of blow. Frontal hematomas, being most often caused by occipital blows, accounted for 46% of their cases. In 64% of cases with lateral blows the hematoma occurred on the same side as the trauma. They also noted that temporal hematomas most often resulted from a lateral blow to the head. The temporal lobes appear to be most commonly involved, followed by the frontal lobes, then parietal and occipital lobes.[9,26]

Posterior fossa hematomas are relatively uncommon.[57,69,74] A high degree of suspicion is necessary for their diagnosis. This level of suspicion should be heightened in the presence of occipital trauma, especially when there is an associated occipital skull fracture.[63,71,84,85] Traumatic basal ganglia hematomas also are uncommon, comprising about 2 to 4% of ICH.[42]

Often, ICH occur in association with other forms of intracranial abnormalities.[14,73] Most commonly, these hematomas are associated with contusions, but 28% are associated with subdural and 10% with epidural hematoma.[70] ICH can occur in multiple locations after head injury[21,80] and can arise in areas that appear normal on CT scans obtained soon after injury.[25,54,70,87]

Making a diagnosis of ICH is extremely difficult on clinical grounds alone, since symptoms depend not only on the size and location of the hematoma, but also on the amount and location of surrounding brain injury caused by the precipitating event. ICH, especially those that involve the frontal or temporal lobes, may produce no abnormal neurologic signs or symptoms. However, hemorrhages can be associated with the presence of a fixed neurologic deficit.[39] This is characterized by the early development of a post-traumatic deficit that remains stable throughout the patient's subsequent clinical course. The development of a progressive neurologic deficit in a patient with an ICH increases the likelihood of hematoma expansion or increasing pressure effects.

One should consider several factors when evaluating patients with ICH, including level of consciousness, intracranial pressure (ICP), size and location of the hematoma, and duration between time of injury and onset of symptoms.

Thirty-three to 50% of patients who have an ICH during their hospitalization, are unconscious on admission (Glasgow Coma Scale 8 or less).[70,82] As many as 20% of these patients demonstrate a classic lucid interval before the onset of coma.[70] Patients who are deeply comatose and have large hematomas soon after injury have a high mortality.[17,20,58,77] In contrast, surgery in patients with only mild disturbances of consciousness results in lower mortality.[59] Obviously, level of consciousness is directly related to the severity of the overall brain injury, but close and regular assessment of neurologic status can lead to planned intervention at the optimal time and may prevent neurologic deterioration.

Because hematomas are space-occupying lesions, they may cause an increased ICP. In an effort to predict which patients would require surgical evacuation, Galbraith and Teasdale[23] reviewed 26 patients with ICH and found that increased ICP correlated with subsequent need for surgery. Patients with ICP below 20 m H_2O in the presence of intracranial hemorrhage, rarely needed surgery. They recommended early evacuation for patients with ICP above 30 cm H_2O; in patients with ICP between 20 and 30 cm H_2O, they suggested close observation with immediate surgery on deterioration. These patients generally were not treated with hyperventilation or osmotherapy to control ICP before the decision was made whether or not to operate.

ICH certainly can cause intracranial hypertension and its removal generally will result in lowering of the ICP, even though outcome may be unchanged.[59,60] ICH can cause marked shifts of intracranial structures; the presence of midline shift has been taken to be evidence of a poor prognosis.[50] Signs of tentorial herniation are also associated with mortality, approaching 100% in decerebrate patients.[29,39] Hematomas involving more than one lobe, that is, the so-called panhemispheric hematoma, have been associated with a survival rate of 20%.[70]

The surgeon also must consider hematoma location and tailor management to the specific area of involvement, several requiring special consideration.[45]

Because of their proximity to the brainstem, expanding lesions within the anterior temporal lobe can cause rapid neurologic deterioration with increased morbidity and mortality. Brainstem compression can occur despite relatively normal ICP recordings.[44] This is undoubtedly responsible for the higher mortality recorded in patients with anterior temporal lobe hematomas compared with that in patients with hematomas elsewhere.

Likewise, cerebellar hematomas, although relatively rare in trauma, are often associated with brainstem compression, rapid deterioration, and death; midline ICH results in a much higher mortality than those in the hemispheres.[84] A delay in diagnosis can affect outcome.[42] High suspicion in patients with occipital trauma, especially those with occipital fractures, can lead to earlier diagnosis. However, despite early diagnosis, mortality remains high in these patients.

Basal ganglia hemorrhage has been associated with severe head injury, with 4% of traumatic ICH occurring in the basal ganglia.[42] Diffuse brain injury accompanying this ICH probably is responsible for the poor prognosis in these patients.

Traumatic intraventricular hemorrhages may result from tears in the ventricular walls or rarely from damage to the choroid plexus. Little or no neurologic deficit may be seen in these patients. Secondary intraventricular hemorrhages result from a rupture of an ICH into the ventricular system. There may often be significant mortality associated with this event, but not always.[3]

Of the lobar hemorrhages, frontal lobe ICH have the lowest morbidity and mortality; this is related to their occurrence in a relatively silent area of the brain.

One study noted that the onset of symptomatic ICH can become evident at various times after injury (Table 5–1). These patients predominantly had had falls and low-velocity injuries. The study emphasizes that hematomas may not be present immediately after injury

Table 5–1 Time After Injury for ICH Development

0–3 hours	20%
3–6 hours	6%
6–24 hours	29%
after 24 hours	46%

or even at the time of initial evaluation but they may develop subsequently. In this series coma was not necessarily associated with the presence or the subsequent development of ICH. Only 17% of the patients who were in coma immediately after injury developed ICH within 6 hours. Thirty-five percent of initially comatose patients, however, developed hematomas after 24 hours.[70] However, in a larger series of 1030 comatose patients the incidence of delayed hematoma, estimated as more than 15 cc by CT scan, was less than 5% (unpublished data from the National Institutes of Health Traumatic Coma Data Bank).

PATHOPHYSIOLOGY

Courville[15] proposed three distinct mechanisms of hematoma formation: (1) blows to the head resulting in a depressed fracture and laceration of the brain, with subsequent hematoma formation; (2) hematomas caused by penetrating wounds. These were seen to lie in the path of the wound canal, but were confined to the brain substance; and (3) hematomas resulting when the head in motion struck a relatively stationary object. Two forms of hematoma may occur in conjunction with this third proposed mechanism. First, overlying cortical-subcortical contusions can form as a superficial collection of blood within the brain, or, second, a primary hematoma may develop deep in the white matter. This third mechanism in the development of an ICH is thought to be due to rotational and angular impact forces. The rotational forces may account for the high association of ICH with falls and motor vehicle accidents.

ICH probably develops from movement of the brain within the cranium, which causes tearing of blood vessels followed by hemorrhage within the brain substance.[3] Significant clots may evolve from the coalescence of many small cortical hemorrhages or from damage to a single blood vessel. After injury there can be necrosis, breakdown of the brain tissue, and subsequent hemorrhage. These hematomas tend to be large in nature, replacing the cerebral substance. The ICH in association with the edema that occurs in the surrounding tissue is responsible for the intracranial hypertension often seen.

In addition to the mass effects and increased pressure often seen with ICH, there are metabolic changes occurring at the cellular level that contribute to the patient's condition and to outcome. Animal studies have demonstrated that the presence of hemorrhage within a hemisphere results not only in profound local ischemia but in ipsilateral hemispheric ischemia as well.[53,68] Both contribute to increased cell death and damage surrounding the hemorrhage. Autoradiographs of the surrounding tissue have given evidence of marked hypoperfusion. Although decrease in global cerebral perfusion pressure has been used as an explanation for these changes, they are more likely due to an increase in surrounding tissue pressure with local compression of the microcirculation. This mechanism was first suggested by Cushing[16] and has been documented by Misukami and Tazawa.[51] In association with perfusion changes there is angiographic evidence of arterial spasm in up to 50% of patients after ICH. This spasm may be global or segmental in nature and associated changes in the local circulation may be seen.[3,12]

Cerebrospinal fluid (CSF) acidosis also occurs after ICH development, due to the metabolic changes that occur in response to tissue hypoxia. Tissue oxygen tension around the hematoma is markedly increased, but there is an associated decrease in oxygen tension in the CSF.[72] These and other factors undoubtedly contribute to the multiple manifestations that occur.

DELAYED TRAUMATIC INTRACEREBRAL HEMATOMAS

Delayed traumatic intracerebral hematomas, (DTICH) first described by Bollinger[8] in 1891, have been thought to be a rare entity following head trauma. It appears that they are more common than once was thought, due to increased use of serial CT scans in the management of the head-injured patient. Incidence has been given variously as 1.3 to 7.4% in patients with severe head injury.[11,18,25,54]

DTICH are described as hematomas occurring after an interval during which no hematoma is found, after which they become evident from hours to days following the head injury.[22] Delayed hematomas occur more frequently in older age groups, with incidence roughly parallel to the age distribution of patients developing subdural hematomas.[4,78] DTICH formation has been linked to the rotational forces involved in falls more commonly than with other traumatic events.[18,30]

The mechanism of DTICH formation most commonly suggested is that of a vessel wall weakness.[18,87] After injury, there is an associated loss of autoregulation leading to a decrease in cerebral vascular resistance with increased blood pressure in the capillary bed that allows hematoma formation by leakage of blood through the damaged vascular walls.[65] Hypoxia and hypotension may contribute to clot development. Other investigators believe that changes in pH resulting from cell damage and metabolic breakdown produce a vessel dilation leading to hematoma formation.[19,25,87]

DTICH can occur after brain decompression by removal of extracerebral hematomas. Damaged vessels may be tamponaded by the pressure from the subdural or epidural hematoma, release of which allows ICH formation.[18,31,52,70,75]

Some investigators have noted a relationship of disseminated intravascular coagulopathy and fibrinolysis to DTICH.[34–37,79] Clotting abnormalities result from thromboplastic substances released into the circulation after brain injury.[1,2,24,47] In the presence of disseminated intravascular coagulation, microthrombi can occlude small vessels, initiating a sequence of events; that is distal infarction, lysis of the thrombi, hemorrhage into the area of infarction, and the development of a delayed ICH. This may occur in the presence of a normal prothrombin time, partial thromboplastin time and platelet count.[34] The relationship of DTICH to coagulopathy, however, was questioned by Saweda et al.[66] who failed to find evidence of coagulopathy in 18 patients who developed delayed ICH.

The clinical picture of the development of a delayed hematoma is that of a patient who has shown improvement or remained stable after head injury and who then rapidly deteriorates.[10,38] Patients undergoing ICP monitoring may show sudden marked intracranial hypertension. Occasionally, DTICH are shown to occur on serial CT scans when no change in neurologic status or ICP has occurred. These hematomas can also be found in patients who fail to improve and may contribute to the patient's poor clinical status.

TREATMENT

Timing and decision for operative intervention in patients with ICH often can be difficult. Certainly, not all ICH require surgical evacuation. The factors favoring surgery must be weighed against the potential risks. The decision to operate will be based on the patient's general condition and associated brain injuries, the site and size of the hematoma, and the perception that ICH removal will improve the neurologic outcome.[81] There is no one right way to treat patients with ICH, and where one physician may be surgically aggressive in hematoma removal, another physician may successfully manage such a patient non-operatively. Both methods can be correct, requiring skillful application of critical judgment.

At our institution, we have adopted an aggressive surgical approach with patients who present with a traumatic ICH. Large ICH are space-occupying lesions, and can contribute to increased ICP. Knowing that their removal often lowers ICP, we tend to operate on patients with large hematomas or those producing mass effect on CT scan. Likewise, patients with ICP above the 25 to 30 torr range that cannot be lowered by medical management or with ICP in the 20 to 25 torr range and increasing are considered strongly for hematoma removal to control intracranial hypertension.[50] If ICP remains below 20 torr consistently, surgery usually is not necessary.[44] Shift of midline structures does not necessarily correspond with the need for surgery.[76] Patients with an ICH who have evidence of progressive neurologic deterioration or who have stabilized at an unsatisfactory level are considered candidates for surgical intervention.[13,48] Coma is not in itself considered an indication for or against surgery; rather, the decision is based on the hematoma size and location, ICP, and evidence of mass effect. When confronted with a patient who has both an intracerebral and a subdural or epidural hematoma, we try to remove both during the same procedure whenever possible.

In each of these cases, logical arguments can be made for managing the patient conservatively.[58] The location of the hemorrhage is a definite factor in management decisions. ICH within the anterior temporal lobe can cause rapid neurologic deterioration, and we tend to operate earlier and to remove smaller hematomas than in most other brain regions.

We also tend to be more aggressive in operating and removing intracerebellar hemorrhages because of their proximity to the brainstem, although some can be managed without surgery.[62] The size of a cerebellar hematoma seems to be a determinant of the severity of brainstem compression or a predictor of outcome only when very large or very small. If the hematoma exerts pressure evenly on all the structures in the posterior fossa, including the brainstem and vermis, it can cause upward herniation of the vermis and is diagnosed by obliteration of the quadrigeminal cistern on CT. This cistern compromise indicates brainstem compression and the need for urgent posterior fossa decompression.[74]

Hemorrhages in the basal ganglia often are accompanied by other severe brain injury and have a high mortality and morbidity rate.[42] Because of size (often small) and associated lesions, we operate on relatively few of these patients. Recently, in a few patients, we have evacuated larger traumatic basal ganglia hemorrhages using stereotactic techniques but do not know if this approach will be useful generally.

Intraventricular hemorrhages, especially in those patients who are neurologically normal, can often be followed with expected gradual resolution of the hemorrhage within the ventricle. Serial CT scans should be used to monitor the possible development of hydrocephalus. Occasionally, ventricular drainage is needed.

If the hemorrhage is old, needle aspiration of a liquefied hematoma, may be effective.[5,64,86] Recent reports have described the use of a stereotactic needle developed by Bocklund and Holst,[7] and others for removal of intracerebral hematomas.[30,46,56] Further experience will be necessary to judge the ultimate usefulness of this procedure.

We generally prefer a craniotomy for ICH removal except when a circumscribed hematoma has been identified and may be removed through a small craniectomy or trephine.

It is often useful to turn a large frontotemporal bone flap using a question mark skin incision, the backward arch of which provides access to the full length of the temporal lobe and to a clot in the parietal region.[73] If the intraparenchymal lesion is not accessible through this frontotemporal craniotomy, an appropriate flap should be turned over the exact location.

Contusions, foci of necrotic brain, and hemorrhage usually appear on the surface of the anterior and inferior frontal lobes and the temporal lobes. Contused brain is irreversibly damaged; it acts as a mass lesion and also may cause further local brain swelling. Surface contusions larger than 1 to 2 cm in diameter incidential to an operative extra-axial clot probably should be removed; often a surface contusion will extend several centimeters or more into the hemisphere and the cortical surface of the contusion is only the tip of the iceberg. The soft necrotic bluish tissue can easily be aspirated, and aspiration should be continued until a circumferential margin of healthy brain tissue is reached.

Multiple small contusions showing the areas of hemorrhage beneath an intact pia-arachnoid do not necessarily indicate that the underlying brain is irreparably damaged and care should be taken not to injure or remove viable brain. Contusions over the more posterior superior temporal lobe or in the region of the central sulcus, and parietal and occipital lobes should be evacuated carefully and only if the brain is clearly necrotic.

ICH, with little admixed brain, are located commonly in the frontal and temporal regions and tend to present deeper in the tissue than do contusions. They are usually relatively easy to remove under direct vision, but the surgeon must be meticulous in achieving absolute hemostasis after clot removal. Sometimes a partial lobectomy is appropriate if a large portion of the lobe has been damaged, especially if it is on the nondominant side. The surgeon should consider the possibility of bilateral diffuse damage; it is unwise to remove largely intact frontal or temporal lobes in order to provide an internal decompression in severely injured patients. Occasionally, sudden, massive brain swelling occurs after the dura is opened, either immediately or sometimes minutes after a clot or contusion has been removed. The hematoma or contusion should quickly be resected as thoroughly as possible and attempts made to reduce brain volume, such as by induced arterial hypotension, mannitol administration, and hyperventilation. A bolus of pentobarbital (10 mg/kg intravenously) may help, but only if the patient is not hypotensive. The brain swelling is usually the result of defective cerebral autoregulation, but new acute intraoperative hemorrhage must be excluded. Intraoperative ultrasound is extremely helpful in identifying new hemorrhage or ensuring adequate removal of the original hematoma.[40,55]

If the brain is relaxed after clot removal, the dural incision should be closed and the bone flap replaced and fixed in place.

When we choose nonsurgical management, we follow the patient carefully with frequent neurologic examinations and serial CT scans as indicated. ICP is monitored and controlled using osmotics, diuretics, and controlled ventilation until ICP is normal and the patient is improving, or until we conclude that surgical removal of the ICH is needed.

Some investigators have pointed out the improved prognosis and the lowered surgical mortality in delaying surgical management of ICH for several days after onset.[58] Undoubtedly, this eliminates as surgical candidates those patients who do not survive the immediate post-traumatic period and thus provides a better selection of patients for surgery. Often, patients may be too unstable from multiple systemic injuries to tolerate early surgery. In these cases, aggressive management aimed at controlling ICP can delay the decision to operate until the patient is better able to tolerate the procedure and may improve outcome.

OUTCOME

Outcome in patients with ICH depends on many factors. Despite an improved ability for early recognition, aggressive management, and close monitoring of patients with ICH, outcome remains unsatisfactory. This poor outcome is closely related to the severity of the injury producing the hematoma as well as to the hematoma itself. Most reports give mortality rates in the range of 25 to 58%.[6,28,29,33,49,61,67]

Level of consciousness, size of hematoma, and site of involvement have already been mentioned as factors that affect outcome. In addition, the age of the patient and the associated systemic disease or trauma must be considered as important contributing factors. Each must be taken into account by the neurosurgeon as overall care and management decisions are made.

REFERENCES

1. Auer L: Disturbances of the coagulatory system in patients with severe cerebral trauma, I. Acta Neurochir (Wien). 43:51–59, 1978.
2. Auer L, Ott E: Disturbances of the coagulatory system in patients with severe cerebral trauma, II. Acta Neurochir (Wien) 49:219–226, 1979.
3. Bakay L, Glasauer F: Intracranial hemorrhage. In Bakay L, Glasauer F (eds): Management of head injury. Boston: Little, Brown 1980, pp 175–262
4. Baratham G, Dennyson W: Delayed traumatic intracerebral hemorrhage. J Neurol Neurosurg Psychiatry, 35: 698–706, 1972.
5. Beatty R, Zervas N: Stereotactic aspiration of brain stem hematoma. Neurosurgery 13:204–207, 1983.
6. Becker D, Miller J, Ward J, et al.: The outcome from severe head injury with early diagnosis and intensive management. J Neurosurg 47:491–502, 1977.
7. Bocklund E, Holst H: Controlled subtotal evacuation of intracerebral hematomas by stereotactic technique. Surg Neurol 9:99–101, 1978
8. Bollinger O: Uber traumatische stat-apoplexie: Ein beitrag zur lehre der hirnerschatterarg, in internationale beitrage zur wissenschaft lichen medizin, vol 2. Berlin: Festschrift, Rudolf Verchow, A Hirschwold, 1891, pp 457–470.
9. Browder J, Turney M: Intracerebral hemorrhage of traumatic origin. NY State J Med, 42:2230–2232, 1942.
10. Brown F, Mullan S, Duda E: Delayed traumatic intracerebral hematomas. J Neurosurg 48:1019–1022, 1978.
11. Clifton G, Grossman R, Makela M, et al.: Neurological course and correlated computerized tomography findings after severe closed head injury. J Neurosurg 52:611–701, 1963.
12. Cohadon F, Richer E, Castel J, et al.: Aspects cliniques et angiographique des lesions parenchymateuses fronto-temporales d'origine traumatique. Neurochirurgie 19:417–430, 1973.
13. Cook A: Traumatic intracranial hemorrhage, NY State J Med 63:699–701, 1963
14. Cooper P, Ho V: Role of emergency skull X-ray films in the evaluation of the head injured patient: A retrospective study. Neurosurgery 13:136–140, 1983.
15. Courville C: Traumatic intracerebral hemorrhages, with special reference to the mechanics of their production. Bull Los Angeles Neurol Soc 27:22–32, 1962.
16. Cushing H: Some experimental and clinical observations concerning status of increased intracranial tension. Am J Med Sci 124:375–400, 1902.
17. Da Pian R, Dulle O, Bricolo A, et al.: Lacerazioni cerebelli traumatiche: Considerazioni su 190 casi operati. Minerva Neurochir, 11:147–153, 1967.
18. Diaz F, York D, Larson D, Rockswold G: Early diagnosis of delayed post traumatic intracerebral hematomas. J Neurosurg 50:217–233, 1979.
19. Evans J, Scheinker I: Histologic studies of the brain following head trauma. J Neurosurg 3:101–113, 1946.
20. Freckman N, Sarter K, Matsumoto K: Angiographic demonstration of vascular injuries following head injury and its significance. Adv Neurosurg 5:116–123, 1978.
21. French BN, Dublin AB: The value of computerized tomography in the management of 1000 consecutive head injuries. Surg Neurol 7:171–183, 1977.
22. Fukamachi A, Nagasoki Y, Kohno K, Wakao T: The incidence and developmental process of delayed traumatic intracerebral hematomas. Acta. Neurochir. (Wien) 74:35–39, 1985.

23. Galbraith S, Teasdale G: Predicting the need for operation in the patient with occult traumatic intracranial hematoma. J Neurosurg 55:75–81, 1981.

24. Goodnight S, Kenoyou G, Rapaport S, et al.: Defibrination after brain tissue destruction. N Engl J Med 290: 1043–1047. 1974.

25. Gudeman S, Kishore P, Miller J, et al.: The genesis and significance of delayed traumatic intracerebral hematoma. Neurosurgery 5:309–313, 1979.

26. Gurdjian E, Gurdjian E: Cerebral contusion: Re-evaluation of the mechanism of their development. J Trauma 16: 35–51, 1976.

27. Gurdjian E. Thomas L: Traumatic intracranial hemorrhage. In Brock S (ed) Injuries of the Brain and Spinal Cord and Their Coverings. New York: Springer 1974, p 282

28. Gurdjian E. Webster J: Traumatic intracranial hemorrhage. In Brock S (ed): Injuries of the Brain and Spinal Cord. New York: Springer, 1960, pp 127–186

29. Heiskanen O, Vapalahti M: Temporal lobe contusion and hematoma. Acta Neurochir (Wien) 27:29–36, 1972.

30. Higgins A, Nashold B: Modification of instrument for stereotactic evacuation of intracerebral hematoma: Technical note. Neurosurgery 7:604–605, 1980.

31. Hirsh L: Delayed traumatic intracerebral hematomas after surgical decompression. Neurosurgery 5:653–655, 1979.

32. Jamieson K, Yelland J: Traumatic intracerebral hematoma. J Neurosurg 37:528–532, 1972.

33. Karimi-Nejad A, Hamel E, Frowein K: Prognosis for traumatic intracerebral hematoma. Nervenarzt 50:432–435, 1979.

34. Kaufman H, Hui K, Mattson J, et al.: Clinical pathological correlations of disseminated intravascular coagulation in patients with head injury. Neurosurgery 15:34–42, 1984.

35. Kaufman H, Mouke J, Olson J, et al.: Delayed and recurrent intracranial hematomas related to disseminated intravascular clotting and fibrinolysis in head injury. Neurosurgery 7:445–449, 1980.

36. Kaufman H, Sadhu V, Clifton G, Hundel S: Delayed intracerebral hematoma due to traumatic aneurysm caused by shotgun wound: A problem of prophylaxis. Neurosurgery 6:181–184, 1980.

37. Kelmowitz R, Annis B: Disseminated intravascular coagulation associated with massive brain injury. J Neurosurg 39:178–180, 1973.

38. Koulouris S, Rizzol H: Delayed traumatic intracerebral hematoma after compound depressed skull fracture: Case report. Neurosurgery 8:223–225, 1981.

39. Levinthal R, Stern W: Traumatic intracerebral hematoma with stable neurological deficit. Surg Neurol 7: 269–273, 1977.

40. Lillehei K, Chandler W, Knate J: Real-time ultrasound characteristics of the acute intracerebral hemorrhage as studied in the canine model. Neurosurgery 14:48–51, 1984.

41. Lobato R, Cordobes F, Rivas J, et al.: Outcome from severe head injury related to the type of intracranial lesion. J Neurosurg 59:762–774, 1983.

42. MacPherson P, Teasdale E, Khaker S, et al.: The significance of traumatic hematoma in the region of the basal ganglia. J Neurol, Neurosurg, Psychiatry 49:29–34, 1986.

43. Martinowitz U, Heim M, Tadmov R, et al.: Intracranial hemorrhage in patients with hemophilia. Neurosurgery 18:533–541, 1986.

44. Marshall LF, El-Hefnawi M: Spontaneous intracranial hemorrhage. Semin Neurol 4:422–429, 1984.

45. Marshall L: Mass lesion location determines the level of ICP which produces brainstem compression. Report at the annual meeting of the American Association of Neurological Surgeons, 1985.

46. Matsumoto K, Hondo K: CT-guided stereotaxic evacuation of hypertensive intracerebral hematomas. J Neurosurg 61:440–448, 1984.

47. McGauley J, Miller C, Pennor J: Diagnosis and treatment of diffuse intravascular coagulation following cerebral trauma. J Neurosurg 43:374–376, 1975.

48. McLaurin R, McBride B: Traumatic intracerebral hematoma: Review of sixteen surgically treated cases. Ann Surg 143:294–305, 1956.

49. Merrin M, Pitts F: Delayed apoplexy following head injury ("traumatische Spät-Apoplexie"). J Neurosurg 33:542–547, 1970.

50. Miller J, Butterworth J, Gudeman S, et al.: Further experience in the management of severe head injury. J Neurosurg 54:289–299, 1981.

51. Mizukami M, Tazawa T: Theoretical background for surgical treatment in hypertensive intracerebral hemorrhage. In Mizukami M, Kogare K, Kanay H (eds): Hypertensive Intracerebral Hemorrhage. New York: Raven Press, 1983, pp 239–247.

52. Modesti LM, Hodge CJ, Barnwell M: Intracerebral hematoma after evacuation of chronic extracerebral fluid collections. Neurosurgery 10:689–693, 1982.

53. Nath F, Kelly P, Jenkins A, et al.: Effects of experimental intracerebral hemorrhage on blood flow, capillary permeability and histochemistry. J Neurosurg 66:555–562, 1987.

54. Ninchoji T, Uemura K, Shimoyama I, Hinokuma K, Bun T, Nakajima S: Traumatic intracerebral hematomas of delayed onset. Acta Neurochir (Wien) 71:69–90, 1984.

55. Ostrup R, Bejar R, Marshall L: Real-time ultrasonography: A useful tool in the evaluation of the craniectomized brain injured patient. Neurosurgery 12:225–227, 1983.
56. Pan D, Lee L, Chen M, Manns A: Modified screw and suction technique for stereotactic evacuation of deep intracerebral hematomas. Surg Neurol 25:540–544, 1986.
57. Papadakis N, Safran A, Ramirez L, Sujatanond M, Mark VH: Traumatic cerebellar hematoma without subdural hematoma. JAMA 235:530–531, 1976.
58. Papo I, Caneschi S: Considerazioni sul trattamento chirurgilo dei focolai lacero contusiui traumatici. Minerva Neurochir 8:86–88, 1963.
59. Papo I, Caruselli G, Luongo A, et al.: Traumatic cerebral mass lesions: Correlations between clinical, intracranial pressure, and computed tomographic data. Neurosurgery 7:337–346, 1980.
60. Papo I, Caruselli G, Scarpelli M: Intracranial pressure time course in intracerebral traumatic hematomas. In Shulman K, Marmarou A, Miller J, et al. (eds): Intracranial Pressure, IV. Berlin: Springer Verlag. 1980, pp 33–35.
61. Piepmeier J, Wagner F: Delayed post-traumatic extracerebral hematomas. J Trauma 22:455–460, 1982.
62. Pozzati E, Piazza G, Padovani R, Gaist G: Benign traumatic intracerebellar hematoma. Neurosurgery 8:102–103, 1981.
63. Pozzati E, Grossi C, Padovani R: Traumatic intracerebellar hematomas. J Neurosurg 56:691–694, 1982
64. Pozzati E, Giukiano G, Guist G, et al.: Chronic expanding intracerebral hematoma. J Neurosurg 65:611–614, 1986.
65. Pretorius M, Kaufman H: Rapid onset of delayed traumatic intracerebral hematoma with diffuse intravascular coagulation and fibrinolysis. Acta Neurochir (Wien) 65:103–104, 1982.
66. Saweda Y, Sadomitsu D, Sakmoto T, et al.: Lack of correlation between delayed traumatic intracerebral hematoma and disseminated intravascular coagulation. J Neurol Neurosurg Psychiatry 77:1125–1127, 1984.
67. Schaible D, Smith L, et al.: Evaluation of the risks of anticoagulation therapy following experimental craniotomy in the rat. J Neurosurg 63:959–962, 1985.
68. Sinar E, Mendelow A, Graham D, Teasdale G: Experimental intracerebral hemorrhage: Effects of a temporary mass lesion. J Neurosurg 66:568–576, 1987.
69. Sokol JH, Rowed DW: Traumatic intracerebellar hematoma. Surg Neurol 10:340–341, 1978.
70. Soloniuk D, Pitts LH, Lovely M, Bartkowski H: Traumatic intracerebral hematomas. Timing of appearance and indications for operative removal. J Trauma 26:787–793, 1986.
71. St. John J, French B: Traumatic hematomas of the posterior fossa. Surg Neurol 25:459–466, 1986.
72. Sussman B, Barber J, Gould H: Experimental intracerebral hematoma. J Neurosurg 41:177–186, 1974.
73. Tandon P, Prakesh B, Bunerji A: Temporal lobe lesions in head injury. Acta Neurochir (Wien) 41:205–210, 1978.
74. Taneda M, Hayakawa T, Mogami H: Primary cerebellar hemorrhage. Quadrigeminal cistern obliteration on CT scans as a predictor of outcome. J Neurosurg 67:545–552, 1987.
75. Taneda M, Irino T: Enlargement of intracerebral haematomas following surgical removal of epidural haematomas. Acta Neurochir (Wien) 51:73–82, 1979.
76. Teasdale G, Galbraith S, Jennett B: Operate or observe? ICP and the management of the "silent" traumatic intracranial haematoma. In: Shulman K (ed): Intracranial Pressure V. Springer-Verlag, 1980.
77. Teasdale G, Galbraith S, Murray L, et al.: Management of traumatic intracranial hematoma. Br Med J 285: 1695–1697, 1982.
78. Tedeschi G, Bernini P, Cerillo A: Indications for surgical treatment of intracerebral hemorrhage. J Neurosurg 43:590–595, 1975.
79. Touho H, Hirakawa K, Hino A, et al.: Relationship between abnormalities of coagulation and fibrinolysis and postoperative intracranial hemorrhage in head injury. Neurosurgery 19:523–531, 1986.
80. Tsukahura T, Nishikawa M, Iwuma M, Kim S: Traumatic intracerebral midline hematoma. Acta Neurochir (Wien) 62:73–77, 1982.
81. Ugrumov V, Zotov Y, Shchedryonok V: Early surgical treatment of traumatic intracranial hematomas and laceration foci as the main factor of favorable prognosis. Acta Neurochir [Suppl] (Wien) 28:199–200, 1979.
82. Van Dongen K, Braakman R: Late computed tomography in survivors of severe head injury. Neurosurgery 7: 14–21, 1980.
83. Vigouroux R, Guillermain P: Hematoma sous-dural aign et attrition cerebrale post traumatique: Technique operatoir. Neurochirurgie 19:481–484, 1973.
84. Wojak J, Cooper P: Traumatic lesions of the posterior cranial fossa. Contemp Neurosurg 8:1–6, 1986.
85. Wright R: Traumatic hematomas of the posterior cranial fossa. J Neurosurg 25:402–404, 1966.
86. Yashon D, Kosnik E: Chronic intracerebral hematoma. Neurosurgery 2:103–106, 1978.
87. Young H, Gleave J, Schmidek H, Gregory S: Delayed traumatic intracerebral hematoma; report of fifteen cases operatively treated. Neurosurgery 14:22–25, 1984.
88. Zimmerman R, Bilaniuk L, Gennarelli T, et al.: Cranial computed tomography in diagnosis and management of acute head trauma. Am J Radiol 13:29–34, 1978.

6

Management of Associated Cranial Lesions

JEFFREY ROBINSON AND PAUL J. DONALD

Because cranial and facial injuries occur often in the same patient, the neurosurgeon should be familiar with some of these injuries and assist in their management jointly with otolaryngologists or plastic surgeons. In this chapter, we address the anatomy, diagnostic evaluation, and treatment of zygomatic, mandibular, frontal sinus, nasoethmoidal, and maxillary trauma to familiarize neurosurgeons with optimal care of these injuries.

FRACTURES OF THE ZYGOMA AND ZYGOMATIC ARCH

The zygoma forms the lateral buttress of the middle third of the face. It occupies a prominent position and can be fractured by a force as low as 50 g.[18] Fractures of the zygoma are second in incidence only to fractures of the nasal bones. Incidence in fractures of the zygoma and of fractures of the midface has shown a marked increase since World War II.[27] In private community hospitals, motor vehicle accidents remain the most common cause; in public hospitals, assault is the most common factor. A smaller number of zygoma fractures occur as a result of sports injuries.

The malar surface of the zygoma forms the prominence of the cheek (Fig. 6–1). A variety of muscles attach to the zygoma, as does the temporalis fascia. When the temporalis fascia attachment is disrupted, downward displacement of the fractured zygoma usually occurs due to the strong downward pull of the masseter. The lateral canthal tendon is attached to the lateral portion of the zygoma. The orbital surface of the zygoma forms part of the floor and lateral wall of the orbit.

Classification of zygomatic fractures correlates the direction of impact with the resultant displacement and stability of the fracture after surgical correction (Table 6–1).[16,28] As in all cases of significant maxillofacial trauma, a complete history and physical examination should be performed. The origin of the injury, the direction of the force, and the site of impact are all important. The specific symptoms of zygomatic fractures may be few.

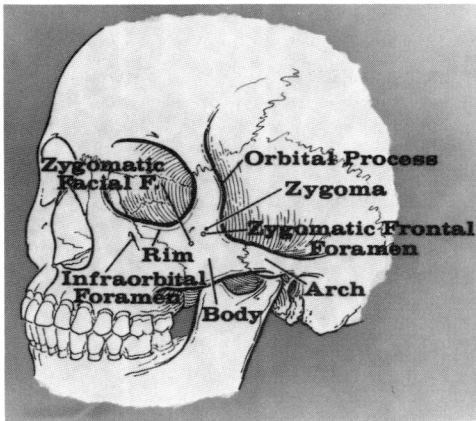

Figure 6–1. Illustration showing the general anatomy of the zygoma. (From Donald.[8] Reprinted with permission.)

Localized swelling, pain, and tenderness are usually present. Numbness in the distribution of the infraorbital nerve is common. Unilateral epistaxis often occurs from bleeding into the maxillary sinus or from concomitant nasal injury. Flattening of the bony contours of the cheek is usually present, but is often disguised by soft tissue swelling. Some drooping of the upper lip and deviation of the philtrum will appear when significant inferior displacement of the origins of the zygomaticus major and minor and levator labii muscles occurs. Intraoral hematoma may be noted and a bony "step-off" palpated within the upper buccal sulcus. Trismus may occur from the pull of the masseter muscle on the fractured arch. Bony step-offs at the zygomaticofrontal suture area and infraorbital rim are seen when a complete tripod fracture occurs. Rarely is subcutaneous emphysema seen.

Subconjunctival hemorrhage is common and a hyphema or ruptured globe may occur.

Table 6–1 Classification of Zygomatic Fractures*

Type I	No significant displacement
Type II	Fracture of the zygomatic arch
Type III	Rotation around the vertical axis
	Laterally
	Externally
Type IV	Rotation around the longitudinal axis
	Medially
	Laterally
Type V	Displacement of the complex—en bloc
	Medially
	Inferiorly
	Laterally (rare)
Type VI	Displacement of the orbitoantral partition
	Inferiorly (blow-out fracture)
	Superiorly (rare)
Type VII	Displacement of the orbital rim segments
Type VIII	Complex comminuted fractures

*Adapted from Rowe and Killey.[28]

Disruption of the orbital floor allows inferior herniation of orbital contents into the maxillary antrum causing enophthalmos and diplopia. The patient may tilt his head to restore a horizontal visual axis. Entrapment of the inferior rectus muscle in the orbital fracture line will cause diplopia on upward gaze. A forced duction test will confirm entrapment. An ophthalmologic consult is mandatory because concomitant global injury is common.

Radiographic evaluation is essential to treatment planning. The three most useful views are the Waters (Fig. 6–2), Caldwell, and submentovertex. Tomograms are useful when more detail is required. Computed tomography (CT) scans are extremely valuable in evaluating complex injuries in the orbital area and are an essential part of the evaluation of patients with altered vision who may need orbital decompression.

The care of life-threatening problems takes precedence in the management of facial trauma. In the absence of more serious injuries, treatment may proceed in an orderly fashion.

Nondisplaced zygoma or zygomatic arch fractures without disruption of the orbital floor or ocular dysfunction require no treatment. Weekly follow-up for 2 weeks and again at 4 weeks should be carried out and photographic documentation is advisable. In cases of minimal displacement without functional disturbance the treatment decision should be the result of discussion between patient and surgeon. Some patients may wish to forego operative treatment and accept a minor contour deformity.

Significant contour deformities should be reduced and adequately fixated (Fig. 6–3). Orbital floor defects and ocular muscle entrapment need surgical correction. Treatment should be carried out within 7 to 10 days before fibrous fixation makes reduction difficult. In children, reduction is carried out within 1 week.

More than 60% of fractures are stable after reduction without fixation.[17] Open reduction with stable fixation, however, allows for more accurate reduction under direct visualization. The orbital floor and infraorbital nerve can be directly inspected, and the risk of later displacement due to the pull of the masseter muscle and other factors is reduced.

When treatment is delayed, the reconstruction is more difficult to manage. Depression

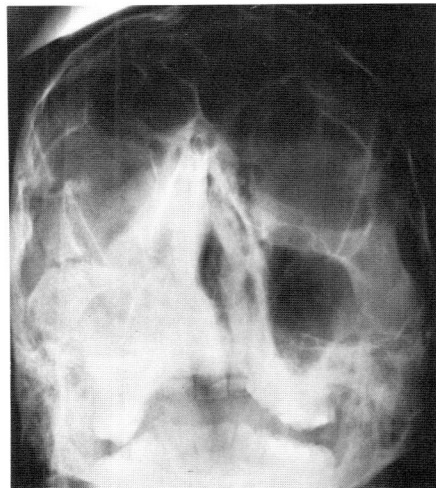

Figure 6–2. A Waters view (x-ray) showing a zygomatic fracture.

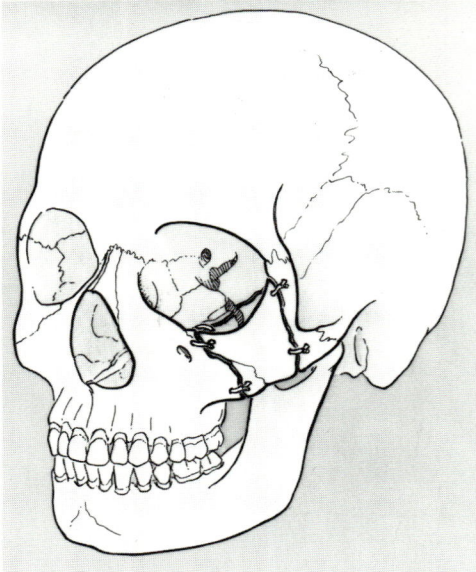

Figure 6–3.   Line drawing of a zygoma body fracture with interosseous wiring at the frontozygomatic and inferior orbital rim fracture sites as well as at articulation with the maxilla.

of the malar prominence may be corrected by onlay calvarial bone graft. More complex ocular problems, diplopia, enophthalmos, ptosis, and reduced visual acuity sometimes result from fractures of the zygoma. In consultation with an ophthalmologist, orbital floor defects are repaired and malunion is corrected by osteotomies, repositioning of the zygoma, and calvarial bone grafts. Surgery on the extraocular muscles is sometimes required to correct persisting diplopia. If the lateral canthal ligament has been inferiorly displaced, the palpebral fissure will develop an antimongoloid slant which may require correction. Posteroinferior displacement of the body of the zygoma may impinge on the coronoid process and limit jaw opening, requiring osteotomy and repositioning of the zygoma for correction.

MANDIBULAR FRACTURES

The mandible is one of the most important bones in the body and its aesthetic form is always evident (Fig. 6–4). In the management of injuries of the mandible, careful attention must be paid to both aesthetics and the restoration of function.

The response to loading of the mandible is similar to an architectural arch. Anterior loading of the mandible over the symphysis menti or one mental foramen results in high tensile strain in the subcondylar area and along the lingual plates of the opposite molar region, common sites of mandibular fracture (Fig. 6–5, 6–6, 6–7).[15] With fractures of the subcondylar region, the strong pull of the lateral pterygoid muscle causes anteromedial displacement of the condyle. If the joint capsule is ruptured, total dislocation may occur.

Ramus fractures are splinted by the strong masseter and medial pterygoid muscles and exhibit little displacement. A fracture through the angle, however, is displaced by the strong forces applied to the posterior fragment by the pterygomasseteric sling, causing medial as well as upward and forward displacement of the posterior fragment. In anterior body

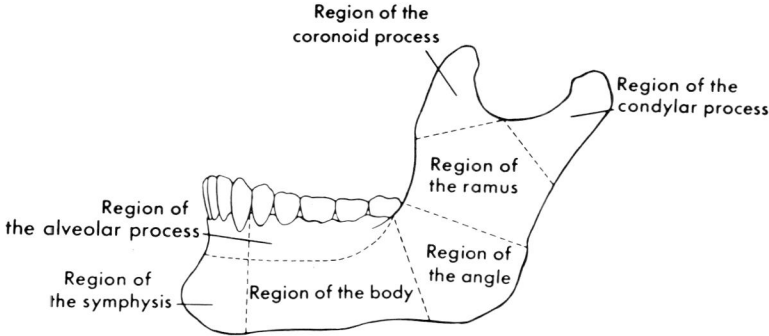

Figure 6–4. Line drawing showing the anatomy of the mandible. (From Dingman and Natvig.[3] Reprinted with permission.)

fractures, the upward pull of the pterygomasseteric sling is counteracted by the downward pull of the mylohyoid muscle. However, the mylohyoid also exerts a medially directed force, which is uncpposed, causing "lingual" displacement.

Radiographic evaluation of mandibular fractures usually includes a posteroanterior view, a Towne's view, and two lateral oblique views. The Towne's view is used for evalation of the mandibular condyles, but is difficult to interpret and it needs to be supplemented by a modified Towne's view or tomography. The two lateral oblique films show the mandibular body, angle, and parasymphyseal area. A panoramic radiograph (Panorex) is frequently ordered and allows a good view of the entire mandibule. It shows the relationship of the fracture line to the teeth and allows an appreciation of dental disease.

An accurate history may give the direction and velocity of the injuring force. A high velocity injury, such as a motor vehicle accident, has a high probability of additional trauma, such as intracranial, visceral, or spine injury. A contrecoup mandibular injury is common in the mandible with fractures occurring opposite the site of impact and maximal contusion. The examiner's attention is drawn to the area of maximal contusion and the opposing mandible fracture may go unnoticed.

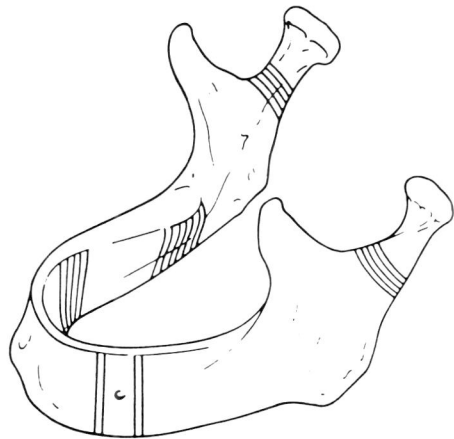

Figure 6–5. Distribution of strain lines as a result of force over the symphysis menti or one mental foramen. (From Rowe and Williams.[29] Reprinted with permission.)

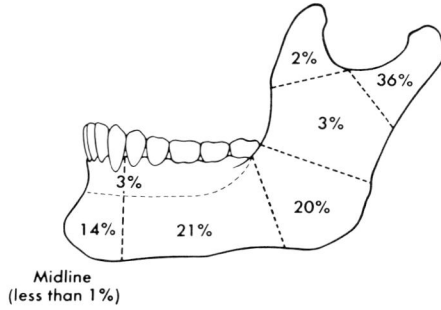

Figure 6–6. Line drawing showing the incidence of fractures at different sites. (From Dingman and Natvig.[3] Reprinted with permission.)

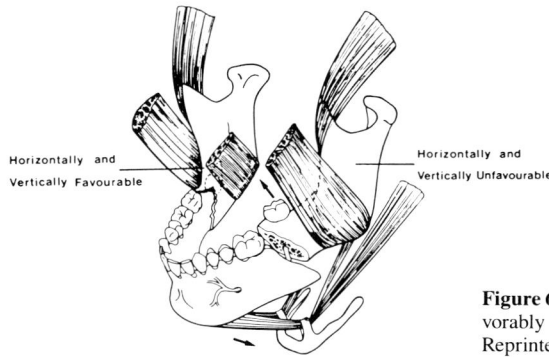

Figure 6–7. Line drawing showing favorably and unfavorably aligned fractures. (From Rowe and Williams.[29] Reprinted with permission.)

The most common symptoms are of pain, trismus, and malocclusion. Anesthesia, swelling, and ecchymosis are also common. The presence of trismus (the inability to open the mouth due to muscle pain) suggests a fracture in the posterior aspect of the mandible. Contusion and ecchymosis will assist in the localization of the site of injury. Numbness suggests damage to the inferior alveolar, mental, or lingual nerves.

Intraoral inspection will detect loose, avulsed, or fractured teeth. Variation in the height of the occlusal surfaces, ecchymosis around a tooth, or a tear in the mucoperiosteum may indicate a fracture site. Occasionally, fractured bone can be seen jutting into the mouth or through the facial skin. An accurate assessment of the dentition and occlusion is an essential part of treatment planning.

Extraoral inspection will identify localized tenderness and the feeling of crepitus, which can assist in localizing fracture sites. Occasionally, there is subcutaneous emphysema as far down as the clavicles. The patient should be examined for anesthesia in the distribution of the inferior alveolar and lingual nerves. Mouth opening should be recorded in millimeters. Deviation of the mandible on opening suggests interference with the translatory movement of the condyle on the side of deviation. Tenderness of the external auditory canal or directly over the temporomandibular joint suggests intracapsular damage or a subcondylar or condylar fracture. Patients are extremely sensitive to minimal alterations in occlusion and will give a history of "altered bite."

The goals of managing mandibular fractures are the restoration of occlusion, the anatomic reduction of fracture fragments and the immobilization of the fracture until adequate healing has occurred. Potential problems are infection, malocclusion, nonunion, and inadequate nutrition. Mandibular fractures are commonly open and are usually multiple.

An operative approach is required in most mandibular fractures. Even in the patient with a minimally displaced fracture who can bite to normal occlusion, the immobilization of the fracture by intermaxillary fixation will lessen the discomfort and the risk of fracture displacement.

The choice of reduction technique (open versus closed) is dictated by the position and nature of the fracture and the patient's dentition. Subcondylar fractures and undisplaced body fractures in patients with good dentition are frequently managed in a closed fashion. Parasymphyseal and angle fractures are more commonly treated by open reduction and internal fixation. The most common closed technique used is the application of Erich-type arch bars and intermaxillary (maxilla to mandible) fixation. Open reduction is almost always accompanied by some form of internal fixation. Most commonly, interosseous wiring, a combination of a simple interosseous wire with a figure-8 basket wire passed through the same two holes provides satisfactory fixation in most instances[14] (Fig. 6–8). Alternatively, four-hole figure-8 wiring can be used. This technique is useful in the parasymphyseal region, but is more difficult in the proximity of the inferior dental canal. In more stable fractures, a figure-8 basket wire alone or a single interosseous wire may be adequate. Recently compression plates have been used to reduce and stabilize mandibular fractures (Fig. 6–9). They are expensive, more time consuming to apply, and require wide exposure and more periosteal elevation than interosseous wires, but reduce the need for postoperative intermaxillary fixation.

External fixation devices, such as the Hall-Morris device[25] (Fig. 6–10 A, B) may be useful in difficult cases where osseous union may take longer than 6 weeks. If bone loss has occurred and delayed grafting is planned, rigid external fixation will maintain the correct

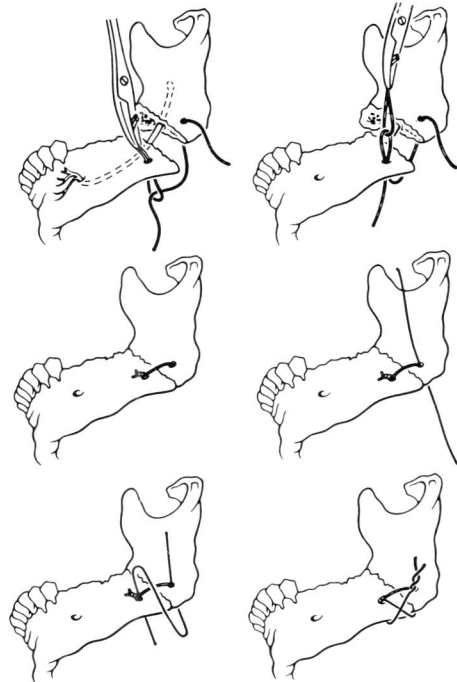

Figure 6–8. Line drawing of transosseous wiring technique of mandibular fracture. (From Rowe and Williams.[29] Reprinted with permission.)

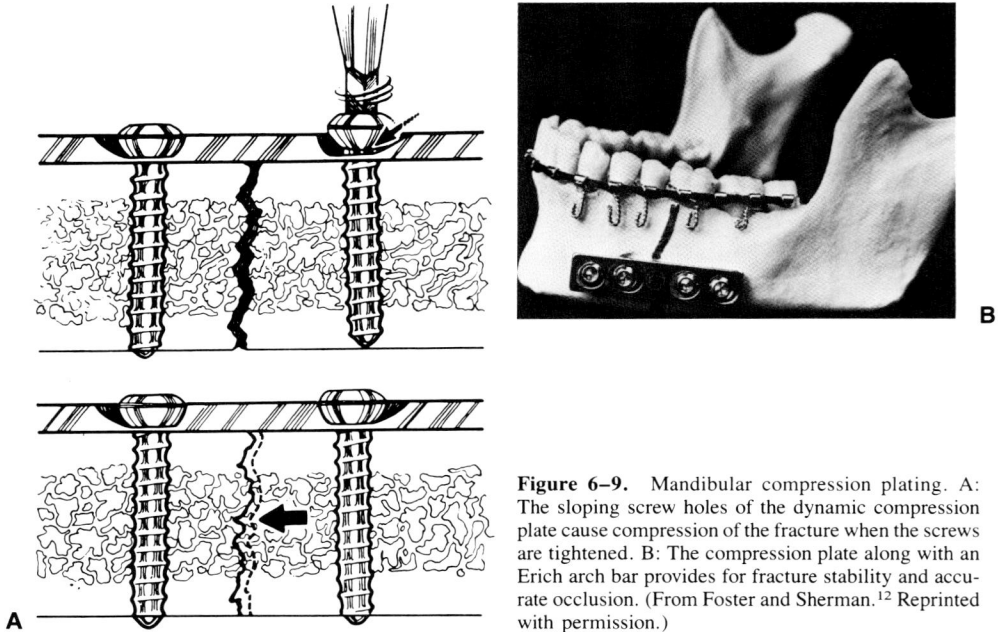

Figure 6–9. Mandibular compression plating. A: The sloping screw holes of the dynamic compression plate cause compression of the fracture when the screws are tightened. B: The compression plate along with an Erich arch bar provides for fracture stability and accurate occlusion. (From Foster and Sherman.[12] Reprinted with permission.)

anatomic relationship of the fragments. Also in grossly comminuted fractures, periosteal stripping from poorly vascularized fragments is avoided.

External fixation predates rigid internal fixation by compression plates. The most commonly used device is the Hall-Morris biphase apparatus.[25] Two percutaneous pins are inserted at least 1 cm apart on each side of the fracture line. The pin ends have self-tapping cortical threads that engage both bony cortices on insertion. The first phase is comprised of an adjustable metallic bar linkage system. After manual reduction of the fracture, the first phase is tightened to rigidly hold the reduction. A cold-cure acrylic bar is fashioned and applied to the percutaneous pins as the second phase (Fig. 6–10 A). Alternatively, the acrylic may be forced into a clear endotracheal tube using a 60 cc syringe. Small cuts are made in the tube at the pin sites and the tube is firmly attached to the pins. Cool irrigation needs to be applied to the pins as the acrylic cures by an exothermic process. Once the acrylic has hardened, the first phase can be removed (Fig. 6–10 B). The external fixation device can be removed at the time of bone grafting or once osseous union has taken place. External fixation is cumbersome and some facial scarring from the percutaneous pins is inevitable; pin tract infection with localized osteitis may occur but is uncommon.

Pediatric mandibular fracutres need even earlier mobilization and rarely require open reduction. Children have excellent potential for healing and remodeling and may even regenerate a new condyle. Unfortunately, growth disturbance resulting in mandibular asymmetry may be a long-term sequela.[22]

The edentulous mandible is often the most difficult to manage. The absence of teeth makes intermaxillary fixation difficult to achieve. Mobile soft tissue on edentulous ridges makes stable fixation using dentures or splints difficult. Dentures broken during the

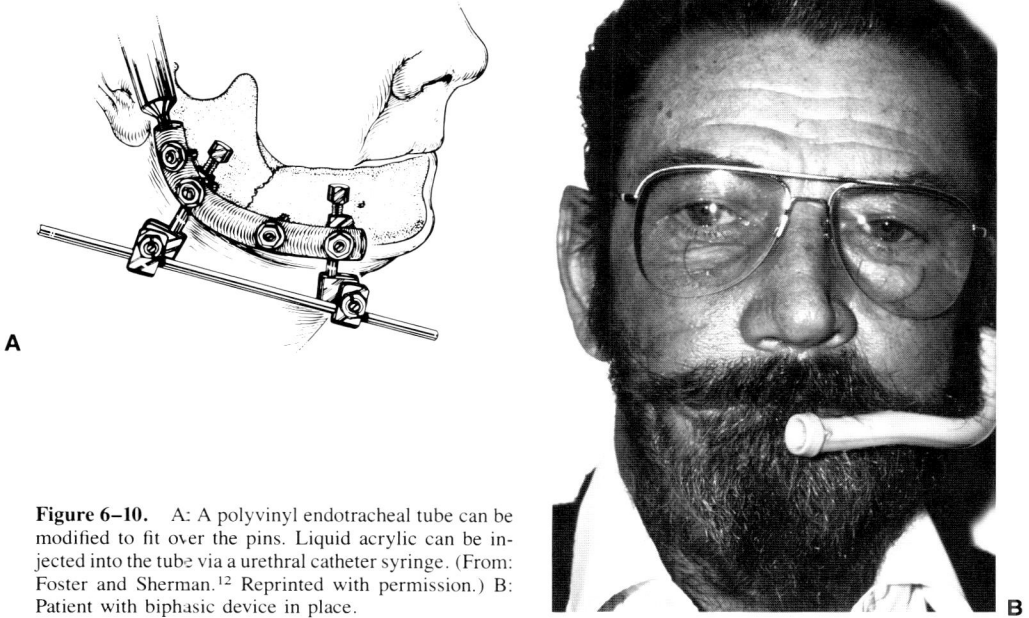

Figure 6–10. A: A polyvinyl endotracheal tube can be modified to fit over the pins. Liquid acrylic can be injected into the tube via a urethral catheter syringe. (From: Foster and Sherman.[12] Reprinted with permission.) B: Patient with biphasic device in place.

traumatic incident should be retrieved and repaired because they make the best splints. The mandible is frequently atrophic with little capacity for repair. Fractures of edentulous mandibles, which are not severely atrophic, may be stabilized by bone plates or interosseous wire fixation. The severely atrophic mandible can be treated by closed reduction and external fixation. Bone grafting is sometimes required to achieve satisfactory union.

Teeth may be fractured, loosened, or avulsed during maxillofacial trauma. Avulsed teeth have an acceptable chance of survival if they are replaced within 4 hours of injury. They should not be sterilized or placed in antiseptic solutions but should simply be washed clean and accurately replaced. Support is obtained by attachment to adjacent teeth or an arch bar with dental wire. A root canal procedure should be performed by an endodontist within 2 to 3 weeks. Dental fractures may involve the enamel alone or expose the pulp. If dental assistance is not available, a temporary dressing should be applied to any teeth with pulp exposure and dental attention sought the next day. Traumatized teeth may become nonvital and require careful dental follow-up.

The most common complication of mandible fractures is infection because of frequent contamination with oral flora. Infection also may spread from a nonvital tooth or an avascular area of bone. Immediate and perioperative antibiotics can reduce the incidence of these infections.[2] Delay in debriding, cleaning, and stabilizing the fracture increases the risk of infection.

When a delayed infection occurs, radiographs should be taken, including occlusal views to look for bone absorption around an infected nonvital tooth. Bony sequestra and retained roots should be removed and the wound carefully debrided and irrigated with antiseptic solution. The patient is kept on systemic antibiotics and the wound is packed or repeatedly irrigated using a Penrose drain and catheter system. Often the intraosseous wires require removal because they act as a foreign body perpetuating the infection. Following debridement and the resolution of infection, an autogenous bone graft is often required to fill the residual defect and obtain bony union.

Postfracture hypomobility of the temporomandibular joint (TMJ) is common after prolonged immobilization. Once intermaxillary fixation is discontinued, the patient is placed on a soft diet, often with the use of nighttime elastics. Progressive mobilization of the jaw may be aided by physiotherapy. The goal is to obtain an interincisal distance of at least 40 mm. The use of a mouth prop is sometimes a useful adjunct. Postfracture hypomobility may be due to muscle scarring or TMJ dysfunction. Intracapsular condylar fractures need early mobilization and good postoperative physiotherapy to avoid hypomobility. Bony or fibrous ankylosis may occur if mobilization is not actively pursued.

Malunion and nonunion are fortunately less common sequelae than infection or hypomobility. Malunion may result from failure to reduce a fracture accurately, inadequate stabilization, or infection and usually causes malocclusion. Minor degrees of malocclusion can sometimes be corrected by occlusal grinding or the prolonged use of strong elastic band traction. More severe malocclusion and malunion may require osteotomies for correction. Nonunion of the mandible is fortunately uncommon. Most cases labeled as being nonunions are, in fact, fibrous unions. The management of nonunions or fibrous union requires the removal of fibrous tissue, autogenous bone grafting, and fixation, usually with an external appliance.

FRONTAL SINUS FRACTURES

In former times, fractures of the frontal sinus occurred principally as a wartime injury. Today, high-speed motor vehicle and industrial accidents are the chief causes. Nahum[26] has shown that a force of between 800 and 2200 lb is necessary to fracture the frontal sinus. The tremendously strong, outwardly convex anterior cranial vault will sustain forces two to three times greater than the other facial bones without fracturing.

The frontal sinus is roughly pyramidal in shape with its apex superiorly. Its outwardly convex anterior wall is exceedingly thick, whereas the base and posterior walls are relatively thin (Fig. 6–11). Near the midline, the two frontal sinuses are separated by a septum. On each side of the base of the septum lie the frontonasal ducts, which commonly are foramena.[23] Frontoethmoid cells surround the ductal area, which drains into the middle meatus of the nose. The posterior wall of the frontal sinus forms the anteroinferior part of the anterior cranial fossa (Fig. 6–11). The superior sagittal sinus lies directly against the posterior wall in its early course, making it vulnerable to injury in penetrating fractures. Fortunately, the dural walls of the superior sagittal sinus are tough, making rupture uncommon.

The paranasal sinuses are lined by ciliated, pseudostratified columnar epithelium that typifies the respiratory tract. Frontal sinus mucosa, however, is not typical in its response to injury.[4] In the other paranasal sinuses, the mucosa usually regenerates after an injury, to resemble closely its preinjury state. In the frontal sinus, areas of cuboidal epithelium develop that are devoid of cilia. The submucosa in these areas is thickened, fibrotic, and infiltrated with chronic inflammatory cells. The mucosa acquires a peculiarly unique tendency for cyst or mucocele formation. Mucoceles are prone to infection, becoming mucopyoceles. With bone erosion and dural exposure, infection of the meninges or brain can occur. Mucocele formation is also induced by obstruction of the frontonasal duct. Stenosis

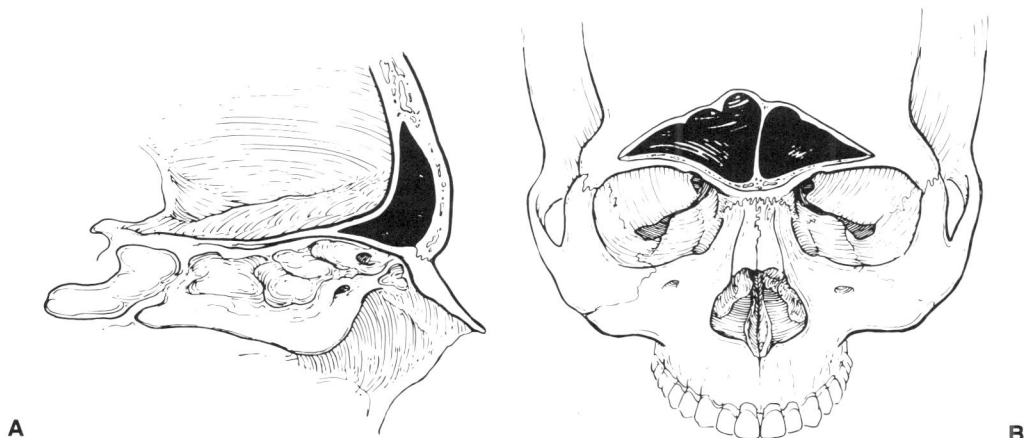

Figure 6–11. Convexity of frontal sinus walls and attenuations both laterally and posteriorly of cavity showing relative thickness of walls and septations. A: Sagittal view. B: Frontal view. (From Donald.[9] Reprinted with permission.)

of the duct occurs after a fracture through the duct or chronic inflammation. Mucosal remnants left after incomplete mucosal excision are prone to form mucoceles. Adequate mucosal removal requires burring of a thin layer of bone from the entire sinus cavity.[10]

The patient with a frontal sinus fracture often will have a concomitant head injury or multiple trauma. Examination may show a bony depression over a depressed anterior wall fracture. Soft tissue swelling soon begins to obscure this finding. Epistaxis is common, as are concomitant facial bone fractures. Cerebrospinal fluid (CSF) rhinorrhea may result from a posterior wall fracture with a dural tear or from an associated fracture of the anterior cranial fossa floor. Epistaxis and CSF will produce a "halo sign," formed when a drop of nasal fluid on a piece of absorbent paper separates into a central blood spot surrounded by a ring of yellow or clear fluid. A conscious patient will complain of pain and swelling over the fracture site and may have forehead numbness.

A standard sinus radiographic series (Waters, Caldwell, lateral, and submentovertical views) is usually ordered, which will show sinus opacification and may reveal a fracture line. A depressed anterior wall fracture is frequently evident on the lateral view. CT is the most valuble study, showing the contents of the sinus, the brain, the frontonasal duct area, as well as the fracture lines. Cervical spine films also should be obtained, since the location and severity of the force necessary to produce a frontal sinus fracture also can cause a cervical spine injury.

Fractures may be divided into the following types: anterior wall—linear, depressed, compound, comminuted; posterior wall—linear, depressed, depressed with CSF leak, extensively comminuted; frontonasal duct; and through-and-through. Fracture management is directed toward preventing external deformity, CSF leakage, chronic sinusitis, and the long-term complications of osteomyelitis, mucopyocele, meningitis, or cerebral abscess. In the patient with several fractures, the treatment plan gives highest priority to the management of the fracture with the most serious sequelae. If an anterior wall fracture is compound, wound exploration will reveal the fracture sites. The wound should be thoroughly irrigated and carefully inspected for embedded foreign bodies. In linear fractures without anterior wall displacement the anterior wall can be safely left alone. Depressed anterior wall fractures should always be opened. Failure to elevate an anterior wall fracture will leave a cosmetically obvious depression in the patient's forehead. In addition, damaged sinus mucosa trapped in the fracture area may predispose the patient to future mucocele formation. The preexisting laceration in compound wounds is used for surgical access. If additional access is required, extension of the laceration along the natural forehead lines can be carried out. In compound fractures, access is gained through either a coronal or a butterfly incision (Fig. 6–12). A coronal incision is cosmetically the most suitable in patients with a normal hairline but is best avoided in the balding male patient. The butterfly incision can produce an unaesthetic appearance, but careful attention paid to incision planning and suture technique can make it an acceptable approach. An incision is made through the inferior hairs of the brow, keeping the blade parallel to the downward slanting line of the hair follicles, reducing the risk of damage to the hair follicles, and creation of a "split-brow" appearance is minimized. The brow incisions are joined by a horizontal incision across the glabellar region. In patients with large frontal sinuses, the access gained through the brow incision is inferior to that gained by a coronal incision.

The depressed fragments are elevated using a small hook or small periosteal elevators. The periosteal attachments are preserved as much as possible. The sinus mucosa adjacent to the fracture lines is incised and the inner table of the underlying bone is burred away. Twenty-eight gauge interosseous wire is used to stabilize the fragments. In comminuted fractures the final result resembles a jigsaw puzzle. Adequate stabilization can usually be achieved by interosseous wiring and the temptation to pack the sinus should be strongly resisted. Packing creates problems by causing further damage to the sinus mucosa as well as increasing the chance of infection. The use of a balloon catheter brought through the frontonasal duct is nearly always an unnecessary and hazardous procedure. A protective guard can be created

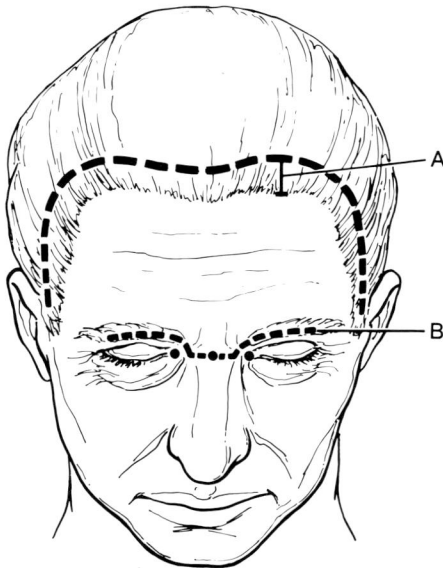

Figure 6–12.   Line drawing showing coronal (A) and butterfly (B) incisions. (From Donald.[9] Reprinted with permission.)

from an appropriately shaped finger splint taped or plastered to the lateral aspects of the forehead.

In comminuted fractures fragments of bone may be missing. Primary calvarial bone grafting in a contaminated field carries the risk of infection and graft absorption. Defects less than 1.5 cm in diameter can be left and corrected secondarily if any cosmetic defect becomes evident.

The management of posterior wall fractures is more controversial than that of anterior wall fractures. An important point to establish is whether there has been any displacement of the fracture. With displacement, a dural tear is more likely and the chance of mucosal ingrowth is much greater. Because of the difficulty in establishing displacement even with CT scanning. these fractures should be explored. (See Editor's note.) If these patients are simply followed, many will be lost to follow-up and the first manifestation of a developing mucocele or mucopyocele may be a fatal meningitis or cerebral abscess.

A coronal or butterfly incision is used for exploration. An osteoplastic flap as described by Montgomery[23] is used for entry into the sinus. The posterior wall is inspected for dural tears or CSF leakage. Dural repair is addressed first with neurosurgical consultation sought for major tears. A craniotomy and a dural graft are often necessary to repair these. With minor tears, the closure can usually be performed directly through the sinus fracture site. Following repair of the dura, all of the mucosa is removed from the sinus cavity. The bone of the sinus interior is then burred away to ensure that there is no mucosal regrowth. Care should be taken to remove all mucosa from the corners and recesses using small diameter diamond burrs. The frontonasal duct mucosa is elevated and turned on itself. An abdominal fat graft is carefully harvested and used to fill the sinus cavity. The fat should be handled atraumatically and carefully inserted to fill all corners of the cavity. When large fragments of the posterior wall are either devitalized or missing, cranialization should be done. Fractures across the frontonasal duct are difficult to diagnose. Plain films rarely show the fracture and even CT scanning may fail to demonstrate the defect. The persistence of a fluid level in the frontal sinus 2 weeks or more after injury is suggestive of duct injury. A trephine through the thin floor of the sinus with the instillation of a vasoconstrictor solution, followed by the contrast material allows radiographic confirmation of ductal patency. An alternative method is to instill methylene blue and look for its emergence in the nose by anterior rhinoscopy.

If only one duct is fractured, the intersinus septum may be removed via an osteoplastic flap procedure or through a large inferior trephination to allow drainage through the other sinus. When both ducts are fractured, fat obliteration of both sinuses is carried out as described previously. An alternative is the performance of a Lynch frontoethmoidectomy. In this procedure, an incision is made from the inferior margin of the brow curving downward to lie midway between the nasal dorsum and the medial canthus. An external ethmoidectomy is performed and the floor of the frontal sinus is removed, creating a wide opening into the nose. A laterally based Sewell-Boyden mucoperiosteal flap can be turned up into the frontal sinus to facilitate mucosal relining of the frontonasal connection.

Through-and-Through Injuries

The through-and-through injury is the most serious frontal sinus injury. Fifty percent of the injured die at the scene of the accident or in transit; another 24% die in the postoperative period.[6] The injury involves an external laceration, a fracture of both the anterior and posterior sinus walls, and usually dural lacerations and contusion of the adjacent frontal lobes. The cerebral injury is the most serious life-threatening component. An urgent craniotomy is often required with removal of necrotic brain, control of any cerebral hemorrhage, and repair of the anterior dural defect. Attention should then be paid to the restoration of the anterior sinus wall to provide protection for the brain and a cosmetically acceptable forehead. When the posterior sinus wall is badly comminuted, the procedure of cranialization is preferred to fat obliteration because of the poor revascularization of fat. Cranialization allows room for the edematous brain to expand, thus eliminating the space occupied by the frontal sinus. It also provides anterior protection for the brain while preserving the normal aesthetic contour of the forehead.

After completion of the intracranial portion of the procedure, the frontal sinus is exposed through the frontal craniotomy. Any loose fragments of bone are saved and residual mucosa removed. A drill and bone-biting forceps are used to remove the remainder of the posterior sinus wall. The bony fragments are stored in antiseptic solution until the end of the procedure. The mucosa is completely removed from the sinus and the inner table of the anterior wall is burred. Temporalis muscle or fascia is used to plug the frontonasal duct after inversion of the duct mucosa and burring with a drill. The previously preserved bony fragments are then wired in place to restore the normal contour anterior wall. Brain swelling may fill part or all of the sinus cavity (Fig. 6–13).

In our experience, cranialization has proved to be a reliable method of managing severe injuires.[6] In 72 consecutive patients followed for up to 9 years, there have been no cases of mucocele, mucopyocele, meningitis, or cerebral abscess.

FRACTURES OF THE NASOFRONTAL-ETHMOIDAL COMPLEX

Fractures of the nasoethmoidal area involve multiple bones and are described under a number of headings (naso-orbital fractures, nasoethmoidal fractures, fractures of the naso-

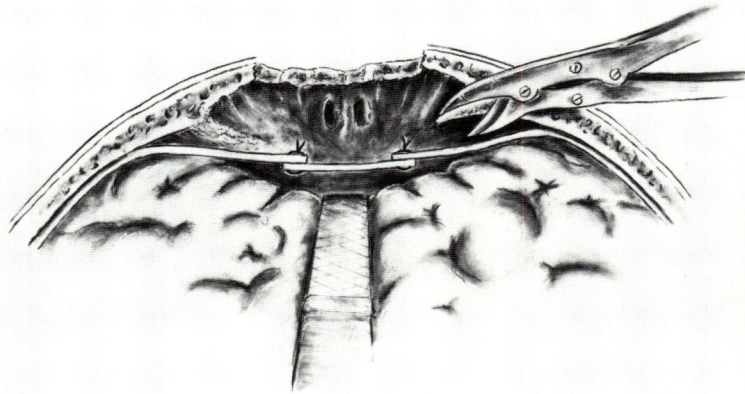

A

Figure 6–13. A: Frontal sinus is cranialized by removing all remnants of posterior sinus wall with rongeur. Walls are drilled flush with anterior fossa with cutting burr. (Figure continued on next page)

B

C

D

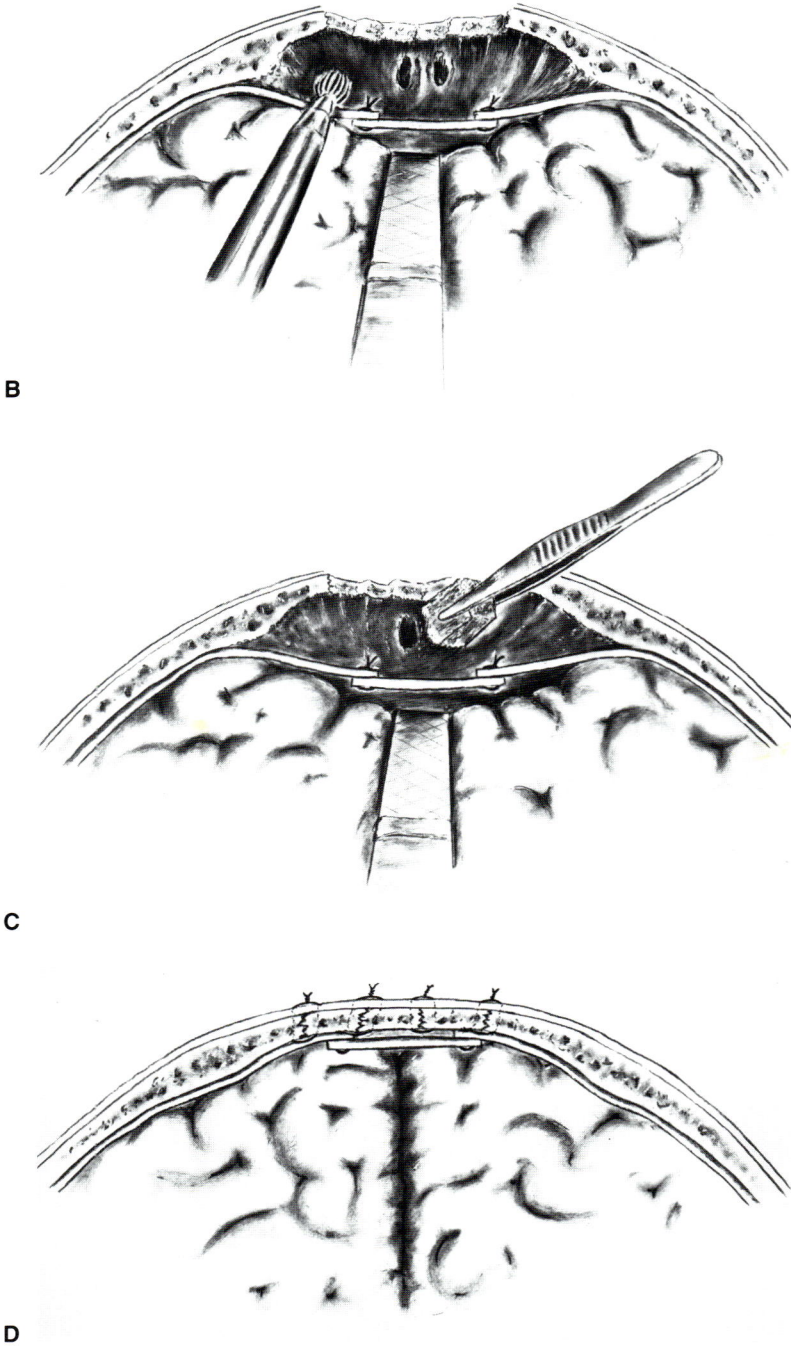

Figure 6–13, cont.   B: Mucosa is meticulously drilled away with cutting burr. C: Temporal muscle plugs are placed in frontonasal ducts. D: Previously cleansed frontal sinus anterior wall fragments are put in place and frontal contour restored. (From Donald PJ.[7] Reprinted with permission.)

ethmoidal maxillo-orbital complex, and fractures of the nasofrontal ethmoidal complex). Fractures in this area are complex, comminuted, and frequently compound.

The nasofrontal ethmoidal complex has a strong triangular outer frame with relatively fragile inner contents. The robust frontal processes of the maxilla meet the nasal process of the frontal bone at the glabella to form the apex of the triangle. The base of the triangle is formed by the upper premaxilla (Fig. 6–14). In its upper portion the triangle contains the nasal bones, the ethmoidal sinuses, the superior and middle turbinates, and the cribriform plate. The intraorbital area contains the ethmoidal sinuses, which are separated from the orbits by the thin bone of the lamina papyracea.

Of considerable clinical importance is the anatomy of the lacrimal system and the medial canthal ligament (Fig. 6–15). The lacrimal bone and frontal process of the maxilla form the lacrimal fossa. Anteriorly, the fossa is bounded by the anterior lacrimal crest formed by the frontal process of the maxilla. The medial canthal ligament anchors the tarsal plates to the medial wall of the orbit and is mainly formed by the tendonous attachment of the orbicularis oculi muscle. This ligament is primarily attached to the anterior lacrimal crest and frontal process of the maxilla. It is also closely associated with the lacrimal sac. A portion of the medial canthal ligament passes posterior to the lacrimal sac and assists the orbicularis oculi muscle in forming a lacrimal pump. The upper and lower lacrimal canaliculi extend 2 mm downward and 8 mm medially to enter the sac as a common stem. The lacrimal sac is 13 to 15 mm in length and occupies the lacrimal fossa before continuing downward to the inferior meatus of the nose as the nasolacrimal duct. Injury to the medial canthal ligament is commonly associated with injury to the lacrimal apparatus. The medial canthal ligament is important in maintaining the configuration of the palpebral fissure.

In the center of the nasofrontal ethmoidal complex is the nasal septum. The bony septum is formed by the vertical plate of the ethmoid, attached in part to the cribriform plate, and the vomer. Projecting forward from the vomer, vertical plate of the ethmoid, maxillary crest, and nasal bones is the quadrangular-shaped septal cartilage. The nasal bones require only a force of 30 to 80 g to produce a fracture. The triangular frame of the nasofrontal ethmoidal complex is stronger but with larger forces will fracture. Little resistance is then offered by the thin medial walls of the orbit and the ethmoidal air cell system to the posterior displacement of the nasal bones and frontal processes of the maxilla. Telecanthus, damage to the lacrimal system, and fracture of the cribriform plate and anterior cranial fossa with CSF leakage may occur.

Nasofrontal ethmoidal complex injuries can be classified as being isolated or com-

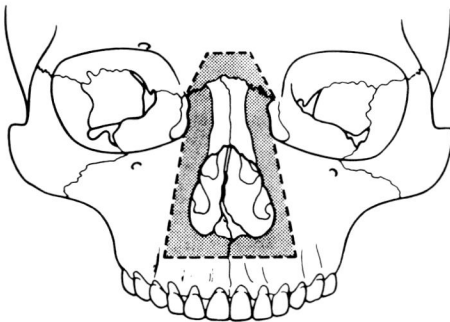

Figure 6–14.   Line drawing showing the strong triangular outer frame. (From Rowe and Williams.[29] Reprinted with permission.)

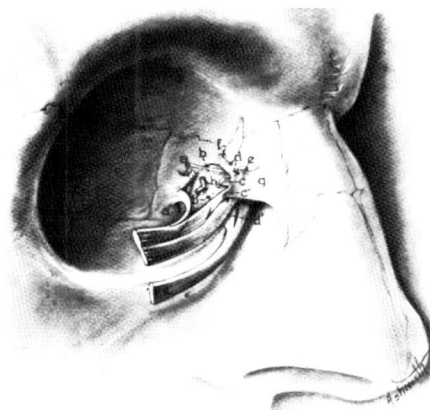

Figure 6–15. Anatomy of the lacrimal apparatus and medial canthal ligament. (From Donald PJ.[5] Reprinted with permission.)

bined. Combined injuries are associated with other midface fractures. A bilateral combined injury is associated with a Le Fort II or III maxillary fracture. This injury frequently involves facial elongation and traumatic telecanthus. A unilateral combined injury is associated with fractures of the orbit and zygomatic complex. Unilateral displacement of the medial palpebral ligament is common with comminution of the orbital rim and displacement of the zygoma. This causes a characteristic antimongoloid slant to the eye and associated globe injury is common.

A useful division of isolated nasofrontal ethmoidal complex fractures into telescope and lateral spread has been proposed by Duvall et al.[11] In telescoped injuries, the nasal bones and central portions of the frontal processes of the maxilla are displaced posteriorly as a unit. They are commonly driven in an upward direction as well, creating an impaction. The medial canthal ligaments are not disrupted. An acute nasofrontal angle with upturning of the nasal tip is characteristic of posterior impaction (Fig. 6–16).

The second type of injury with lateral spread of the fractured components is more common. A posteriorly displaced fracture complex is not maintained as a unit. The frontal processes of the maxilla and nasal bones are comminuted and laterally displaced. Disruption of the medial canthal ligaments occurs usually with disruption of the lacrimal apparatus.

Nasofrontal ethmoidal complex fractures are often associated with Le Fort II and III fractures, orbital fractures, and zygomatic complex fractures. The patient may or may not have been unconscious. There is frequently a laceration over the glabellar region or nasal dorsum. An acute nasofrontal angle is evident initially, and there is marked loss of projection of the nasal dorsum. This quickly becomes obscured by soft tissue swelling. The tip of the nose is more upturned and the philtrum of the lip appears stretched. Ecchymosis is present in the medial canthal and periorbital areas. Conjunctival edema and subconjunctival hemorrhage are common. Medial canthal ligament injury often occurs, resulting in an increased intercanthal distance. An intercanthal distance of 35 mm is at the upper limit of normal and an intercanthal distance of 40 mm is diagnostic of injury. As a useful clinical guide, the intercanthal distance should approximate the width of one eye. Traumatic telecanthus occurs in 15 to 20% of midfacial fractures.[1] In addition to the increased intercanthal distance, there are several other clinical signs. The involved eye becomes almond shaped with rounding of

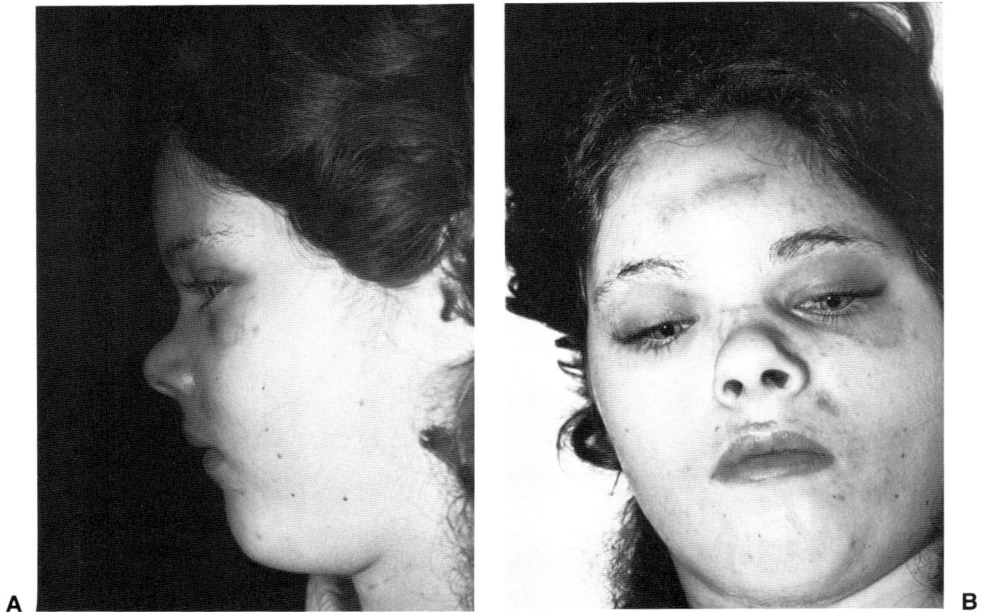

Figure 6–16. Patient with a nasofrontal ethmoidal complex fracture. A: Lateral view. B: Frontal view.

the medial canthal angle and shortening of the palpebral fissure. The eyelids become lax and the epicanthal fold more prominent. Lateral traction is placed on the lateral canthus and "bowstringing" (Furnas test) of the medial canthal tendon can be palpated if the tendon is intact. Associated epiphora and diplopia are common findings but are not diagnostic of medial canthal ligament injury.

CSF leakage often occurs with nasofrontal ethmoidal complex fractures. A history of a clear nasal discharge or salty postnasal drip should be sought. Epistaxis is common, with brisk bleeding occurring from the anterior and posterior ethmoidal arteries. A mixture of blood and CSF often can be detected by a halo sign. Intranasal examination to exclude a septal hematoma should always be performed. Anosmia can occur from cerebral injury or from a fracture of the cribriform plate area or ethmoidal roof.

Radiographic evaluation includes a standard sinus series (Waters, Caldwell, lateral, and submentovertical views). Sinus views will show clouding in the ethmoid sinuses and often in the maxillary sinuses if an associated medial maxillary, orbital, zygomatic, or Le Fort fracture is present. The lateral view will show retrodisplacement of the nasal root; air may be present in the orbit or eyelids. Plain skull films can identify a pneumoencephalocele or skull fracture. A CT scan gives the best appreciation of the fracture complex and of cerebral injury and allows accurate surgical planning.

A systematic approach involving careful clinical assessment, preoperative planning, and surgical repair produces the best results. Closed reduction, even when used in conjunction with lead plates and transosseous wires, produces variable results. Vertical separation of the nasal bones from the frontal bone is unaddressed by closed techniques. Intercanthal spread is often inadequately corrected and the incidence of post-traumatic telecanthus is unacceptably high.

Open reduction can be performed by several approaches. The area can be exposed through an existing laceration, a medial orbital incision, H- and W-shaped incisions for bilateral access, or the coronal incision and forehead flap for severe bilateral injuries. The lacrimal canaliculi are irrigated with saline or dilute methylene blue and the medial canthal tendon is carefully inspected. An ophthalmologist should examine the eye preoperatively, because the incidence of associated globe rupture and other intraocular injuries are high. If CSF leakage is suspected, neurosurgical consultation is also sought. The fracture complex should be disimpacted and reduced. An initial downward movement is required to disimpact the fracture before anterior reduction is possible. The comminuted bone fragments should be carefully replaced in position and interosseous wiring done.

Careful attention must be paid to the lacrimal apparatus; the lacrimal sac is best repaired early, since subsequent scarring makes secondary repair more difficult (Fig. 6–17). Medial canthal ligament avulsion should also be addressed at the time of primary repair. Fortunately, a segment of bone is often avulsed with the ligament, and the bone can be used as an anchor to stabilize the ligament. Because ipsilateral bony comminution may be so severe that stable bone cannot be found, the ligament may require attachment to the opposite medial canthus or to the nasal bone.[21] When both medial canthal ligaments have been avulsed, two transnasal wires are passed, each ligament is secured, and the ends of the wires are twisted down upon a small Teflon felt bolster to prevent tear-through of the wires (Fig. 6–18).

Fractures of the nasofrontal ethmoidal complex may involve fractures of the frontal sinus, orbital roof, or cribriform plate area. Anterior basicranial injuries can be managed via

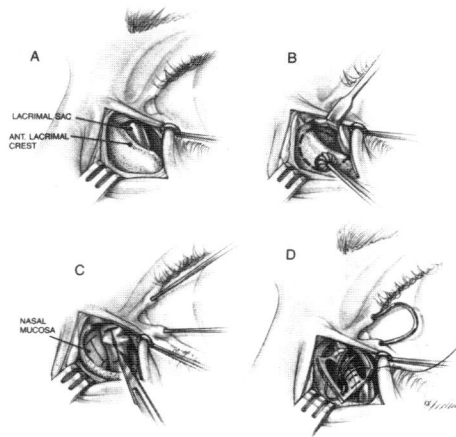

Figure 6–17. Technique of dacrocystorhinostomy. A: The curvilinear incision is created in the medial canthus, which extends from the medial canthal tendon and curves down around the infraorbital rim. The anterior lacrimal crest is exposed after the periosteum is elevated. B: An osteotomy is created by removing the anterior lacrimal crest. The osteotomy is placed inferonasal to the medial canthal tendon and extends down to the entrance of the nasolacrimal duct. The bony defect should approximate the size of the surgeon's thumb. The osteotomy can be created with a Hall drill and burr or a Kerrison punch. C: The nasal mucosa is tented, and an H incision is made into the nasal mucosa to develop anterior and posterior nasal flaps. The lacrimal sac is tented with Bowman probes to identify the sac and create similar anterior and posterior sac flaps in the form of the letter H. D: The posterior flaps of nasal mucosa and lacrimal sac are sutured with 4-0 chronic microtubes, and silicone microtubes are threaded over the posterior flap before closure of the anterior nasal and lacrimal sac flaps. The microtubes are tied together within the nose with 6-0 silk sutures and left to dangle freely. (From Foster and Sherman.[12] Reprinted with permission.)

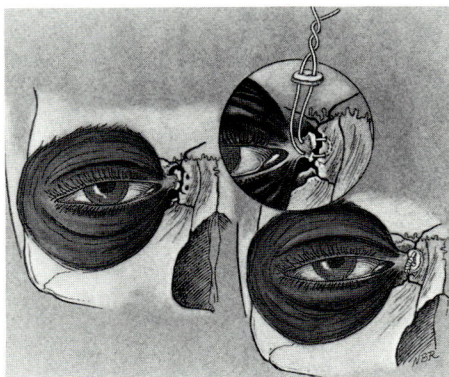

Figure 6–18. Transnasal writing of medial canthal tendon. Inset shows wire with attached Dacron feet bolster securing tendon to adjacent lacrimal and maxillary bone.

a frontal craniotomy. Retraction of the frontal lobes allows evaluation of any injury to the dura, brain, and anterior cranial fossa floor. Necrotic cerebral tissue is debrided, the dura is sutured and reinforced if necessary with pericranium or other tissue from the temporoparietal region, the nasal mucosa is inverted into the nose and the bony defect is repaired using a cancellous bone graft.

Injury of the nasal septum is an integral part of nasofrontal ethmoidal complex fractures. Careful intranasal inspection is required to exclude a septal hematoma and to assess the extent of intranasal injury. Septal hematomas should be dealt with promptly by adequate incision and drainage, intranasal packing, and use of antibiotics. Silastic splints are inserted when lacerations in the nasal mucosa have occurred to prevent the formation of synechiae. The splints should be sutured in place and left for a period of 7 to 10 days. Delayed septoplasty may be required to correct nasal obstruction due to persistent septal deviation.

Primary repair of nasofrontal ethmoidal complex injuries are much more successful than those achieved later. Nevertheless, modern techniques of delayed craniofacial reconstruction can give pleasing results. Osteotomies are used to correct malunion in conjunction with bone grafts for stabilization and the replacement of missing bone. Delayed correction of traumatic telecanthus is more difficult than primary repair. In addition to transnasal canthoplasty, complete mobilization of the anterior orbital contents from the rim and walls and lateral cantholysis are required. Delayed repair of the lacrimal apparatus may require dacrocystorhinostomy or conjunctivorhinostomy. Webbing in the medial canthal region or the development of an epicanthal fold requires surgical correction using a double Z-plasty or Mustarde technique.

MAXILLARY FRACTURES

Fractures of the middle third of the facial skeleton usually result from motor vehicle accidents or altercations. The anterior maxilla tolerates trauma poorly; a force of only 140 to 455 g will fracture the maxilla.[26] The incidence of maxillary fractures varies from 6 to 25% of all facial fractures.[30] They may occur alone but are often associated with fractures of the zygoma, mandible, orbit, or nasofrontal ethmoidal complex. Accurate reduction and stabilization are required to restore good dental occlusion and facial aesthetics.

Most maxillary injuries in reality are fractures of the midfacial skeleton. The two pyramidal-shaped maxillae form a major part of the midface and contribute to the bony skeleton of the orbit, nose, palate, and alveolar ridge. Each maxilla has a pyramidal-shaped body within which is the maxillary sinus. The sinus is very small in children but enlarges as the permanent teeth descend, allowing the available space to pneumatize and expand the sinus. The alveolar process of the maxilla contains the teeth. In the edentulous patient, resorption occurs and there may be little remaining space between the anterior nasal spine and alveolar ridge. The palatine process joins with the palatine bone posteriorly to form the hard palate. The medial wall of the maxillary body forms part of the lateral wall of the nose. A major part of the inferior orbital rim and orbital floor is formed by the maxilla. The frontal process supports the nasal bones and articulates with the nasal process of the frontal bone in the glabellar region. The zygomatic process articulates laterally with the zygoma. Three paired buttresses attach the maxillae to the cranium: anterior, nasomaxillary, middle zygomatic, and posterior pterygomaxillary (Fig. 6–19).

Strong vertical forces can be applied to the maxilla without fracture because of these buttresses. Most fractures of the maxilla are transversely oriented.

The nerve supply to the maxilla arises from the second division of the trigeminal nerve. Superior alveolar nerves course through the thin sinus walls to supply the maxillary teeth and gingiva. The infraorbital nerve arises from the maxillary nerve in the pterygopalatine fossa and supplies sensation to the upper lip, medial face, cheek region, and the lateral aspect of the nose. The abundant blood supply to the maxilla from the maxillary artery and numerous collaterals generally prevents avascular necrosis of bone after trauma. Profuse bleeding after midface fractures may require nasal packing or ligation of the maxillary or external carotid arteries.

Displacement in maxillary fractures occurs chiefly as a result of the original injury, although the medial pterygoid muscles can displace the maxilla toward the angles of the mandible. Much of the maxilla is clothed by nasal, sinus, or oral mucosa and fractures of this region are often contaminated from the nasal or the oral cavity, or both.

The most common maxillary fracture is one involving a segment of alveolus and teeth. Although not as common as mandibular alveolar fractures, the prognosis is better because of the excellent blood supply. Alveolar fractures may occur alone or in combination with other maxillary fractures.

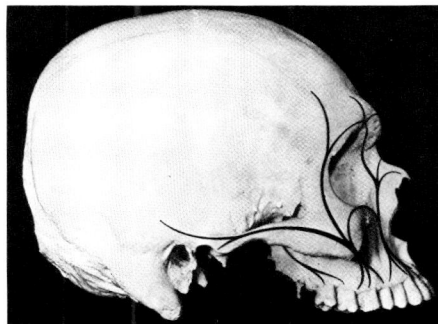

Figure 6–19. Midfacial buttresses. (From Dingman and Natvig.[3] Reprinted with permission.)

In 1901, Rene Le Fort described the patterns of maxillary fracture produced by striking cadaver heads with a wooden club.[18,20] Le Fort found that there was a close relationship between the area of impact and the type of fracture produced. He also found that the fracture patterns, which were usually bilateral in type, were reproducible, leading to the Le Fort classification of three maxillary fractures patterns (Fig. 6–20).

The Le Fort I fracture is a horizontal fracture passing above the floor of the nose and through the lower third of the nasal septum. The mobile segment includes the palate, the maxillary alveolar process, and the lower third of the pterygoid plates.

The Le Fort II fracture line is pyramidal in shape passing across the nasal bridge and entering the medial orbit on each side. The fracture continues inferiorly, passing across the inferior orbital rim and the face of the maxilla near the zygomaticomaxillary suture. The fracture then traverses the lateral wall of the antrum and passes back horizontally through the pterygoid plates. The zygomatic bones remain firmly attached to the skull base and are uninvolved in the fracture.

The Le Fort III fracture causes a craniofacial dysjunction. The fracture line essentially parallels the skull base, passing across the root of the nose backward along the medial wall and floor of the orbit into the pterygopalatine fossa and across the root of the pterygoid plates. The fracture line continues upward and laterally from the inferior orbital fissure to separate the greater wing of the sphenoid and the zygoma and reach the frontozygomatic suture. Fracture of the zygomatic arch near the zygomaticotemporal suture also occurs, resulting in complete craniofacial separation.

The isolated "pure" Le Fort fracture is uncommon, but the classification is useful for treatment planning. Le Fort fractures are commonly associated with other fractures of the facial skeleton. Comminution may be severe and combinations usually occur. An example of this is a fracture combining a Le Fort I on the left with a Le Fort II or III on the right.

A less common fracture is the hemimaxillary fracture or split palate (Fig. 6–21). This fracture divides the palate in the sagittal plane passing within 1 cm of either side of the vomer.

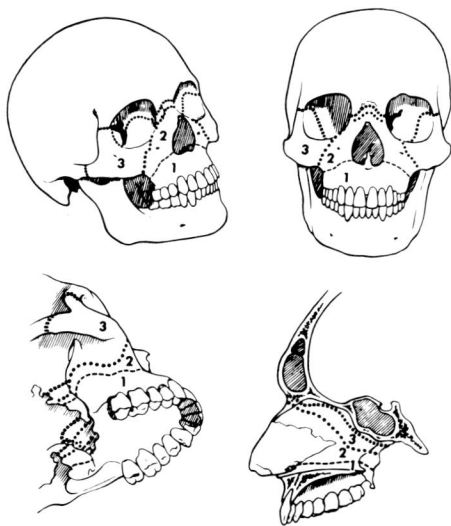

Figure 6–20.   Illustration showing the three classic Le Fort fracture patterns. (From Dingman and Natvig.[3] Reprinted with permission.)

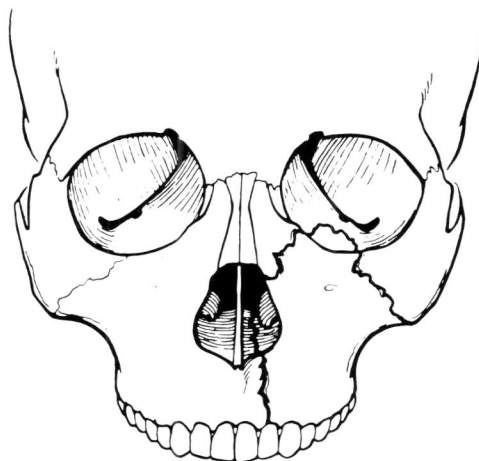

Figure 6–21. Hemimaxillary fracture. (From Foster and Sherman.[12] Reprinted with permission.)

Isolated hemimaxillary fractures are uncommon because a stable zygomatic attachment tends to prevent this fracture from occurring. Hemimaxillary fractures are almost always found with Le Fort II or III fractures. They are thought to be caused by a lateral blow.

Immediate attention is always given to the patient's airway, circulatory status, neurologic status, and cervical spine. Patients with maxillary fractures frequently have multiple trauma. A careful assessment must be made looking for ocular trauma, enophthalmos, CSF rhinorrhea, and otorrhea. The nose should be inspected for septal lacerations, septal fracture, or hematoma, and the source of any bleeding. Massive hemorrhage may occur from severance of one or both internal maxillary arteries. Intraoral inspection should include examination of the teeth, the palate, and the oral mucosa for lacerations or submucosal ecchymosis. The patient's occlusion is always closely examined. The maxilla is typically displaced in a backward and downward direction. This causes elongation and flattening of the midface or a "dish face" appearance. Premature contact of the molar teeth causes an anterior open bite deformity. Malocclusion is usually apparent on inspection; however, with Le Fort III fractures occlusal changes may be slight. The palate should be checked for mobility using the thumb and forefinger of one hand, while the forehead is stabilized with the other. If the fracture is impacted, mobility may not be detected. The mandible is always carefully examined because mandible fractures occur with an incidence of between 20 and 55% in association with Le Fort fractures.[20]

Careful inspection of the face is performed looking for ecchymosis, crepitus, and swelling in suspected fracture sites. The infraorbital rims should be palpated for step deformities. Anesthesia of the upper lip, gingiva, or teeth commonly occurs due to interosseous nerve damage.

Initial radiographic evaluation should include a facial series and a Panorex. The Waters view gives an oblique view of the upper facial bones and is the single most useful plane radiograph. A high Panorex visualizes not only the mandible, but also the maxillary teeth and lower maxilla. Occlusal views are useful for hemimaxillary and alveolar fractures. CT scans will show the extent of the fractures most clearly. Cervical spine views should be obtained during the initial evaluation.

Severe midface fractures can be life threatening with airway management and the control of acute hemorrhage of immediate concern. A tracheostomy is usually required immediately or subsequently. Prolapse of the fractured midface as it is drawn inferoposteriorly by the pull of the medial pterygoid muscles severely jeopardizes the airway. Epistaxis is initially controlled by cautery or nasal packing. If this is inadequate, ligation or embolization of the maxillary or external carotid artery may be required.

Approximately 20% of Le Fort fractures are accompanied by an alveolar fracture.[31] If the maxilla on either side of a displaced alveolar fracture is stable, the fracture is reduced and stabilized by ligation to the adjacent teeth. Stabilization can also be achieved by applying an arch bar to the upper dentition. When there are other fractures of the maxilla, intermaxillary fixation is usually required. A palatal acrylic splint may help stabilize difficult or large segment fractures. In edentulous patients, the upper denture can be wired in place to stabilize the fractured segment. Most alveolar fractures are managed in a closed fashion, but open reduction via a label-buccal sulcus incision is occasionally required. The recommended immobilization period for alveolar fractures is 4 weeks.

Reestablishment of a patient's pretraumatic occlusion is the first step in Le Fort fracture treatment. Restoration of the orbital floors and rims comes next and finally the reconstitution of the aesthetic form of the midface. Arch bars and intermaxillary fixation are usually used to stabilize the patient in occlusion following fracture reduction. Digital pressure alone often reduces the fracture but disimpaction forceps may need to be used. In general, once the correct dental occlusion has been established, the highest maxillary fracture is stabilized first. Direct interosseous wiring or miniplate fixation may be used and can reduce the duration of intermaxillary fixation and the incidence of postoperative maxillary retrusion. Protagonists of open reduction and plating believe that virtually all fracture combinations can be repaired without external fixation. External fixation, however, is useful when marked comminution makes internal fixation difficult. However, in the senior author's experience of greater than 300 Le Fort fractures, external fixation was required only twice. Also, if a Le Fort fracture is associated with a fracture of the cranium, stabilization can be achieved using a halo frame (Fig. 6–22), the Levant frame, and box frames. Plaster of Paris headcaps have also been used, but these give poorer stabilization and more discomfort than halo frames. External fixation devices are cumbersome and poorly suited for use with the confused patient.

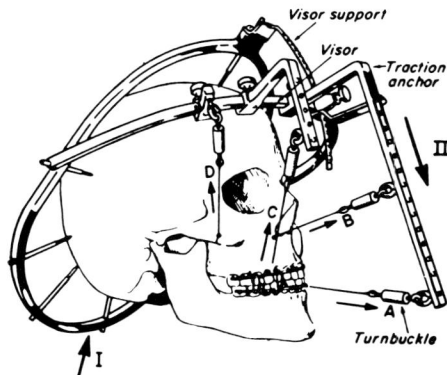

Figure 6–22. Illustration showing a Georgiade or halo frame. (From Georgiade and Nash.[13] Reprinted with permission.)

A Le Fort I fracture is usually the result of a blow to the upper lip at or below the level of the anterior nasal spine. Under general anesthesia, fracture reduction can usually be achieved by digital pressure or with disimpaction forceps. Arch bars, or in edentulous cases, relined dentures or splints, are used to achieve intermaxillary fixation. Suspension wires are then added. The base of the piriform aperture on each side provides a stable suspension point in bilateral Le Fort I fractures. The zygomatic arch may also be used, although this provides a posterosuperiorly directed force and may contribute to midface retrusion. In the presence of significant comminution, interosseous wiring or plating at the base of the zygomatic buttress or piriform aperture reduces the risk of midface shortening (Fig. 6–23). Rigid internal fixation with miniplates can reduce the need for intermaxillary fixation.

In Le Fort II fractures the midface is usually retruded. After the airway is secured and any hemorrhage controlled, the fracture is disimpacted and reduced. The Rowe-Killey disimpaction forceps are well designed for disimpacting even those fractures that are firmly stuck (Fig. 6–24). Arch bars and intermaxillary fixation are applied. Interosseous wires or miniplates are used to stabilize the orbital rim fractures. Inspection and repair of any orbital floor defect is performed at the same time. Additional fixation may be applied at the zygomatic buttresses and the nasofrontal suture (Fig. 6–25). Le Fort II fractures can be suspended from the zygomatic arches. Suspension wires are passed over the zygomatic arch on each side and are attached to the maxillary arch bar. Intermaxillary fixation and suspension is typically maintained for 6 weeks. The patient is always carefully examined to exclude traumatic telecanthus.

Reduction and immobilization of Le Fort III fractures are performed in the same way as described for Le Fort II fractures. The patient is placed in intermaxillary fixation and the frontozygomatic area is stabilized by plating or interosseous wire fixation. A fracture of the zygomatic arch always occurs and if displaced requires reduction. Craniomaxillary suspension wires are applied from the superolateral orbital rim to the maxillary arch bar on each side. Interosseous wiring of the nasofrontal suture may also be performed (Fig. 6–26). The inferior and lateral orbital wall should always be inspected. A good preoperative CT scan

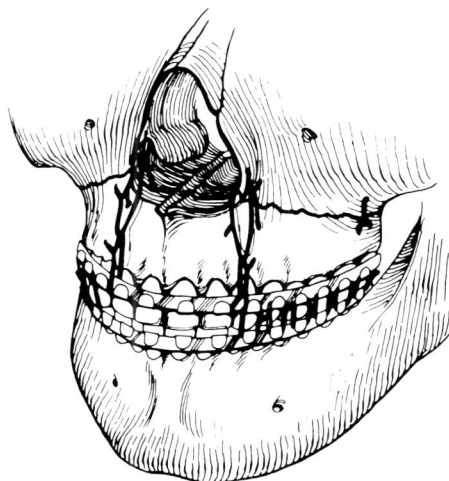

Figure 6–23. Open reduction and internal fixation of Le Fort I fractures. (From Foster and Sherman.[12] Reprinted with permission.)

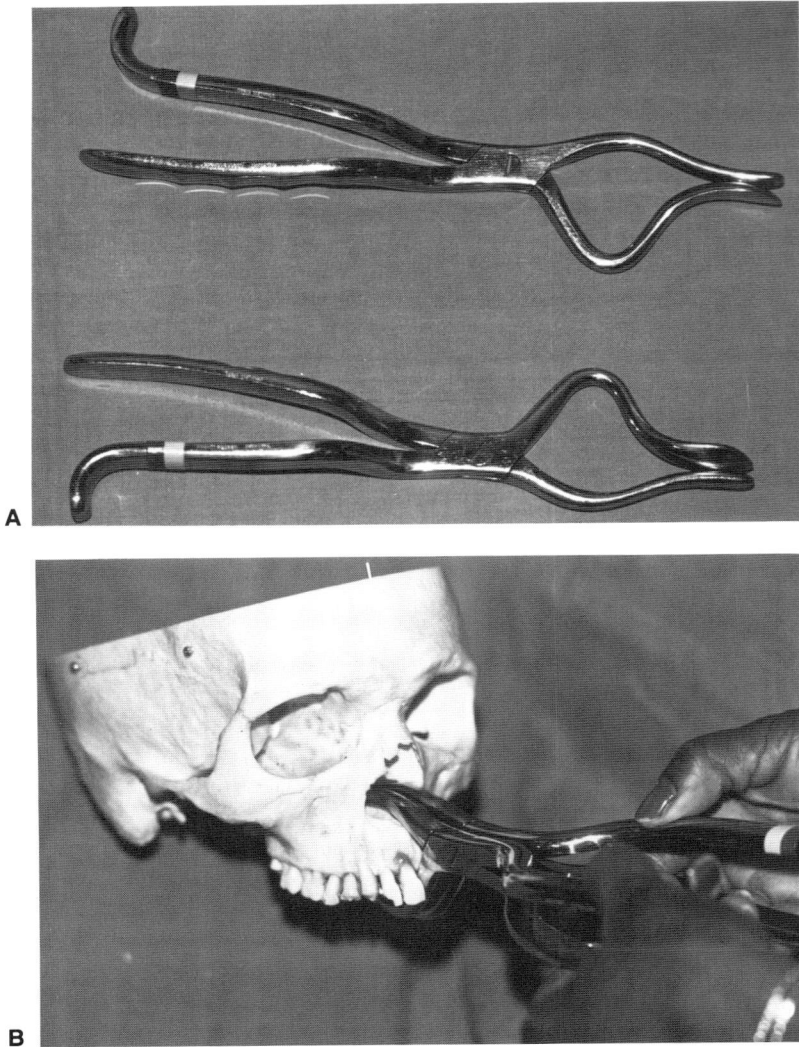

Figure 6–24. A: The Rowe-Killey disimpaction forceps. B: Forceps applied for maxillary disimpaction.

and ophthalmologic examination are invaluable. Once again, intermaxillary fixation is maintained for a period of 6 weeks.

Hemimaxillary fractures are parasagittal, with the fracture line lying within 1 cm of the midline. The application of arch bars and intermaxillary fixation will usually provide adequate stabilization in the patient with a good complement of teeth. There is, however, a tendency for angulation due to rotation of the palatal halves toward the midline. This can be combatted by the fabrication of a palatal splint. Additional stabilization can be gained by direct interosseous wiring at the piriform aperture and occasionally at the posterior end of the hard palate. Intermaxillary fixation is maintained for 6 weeks.

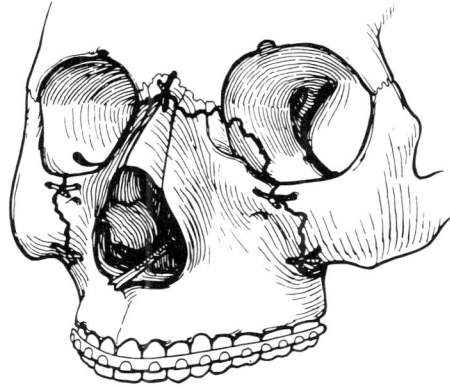

Figure 6–25. Illustration of internal fixation of a Le Fort II fracture. (From Foster and Sherman.[12] Reprinted with permission.)

Early complications of airway compromise and bleeding have already been discussed. CSF rhinorrhea occurs in at least 25% of Le Fort II and III fractures.[24] Most CSF leaks will close within a few days and more than 90% within 3 weeks. Many stop once the fracture is reduced. The role of surgery and antibiotics remains controversial. The value of antibiotics to prevent meningitis has not been clearly demonstrated and many surgeons fear the effects of changes in bacterial flora. Surgery to reduce the maxillary fractures should be performed and CSF leakage into the frontal sinus controlled at the time of frontal sinus repair. Occasionally, simply reducing facial fractures will stop the leak. Bed rest with the head elevated and a lumbar drain are commonly used. Surgical repair is usually reserved for recurrent, delayed onset and spontaneous CSF fistulas. Post-traumatic fistulas continuing beyond 2 to 3 weeks are also considered for surgical repair.

Nonunion of maxillary fractures is uncommon but can occur when there has been severe comminution and inadequate stabilization. Bone grafting of the fracture site and refixation are usually successful. Malunion is more common than nonunion after maxillary fractures. Minor degrees of malocclusion are often seen and in most cases can be managed by nonsurgical means. If the patient's occlusion is satisfactory, onlay bone grafts may be

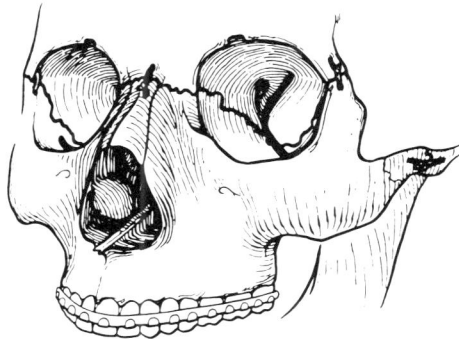

Figure 6–26. Illustration of internal fixation of a Le Fort III fracture. (From Foster and Sherman.[12] Reprinted with permission.)

applied to the depressed area rather than performing osteotomies. Severe deformities such as marked facial elongation or maxillary retrusion can be corrected by Le Fort osteotomies. The "short face" deformity is more difficult to correct and has a high recurrence rate.

Post-traumatic epiphora due to damage to the lacrimal system may occur after Le Fort II and III fractures and may be treated with a dacrocytorhinostomy or conjunctivorhinostomy. Diplopia following Le Fort fractures is not uncommon. In most cases, spontaneous resolution occurs, but extraocular muscle surgery may be required. Blindness is usually an early complication and is most commonly due to laceration of the optic nerve by a bony fragment.

CONCLUSION

The preceding descriptions of facial injuries are fairly detailed in the text because of neurosurgeons' general unfamiliarity with these injuries. Consultation with and treatment by a surgeon skilled in management of craniofacial trauma will provide the patient with the best possible functional and cosmetic results.

EDITOR'S NOTE

Not all fractures of the frontal sinus posterior wall require exploration. If fracture displacement appears to be only a few millimeters and the resultant sinus contour is generally smooth, and there is no apparent CSF leak, the dura usually is intact and exploration unnecessary. If the posterior sinus wall is jagged or a comminuted fragment protrudes intracranially more than 3 to 4 mm or if CSF rhinorrhea accompanies a disrupted posterior frontal sinus wall, then exploration and repair is warranted. Patients treated without operation require close follow-up to ensure that frontal sinus opacification clears within 2 to 6 weeks of injury, thus verifying a patent frontonasal duct. Persistent sinus clouding increases the risk of mucopyocele and subsequent intracranial infection.

RESPONSE TO EDITOR'S NOTE

1. Because of the thin wall of the posterior wall of frontal sinus and the proclivity of damaged frontal sinus mucosa to regrow vigorously and in an abnormal way tends to encyst, a 3 to 4 mm displacement is unacceptable.

2. Close follow-up in trauma patients is exceedingly difficult.

3. Late complications of frontal sinus fractures commonly occur many months and years after the initial injury.

4. Persistent frontal sinus opacification 2 to 6 weeks later may indicate: (1) markedly swollen mucosa; (2) retained fluid secondary to nasofrontal duct fracture, (3) CSF leak without retained fluid secondary to nasofrontal duct fracture; (4) herniated orbital soft tissue (CT scan).

5. Persistent frontal sinus opacification would unlikely indicate a forming mucocele because even experimentally it generally takes months to form (in the cat), and it commonly takes many months to years to be clinically evident.

EDITOR'S SECOND NOTE

Fractures of the posterior wall of the frontal sinus clearly are controversial. When treatment is unclear in the neurosurgeon's judgement, such fractures probably are best managed by joint consultation between neurological and ENT surgeons.

REFERENCES

1. Beyer CHK, Smith B: Naso-orbital fractures, complications and treatment. Ophthalmologica 163:418–427, 1971.
2. Chole RC, Yee J: Antibiotic prophylaxis for facial fractures: A prospective randomized clinical trial. Arch Otolaryngol 113:1055–1057, 1987.
3. Dingman RO, Natvig P: Surgery of Facial Fractures. Philadelphia: WB Saunders, 1969, pp 144, 247, 248.
4. Donald PJ: The tenacity of the frontal sinus mucosa. Otolaryngol Head Neck Surg 87:557–566, 1979.
5. Donald PJ: Frontal Sinus and Nasofrontoethmoidal Complex Fractures. SI Pac #80400. Washington, DC: American Academy of Otolaryngology-Head and Neck Surgery Foundation, 1980, p. 44.
6. Donald PJ: Frontal sinus ablation by cranialization. A report on 21 cases. Arch Otolaryngol 108:142–146, 1982.
7. Donald PJ: Frontal sinus fractures. In Cummings CW, Frederickson JM, Harker LA, et al.: Otolaryngology—Head and Neck Surgery, vol 1. St. Louis: CV Mosby, 1986 p 918.
8. Donald PJ: Fractures of the zygoma. In English GM (ed): Otolaryngology. Philadelphia: JB Lippincott. In press.
9. Donald PJ: The Frontal Sinus. Philadelphia: Lea & Febiger. In press.
10. Donald PJ: Ettin M: The safety of frontal sinus fat obliteration when sinus walls are missing. Laryngoscope 96:190–193. 1986.
11. Duvall AJ, Foster CA, Lyons DP, Letson RD: Medial canthoplasty: Early and delayed repair. Laryngoscope 91:173–183, 1981.
12. Foster CA, Sherman JE: Surgery of Facial Bone Fractures. New York: Churchill Livingstone, 1987, pp 152, 160, 162, 165, 198, 208.
13. Georgiade N, Nash T: A external cranial fixation apparatus for severe maxillofacial injuries. Plast Reconstruct Surg 38:142–146, 1966.
14. Hayton-Williams DS: Delayed jaw fracture therapy: A review of results. Br J Plast Surg 12:378–384, 1959–60
15. Huelke DF: Mechanics in the production of mandibular fractures: A study with the stresscoat technique. I. Symphysea impacts. J Dent Res 40:1042–1056, 1961.
16. Knight JS, North JK: The ossification of malar fractures: An analysis of displacement as a guide to treatment. Br J Plast Surg 13:325–359, 1961.
17. Larsen OD, Thomsen M: Zygomatic fractures: II. A follow-up study of 137 patients. Scand J Plast Reconstr Surg 12:59–63, 1978.
18. Le Fort R: Experimental study of fractures of the upper jaw, Part III. Rev Chir de Paris 23:479–567, 1901. Translated by P. Tessier in Plast Reconstr Surg 50:600–605, 1972.
19. Luce EA, Tubb TD, Moore AM: Review of 1000 major facial fractures and associated injuries. Plast Reconstr Surg 63:26–30, 1979.
20. Manson RN, Hooper JE, Su CT: Structural pillars of the facial skeleton: An approach to the management of Le Fort fractures. Plast Reconstr Surg 66:54–61, 1980.
21. Mathog RH: Post-traumatic telecanthus. In Mathog RH: Maxillofacial Trauma. Baltimore: Williams & Wilkins, 1984, p. 310.
22. McGuirt WF, Salisbury PL: Mandibular fractures: Their effect on growth and dentition. Arch Otolaryngol Head Neck Surg 113:257–261, 1987.
23. Montgomery WW: Surgery of the Upper Respiratory System, vol. 1. Philadelphia: Lea & Febiger, 1971.
24. Morgan GDG, Madan OK, Bergerot JPC: Fractures of the middle third of the face: A review of 300 cases. Br J Plast Surg 25:147, 1972.
25. Morris JH: Biphase connector, external skeletal splint for reduction and fixation of manidbular fractures. Oral Surg. Oral Med. & Oral Path. 2:1382–1398, 1949.
26. Nahum AM: The biomechanics of maxillofacial trauma. Clin Plast Surg 2:59–64, 1975.
27. Rowe NL: Maxillofacial Injuries, vol. 1. New York: Churchill Livingstone, 1985, p 455.
28. Rowe NL, Killey HC: Fractures of the Facial Skeleton, 2nd ed. New York: Churchill Livingstone, 1968.
29. Rowe NL, Williams JL: Maxillofacial Injuries. New York: Churchill Livingstone, 1985, pp 6, 13, 299, 376.
30. Schultz RC, Carbonell AM: Midfacial fractures from vehicular accidents. Clin Plast Surg 2:173–189, 1975.
31. Toomey J: Low Maxillary Fractures in Maxillofacial Trauma. Baltimore: Williams & Wilkins, 1984, p 235.

7

Intensive Care Management of the Head-Injured Patient

JOHN D. WARD

It is imperative to realize that a severe head injury is not a simple or routine problem that will respond to a standard recipe. The clinical problems faced by a head-injured patient are a composite of the injury that the brain has sustained, associated injuries, and subsequent insults that occur when there are serious systemic derangements. The purpose of this chapter is to enable the clinician to anticipate, recognize, and treat those medical problems that occur in the course of managing a patient with a severe head injury.

Although intracranial pressure (ICP) monitoring and management is important in the intensive care of the head-injured patient, it is covered in another part of this book; therefore this topic will not be addressed in this chapter. However, it should be recognized that ICP and other aspects of intensive care are closely connected and often influence one another.

The chapter will be divided into three areas. The first will describe several basic concepts that are important in the management of a patient with a severe head injury. The second will cover the various systemic, metabolic, and neurologic monitoring that is required, and the third will cover common medical problems.

BASIC CONCEPTS

There are several basic concepts known to all of us who deal with neurologic disease but are basic to the care and protection of the brain and bear repeating. The first is that for practical purposes central nervous system (CNS) repair after injury is usually poor and incomplete; injury to it is therefore best prevented rather than repaired, and every attempt should be made to prevent infection, shock, hypoxia, and ischemia, all of which can cause further neurologic damage. The next concept is that a damaged CNS is less able to protect itself than one in which all protective mechanisms are operative. The brain demands a constant availability of oxygen, glucose, and other metabolic substrates to function properly, supplied by sufficient cerebral blood flow (CBF) to meet metabolic demands. There are four variables that affect CBF: mean arterial pressure (MAP), arterial blood gases, metabolic demands, and ICP. The cerebral perfusion pressure (CPP) is the difference between MAP and ICP (CPP = MAP − ICP).[10] Under normal circumstances, a CBF will remain fairly constant with CPP of 60 to 150 mmHg by autoregulation. However, this may be impaired with brain trauma and therefore the patient's CBF can vary directly with CPP. Thus, any disease process that lowers MAP may cause cerebral ischemia and further neurologic damage. Signs of cerebral ischemia occur when CBF decreases below 50 to 60% of normal. As a general rule, it is best to maintain a CPP of at least 50 to 60 mmHg.

The effect of arterial carbon dioxide pressure ($PaCO_2$) on the cerebral vasculature is well known and will not be discussed in any great detail. With CNS injury the $PaCO_2$ should be kept at least in the normal range and perhaps less if there is a problem with elevated ICP.

If the brain is to protect itself from subsequent insult, it is important to ensure that the metabolic needs of the brain are kept to a minimum. Fever, seizures, and other phenomena that increase cerebral metabolism may cause a marginally perfused brain to become ischemic if flow cannot keep pace with metabolism. This is expressed in the relationship

$$CMRO_2 = CBF \times AVDO_2$$

where $CMRO_2$ is the cerebral metabolic rate for oxygen and is dependent on the flow of blood through the brain and the brain's need for oxygen; $AVDO_2$ is the arteriovenous oxygen content difference. CBF can be measured directly, but this is difficult and expensive, whereas $AVDO_2$ can easily be determined by an arterial line and a jugular line passed retrograde up to the jugular bulb. Differences in oxygen content can then be determined. A low $AVDO_2$ reflects either a low metabolic need as seen with a badly damaged brain, hypothermia, or barbiturate coma, or greater than adequate blood flow where low extraction is needed. A high $AVDO_2$ (greater than 7) usually means that need has outstripped flow as a result of either excessive metabolism or low CBF.

The final concept is that there is a complex interaction between the brain and other systems. What is good systemically may not necessarily benefit the brain. For example, a vasodilator may decrease the afterload to the heart and improve cardiac function. However, if it vasodilates the vessels in the cerebral vasculature and if cerebral compliance is decreased, cerebral ischemia due to an increased ICP and lowered CPP may occur. Therefore, any treatment for a systemic problem must be considered in the light of its simultaneous effect on a damaged nervous system.

MONITORING

Adequate intensive care results, in part, from adequate monitoring of those systems that are either likely to be impaired and require support and those that can be altered to enhance care and brain recovery further. Monitoring can be divided into cardiopulmonary, metabolic, neurologic, and neuroelectrical. Some of this monitoring will be continuous and some, such as that of arterial blood gases, will be intermittent. The frequency of intermittent monitoring will depend on the patient's clinical condition and the rapidity with which clinical decisions need to be made. The physician must also balance the expected benefit of having more complete information with the sometimes considerable risk that monitoring poses.

Cardiopulmonary monitoring, in the acute phase of head injury, usually consists of an indwelling arterial catheter and some means of estimating circulating blood volume. In a younger person this may be a central venous pressure line. However, in the patient with cardiac or pulmonary injury or disease or in the older patient, a pulmonary artery catheter with measurements of pulmonary capillary wedge pressure may be required. The advantage of an arterial line is that it provides immediate warning if there is any problem with hypotension and therefore compromise of CPP. A further advantage of an arterial line is the ease with which blood samples can be obtained.

Continuous electrocardiographic monitoring is fairly routine in most intensive care units. Recently, the use of pulse oximetry has become more common. The advantage of this technique is that it provides a minute-by-minute estimation of the adequacy of oxygen saturation of the tissues and therefore tissue perfusion. The technique is especially useful in those patients whose oxygenation may change rapidly and may not be noticed until there is a change in vital signs or in arterial blood gases. Examples are patients with spinal cord injuries whose ventilation is compromised and head-injured patients who have associated pulmonary injury such as a pneumothorax, which may be of sudden onset, or acute respiratory distress syndrome (ARDS).

In most patients with head injuries, it is not necessary to determine the full range of cardiac and pulmonary parameters, such as cardiac output, systemic vascular resistance, pulmonary vascular resistance, or shunt. However, in some patients it will be, and for these patients it must be recognized when additional data are needed to make proper therapeutic decisions.

By the term "metabolic monitoring," we mean following those parameters that reflect the adequacy of systemic homeostatic mechanisms. These include electrolytes, indicators of renal and liver function, and indicators of sufficient nutritional support.

"Neurologic monitoring" means assessing the brain's ability to function. Most commonly, this involves periodic neurologic examinations that assess mental status, cranial nerve function, and motor function. This can also take the form of the Glasgow Coma Scale (GCS)[17] coupled with evaluation of pupillary and motor function. If the neurologic examination cannot be performed because of extensive limitations such as paralysis, then other forms of monitoring are required, such as ICP or neuroelectrical monitoring. ICP monitoring is considered in Chapter 8.

Electrical monitoring of the brain can be divided into two main areas; electroencephalography (EEG), or some processed variant, and evoked potentials acquired either at intervals or continuously. These techniques have been introduced slowly in the intensive care environment for a number of reasons. Continuous electrical monitoring produces an enormous amount of information. It is not always clear what variations in electrical activity mean and what data should be acquired. The most important problem now is to determine what the changes in the electrical variables mean in terms of neurologic function. At present, electrical monitoring has several indications. If it is suspected that a patient is in status epilepticus or is having repeated seizures, then the EEG should be assessed at frequent intervals until the seizures are stopped. If an attempt is being made to decrease cerebral metabolic rate, that is, using barbiturate administration for control of ICP, EEG can be used to monitor the depth of metabolic suppression.

The use of evoked potentials in the intensive care setting so far has limited use. Some physicians have attempted prognostication of outcome based on the evoked potentials;[9,14] others have used the central conduction time as a measurement of recovery.[11] However, for the day to day evaluation of brain function, neuroelectrical monitoring is still in the developmental stages.

SPECIFIC PROBLEMS

This section examines common problems that occur during the intensive care of a severely head-injured patient, including pulmonary difficulties, coagulopathy, nutritional problems, disorders of sodium metabolism, and sepsis. Each problem will be addressed, and its recognition and treatment will be discussed in light of the severely head-injured patient.

Pulmonary Disorders

It is imperative that an adequate airway be established as soon as possible after a head injury has occurred. There is significant evidence that hypoxia and hypoventilation commonly occur after a severe head injury, either from the head injury itself or from associated multiple trauma.[8,12] All patients who have a GCS of 8 or less should be intubated, preferably close to the scene of the accident, depending on the skill of the paramedics involved in the initial care of the patient. Once the patient arrives in the emergency room and certainly in the intensive care unit, the comatose patient should have secure airway control. An early problem in the patient with multiple trauma is a missed or delayed pneumothorax; this may be manifested by changes in the vital signs and arterial blood gases. The pneumothorax may be the result of a percutaneous line insertion, institution of ventilatory assistance and resultant barotrauma, or lung perforation from associated rib fractures. Regardless of the cause, if the blood pressure is unstable, oxygenation decreases, or respiratory insufficiency occurs, especially early in the patient's course, a pneumothorax should be considered. If the patient has severe cardiopulmonary distress and there are unequal breath sounds, the side of the chest with distant breath sound should be aspirated to evaluate and treat pneumothorax. If the patient is otherwise stable, a portable chest film and arterial blood gases should be obtained. Once the diagnosis is made, a chest tube is inserted and usually is left in place until the patient is weaned from the ventilator. We emphasize that a pneumothorax can occur suddenly any time after the institution of positive end-expiratory pressure (PEEP).

Another common problem in the head-injured patient is that of ARDS. This syndrome has multiple causes, among which are aspiration, pulmonary contusion, fat emboli pneumonia, bacteremia, and gram-negative sepsis.[18] With these multiple and diverse etiologies, ARDS can be a significant problem in the head-injured patient. This disease has four phases. The first is a latent phase, when the initial insult occurs; the patient may show no sign of respiratory problems. The next phase is one of acute interstitial edema where the arterial oxygen pressure (PaO_2) falls.

The chest radiograph at this time may be normal, and there is a decrease in lung compliance. Next, there is the accumulation of intra-alveolar edema causing severe arterial hypoxemia even with supplemental oxygen. Chest films show a fluffy infiltrate. If recovery does not occur within a few days, pulmonary fibrosis can begin. Alveolar capillary structures are destroyed and replaced with fibrous tissue, causing further decrease in lung compliance and the need for increased ventilatory pressures. When this stage occurs, the mortality is quite high, reaching between 60 and 80%, depending on age and on the number of organ systems involved.[18] The low PaO_2 that can result from ARDS can worsen preexisting neurologic damage. Consequently, prevention or early treatment is crucial.

Treatment of ARDS requires correction of the initial cause, such as, antibiotics for sepsis or pneumonia and volume replacement for shock as soon as possible. Further measures are aimed at maximizing oxygen saturation. Despite ongoing research, there is no effective therapy to block the alveolar capillary damage. The pulmonary edema is treated with diuretics and ionotropic agents as indicated. The gas exchange derangement is corrected by the use of oxygen, mechanical ventilation, and PEEP. Elevated inspired oxygen is often required, but levels above 50% can also damage lung vascular endothelium.

PEEP is often required to improve oxygenation and although it is controversial whether it actually "pushes" fluid from the alveoli, it does open collapsed alveoli, increases the functional residual capacity of the lung, and improves oxygenation. However, the use of PEEP in a critically ill patient can be injurious. Low levels of PEEP (3 to 5 mmHg) are probably physiologic and cause no problem. If higher pressures are needed, significant physiologic consequences can occur. If the patient is hypovolemic, cardiac output can decrease, with a decrease in MAP and CPP. Therefore intravascular volume needs to be adequate before high levels of PEEP (12 to 20 mmHg) are used. In addition, increased PEEP may be transmitted through the pulmonary vasculature and intrathoracic vessels to cause increased ICP.[1,6] Transmission of pressure through diseased lungs seems to be less than that through normal lungs, and higher levels of PEEP may not increase ICP. However, there is a general consensus that all patients who have a severe brain injury and require levels of PEEP greater than 10 mmHg should have simultaneous ICP monitoring in case ICP is affected. Certainly, all patients with significant ARDS should also have an arterial line, a pulmonary artery catheter, and frequent blood gas determinations.

The other common pulmonary problems that head-injured patients may have are those of aspiration and pneumonia. Aspiration can occur in comatose patients who have poor airway protection with inhalation of blood or stomach contents at the scene of the accident or subsequently when hospitalized. Awareness of the problem, frequent suctioning, and proper technique of enteral feeding can help reduce the problem.

Pneumonia is common in head-injured patients. The diagnosis rests on a combination of fever, positive sputum culture, a Gram's stain of the sputum that shows white blood cells and bacteria, a positive chest film, and blood gas abnormalities. Not all are required for the diagnosis of pneumonia, but a sufficient number should be confirmed before a diagnosis is made and treatment started. If pneumonia is suspected, antibiotic treatment is started after adequate cultures are obtained. However, indiscriminant use of antibiotics when a patient presents only with fever is discouraged. Comatose patients generally do not move much and blood flow to the lungs is shunted to the dependent portions. In addition, secretions collect in dependent lung regions when the upper and anterior lung segments are ventilated better. There are reports that some of these problems can be corrected or avoided by the use of the Roto bed, also called kinetic therapy. Pulmonary shunting appears to improve when the patient is rotated. This can be done manually by turning and repositioning the patient frequently, but use of the automatically turning bed ensures that frequent change in position will occur. When the Roto bed is used, care should be taken that ICP is not adversely affected as the patient turns from side to side.

The final pulmonary problem is that of pulmonary embolism, occuring in up to 15% of patients with neurologic difficulties.[5] This diagnosis can be very difficult in the comatose patient. Frequently, the only indication may be a sudden tachycardia, along with a deterioration in arterial oxygenation. The initial workup consists of a chest radiograph and an electrocardiogram to assess a possible pleural effusion or a wedge-shaped infiltrate and right ventricular strain or right bundle branch block. However, a normal chest film with hypoxemia does not rule out a pulmonary embolism. A ventilation-perfusion scan followed by a pulmonary arteriogram may be needed to confirm the diagnosis.

Coagulopathy

Normal coagulation is critical in the head-injured patient. If coagulation is hypoactive, the patient will bleed, and, if hyperactive, will cause unwanted clotting followed by hemorrhages. Normal homeostasis requires a normal vessel wall, functioning platelets, coagulation factors, and a system of fibrinolysis. We will examine two problems that can occur in the head-injured patient: disseminated intravascular coagulation (DIC) and deep vein thrombosis (DVT).

DIC occurs when, for whatever reason (trauma, sepsis, shock), there is activation of intrinsic or extrinsic coagulation pathways so that clotting factors are consumed and depleted and thrombi are formed within the microvasculture.[2] True DIC probably involves some sort of bleeding and severe abnormality of coagulation tests. A number of the usual laboratory screening tests for coagulopathy (prothrombin time [PT], partial thromboplastin time [PTT], fibrinogen, fibrin split products, and platelets) are abnormal in severely head-injured patients, ranging from 72% with only one abnormal test to 32% with three or more abnormal tests;[13] whether this is a mild form of DIC or not is unclear. However, the physician cannot wait until frank bleeding occurs before attempting to correct coagulation abnormalities. We try to keep the platelet count above 50,000 to 60,000/mm^3 and transfuse platelets if the platelet count falls below these values. If the PTT or PT becomes prolonged, then fresh frozen plasma is given. Administration of these products is continued until coagulation studies become normal. If severe DIC occurs, with abnormalities in the majority of coagulation tests and with bleeding, the patient's outlook is poor. Treatment should try to correct the primary cause if possible and to correct coagulation abnormality by administration of fresh frozen plasma and platelets. The use of heparin or epsilon-aminocaproic acid is controversial but in a desperate situation may be required. It should not be undertaken without appropriate consultation or a knowledge as to the exact cause of the DIC.

The second disturbance of coagulation, venous thrombosis, results from increased coagulability. DVT is a significant problem in the neurosurgical patient. DVT in the calf of neurosurgical patients has been estimated to occur from 29 to 43%, as estimated by injection of radiolabeled fibrinogen. A variety of risk factors predispose the patient to a DVT. Surgery that lasts more than 4 hours increases the risk from 24 to 50%. Other factors are age over 40 years, heart failure, a previous history of DVT, direct trauma to the leg, obesity, malignancy, and pregnancy. Limb weakness may increase the incidence of DVT to as high as 60%.

The best way to treat DVT is to prevent it; two methods are the use of low-dose heparin or of external pneumatic compression devices.[16] Several studies have shown that heparin is probably safe in doses of 5000 U two or three times a day subcutaneously and does lower the incidence of DVT. However, there has been no prospective controlled trial in neurosurgical patients. If low-dose heparin is used, it should be reserved for patients older than 40 years or those less than the age of 40 years who have two or more risk factors. The use of external pneumatic compression stockings has been shown in two studies to decrease the occurrence of DVT. It is important to apply them as soon as possible after admission and to use them until the patient is no longer at risk and, if possible, is up and walking. Compression stockings are used more commonly than low-dose heparin if there is a concern about bleeding or if there are abnormal coagulation studies. However, there are centers that give low-dose heparin immediately after surgery without an increase in bleeding complications.

It can be very difficult to diagnose DVT in an unconscious patient; one must be suspicious and search for DVT diligently. A persistent fever in the absence of a demonstrable infection can be the first clue. Once there is a suspicion, Doppler ultrasound and venography can confirm the diagnosis.

Once DVT has occurred, the patient is anticoagulated with heparin, then converted to oral warfarin. We do not know when it is safe to anticoagulate fully a post-trauma or postsurgical patient. For this reason when a significant DVT occurs in a patient in whom we believe anticoagulation might be unsafe, we use a Greenfield filter inserted into the inferior vena cava; it is fairly easily inserted and is reasonably effective in preventing pulmonary emboli but can cause lower extremity swelling. There are no prospective studies that demonstrate that these filters are effective when used prophylactically.

Nutritional Management

Trauma to the brain initiates a complex series of neuroendocrinologic responses whose goal is to restore body tissue to a normal state. The patient with a severe head injury is significantly hypermetabolic and catabolic soon after injury. If trauma to other systems or sepsis occurs, the hypermetabolism and catabolism is even more pronounced.[4] Our treatment goal is to meet these increased needs with appropriate enteral or parenteral feeding.

Nutritional support should be started within 48 to 72 hours after injury. Calorie and nitrogen requirements can be determined by estimations of the patient's needs, based on age, sex, size, and severity of injury, or directly, which is more accurate but more complex.

Usually, the patient is fed enterally, if this is possible.[3] Various preparations are available for tube feeding, depending on the patient's needs and on associated diseases, such as renal or respiratory failure. A nutritional consultation from a dietician is invaluable in selecting the appropriate formula. There are several principles to follow in enterally feeding a comatose patient. First, it is common for these patients to have difficulty with gastric emptying; therefore care must be taken to not overload the stomach, which can result in vomiting and aspiration. To prevent this, small boluses of feeding with checks for residual volume or continuous feeding via a pump should be used. A small feeding tube placed in the duodenum will also reduce the chance of aspiration. If the patient will require long-term feedings, percutaneous endoscopic gastrostomy may be the best method. In skilled hands, this is a relatively safe and quick procedure that can be done at the bedside. However, like any surgery, it does have some risk. The second problem with enteral feeding is diarrhea secondary to either decreased intestinal absorption or the use of hypertonic solutions or both. The diarrhea can usually be controlled with a combination of drugs, such as Lomotil, or varying the concentration of the formula.

If enteral feeding cannot be started within the first 2 to 3 days and it appears that enteral feeding will not be tolerated for 1 to 2 weeks, then parenteral nutrition should be considered.[15] This is best accomplished by a nutritional support team experienced in the use of hyperalimentation. Hyperglycemia and electrolyte imbalance should be avoided. In addition, high carbohydrate loads can increase carbon dioxide production making weaning from ventilation more difficult. There is no one parameter than can be followed; serum ablumin, serum transferrin, patient weight, skin-fold thickness, delayed hypersensitivity, and the meeting of estimated metabolic needs together can be used to ensure adequate patient nutrition.

Water and Sodium Balance

Brain trauma frequently upsets water and sodium balance, possibly by inappropriate antidiuretic hormone (ADH) secretion.[7] ADH secretion is characterized by a low serum sodium (<135 mEq/L), a low serum osmolality, a urine osmolality that is greater than serum, and an elevated urinary sodium. To treat this, fluid is restricted to about 600 to 800 cc/24 hours. Care must be taken not to reduce circulating volume to the point where hypotension ensues, since this would only aggravate neurologic damage. If the patient does not respond to fluid restriction or if restriction is not feasible and sodium decreases to less than 125 mEq/L, the patient can be carefully given 3% saline. A diuretic (such as furosemide 20 to 60 mg) can help excessive volume accumulation. Other medical therapies for a more chronic hyponatremia are the use of salt tablets, flurocortisone, or demeclocycline. The goal is to keep serum sodium between 135 and 145 mEq/L.

The other difficulty that can arise with water balance is diabetes insipidus. In the head-injured patient, diabetes insipidus is usually secondary to damage to the pituitary gland or stalk and is characterized by an increasing serum sodium level and a large urinary output that has a low specific gravity and osmolality. Sometimes, patients can be fluid overloaded, especially in the immediate postoperative period. However, these patients usually, once they have diuresed the excess fluid, will have a decreasing urine output and a sodium that stays in the normal range. If the patient continues to put out a dilute hypotonic urine with an increasing serum sodium level (greater than 150 mEq/L) then he probably has diabetes insipidus and should be treated. Treatment consists of either acqueous vasopressin 2 to 5 U, subcutaneously, or more recently, the use of desmopressin acetate (DDAVP) either nasally or parenterally. Its duration is usually 8 to 24 hours. In especially refractory cases, a continuous acqueous vasopressin drip may be of value but should be used with caution to avoid water intoxication.

Sepsis

Severely head-injured patients often have associated injuries and need invasive monitoring and surgery, and it is not surprising that infection and sepsis are common. It is impossible to discuss each type of infection and antibiotics, but some general comments are in order. It is important to remove all catheters that are not needed. Invasive monitors are a major source of sepsis in these patients and their use should be given careful consideration. If the lines, especially intravascular lines, cannot be discontinued in 3 days, then they should be changed over a guide wire or the site should be rotated. Foley catheters should be removed as soon as continuous urine output monitoring is no longer required. The patient can then be switched to an external urinary collection device or intermittent catheterization.

Except for certain circumstances, such as the insertion of a shunt or an operation that carries a risk of infection, prophylactic use of antibiotics is to be discouraged. Perioperative antibiotics have been advocated by some surgeons. If used, they should be given only for a brief period of time, usually less than 24 hours. If antibiotics are used unnecessarily or indiscriminately, the normal flora can be eliminated, superinfections can occur, and resistant strains will emerge. This makes even more difficult the treatment of infections that do occur. Fever is common in the comatose patient and should not be treated with antibiotics until an infection has been identified. Cultures should be done frequently of blood, urine, and sputum, and perhaps of wound and cerebrospinal fluid if there is fever and suspicion of infection. Once a specific infection with a specific organism is identified, then those antibiotics that can best treat the infection are used. There are two exceptions to this. The first is that if a significant infection can be shown on clinical grounds (such as positive chest radiograph, fever, and infected sputum seen under the microscope), a presumptive diagnosis of pneumonia can be made, cultures taken, and fairly broad treatment for common organisms started. This is then tailored to more specific treatment when the results of the cultures become known. The second circumstance in which antibiotic treatment needs to be started empirically is when the patient presents with hypotension, decreased systemic vascular resistance, fever, and tachycardia, and a diagnosis of sepsis is made. An aminoglycoside and one other agent, either one of the newer penicillins, such as piperacillin, or one of the third generation cephalosporins, are administered along with fluids and vasopressers, as needed. Corticosteroids are no longer indicated. Again, once specific bacteria are identified, a more specific drug regimen can be instituted.

As can be seen from the foregoing discussion, the care of the severely head-injured patient extends far beyond the brain injury. Continuous attention must be focused not only on the CNS but also on all bodily systems. They should be monitored aggressively but appropriately, and any derangement should be identified and treated before systemic insults can cause further neurologic injury.

REFERENCES

1. Apuzzo MLJ, Weiss MH, Robison V, Small RB, Kurze T, Heiden JS: Effect of positive end expiratory pressure ventilation on intracranial pressure in man. J Neurosurg 46:227–232, 1977.
2. Clark JA, Fimelli RE, Netsky MG: Disseminated intravascular coagulation following cranial trauma. J Neurosurg 52:266–269, 1980.
3. Clifton GL, Robertson CS, Constart CF: Enteral hyperalimentation in head injury. J Neurosurg 62:186–193, 1985.
4. Clifton GL, Robertson CS, Grossman RG, Hodge S, Foltz R, Garza C: The metabolic response to severe head injury. J Neurosurg 60:687–696, 1984.
5. Coon WW: Risk factors in pulmonary embolism. Surg Gynecol Obstet 143:385–390, 1976
6. Frost EAM: Effects of positive end-expiratory pressure on intracranial pressure and compliance in brain injured patients. J Neurosurg 47:195–200, 1977.
7. Fox JL, Falix JL, Shalhoub RJ: Neurosurgical hyponatremia: The role of inappropriate antidiuresis. J Neurosurg 34:506–513, 1971.
8. Gildenberg PL, Makela ME: The effect of early intubation and ventilation on the outcome following head trauma. Dacey RG, Wimm HR, Rimel RW, Jane JA (eds): Trauma of the Central Nervous System. Seminars in Neurosurgery. New York: Raven Press, 1985, p 79–90.
9. Greenberg RP, Becker DP, Miller JD, et al.: Evaluation of brain function in severe human head trauma with multimodality evoked potentials. Part II: Localization of brain dysfunction and correlation with post-traumatic neurologic conditions. J Neurosurg 47:163–177, 1977.
10. Harper AM: Autoregulation of cerebral blood flow: Influence of arterial blood pressure on the blood flow through the cerebral cortex. J Neurol Neurosurg Psychiatry 29:398–403, 1966.
11. Hume AL, Cant BR: Central somatosensory conduction after head injury. Ann Neurol 10:411–419, 1981.
12. Miller JD, Sweet RC, Narayan R, et al.: Early insults to the injured brain. JAMA 240:439–442, 1978.
13. Miner ME, Kaufman HH, Graham SH, Haar FL, Gildenberg PL: Disseminated intravascular coagulation and fibrinolytic syndrome following head injury in children: Frequency and prognostic implications. J Pediatr 100:687–691, 1982.
14. Newlon PG, Greenberg RP, Hyatt MS, et al.: The dynamics of neuronal dysfunction and recovery following severe head injury assessed with serial multimodality evoked potentials. J Neurosurg 57:168–177, 1982.
15. Rapp RP, Young B, Twyman D, et al.: The favorable effect of early parenteral feeding on survival in head injured patients. J Neurosurg 58:906–912, 1983.
16. Swann KW, Black PMcL: Deep vein thrombosis and pulmonary emboli in neurosurgical patients: A review. J Neurosurg 61:1055–1062, 1984.
17. Teasdale G, Jennett B: Assessment of coma and impaired consciousness—a practical scale. Lancet 2:81–84, 1974.
18. Wilson RS, Pontoppidan H, Rie MP: Acute respiratory failure. In: Ropper HH, Kennedy SK, Zervas NT (eds): Neurological and Neurosurgical Intensive Care. Baltimore: University Book Press, 1983, p 87.

8

Intracranial Pressure Monitoring and Treatment

THOMAS G. SAUL

High morbidity and mortality follows primary and secondary brain injury after cranio-cerebral trauma. Primary injury involves direct tissue damage incurred at the moment of impact, such as concussion, cerebral contusion, or laceration. Secondary injury results from shock, hypoxia, hypercapnia or the compressive effects of expanding intracranial hemorrhage.

Increased intracranial pressure (ICP) can follow either primary or secondary brain injury and is common after severe head injury. If uncontrolled, increased ICP is associated with extremely high mortality. Normal ICP is 15 mmHg or less; mortality increases substantially when ICP exceeds 20 to 25 mmHg. Therefore there is not a large margin of safety. This relationship of elevated levels of ICP and mortality is important and is the main justification for monitoring and treating intracranial hypertension.

RATIONALE FOR MONITORING

A number of investigators have reported the adverse effect of intracranial hypertension on outcome after severe head injury. Marshall et al.[23] described that among 75 patients with diffuse head injury, 77% of those with ICP below 15 mmHg had a good recovery (GR) or were moderately disabled (MD). In the 40 patients with ICP above 15 mmHg, only 43% had similarly satisfactory outcomes.[23] Miller et al.[26] noted that among 196 patients with severe head injury, those in whom ICP was never more than 20 mmHg had outcomes of GR or MD 74% of the time, and 18 died. Those patients whose ICP went above 20 mmHg, but could be lowered by aggressive treatment, had a mortality rate of 26% and GR to MD outcome of 55%. However, if the ICP went above 20 mmHg and was not reducible, mortality rate was 92% and the GR or MD outcome was only 3%. They concluded that "virtually all patients in whom ICP cannot be controlled died."[26] Saul and Ducker[32] reported that 69% of their 106 patients died in whom ICP was 25 mmHg or greater, compared with a mortality rate of 15% if the ICP remained less than 25 mmHg.

In addition to documenting that elevated ICP results in a worse outcome, there is mounting evidence that early aggressive treatment of ICP elevations improves outcome. Marshall et al.[24] contended that better outcome was due to early diagnosis, intervention, and aggressive neurosurgical intensive care, including ICP monitoring. They found that aggressive treatment did not produce more vegetative survivors and reported a 28% mortality rate with 60% of their patients having outcomes of GR to MD.[24] Jennett and colleagues[15] described earlier that in the International Data Bank (IDB), including patients from Glasgow, the Netherlands, and Los Angeles, 50% of their patients died and only 39% had a GR or MD outcome.

Bowers and Marshall[3] reported an expanded series from San Diego of 200 patients with severe head injury of whom 52% had GR or MD outcomes with aggressive treatment. They evaluated the effect that ICP monitoring had on the mortality rate in a subgroup of 86 patients with Glasgow Coma scores equal to or less than 5. Forty-nine of these had the ICP monitored and had a mortality rate of 39% compared with a mortality of 62% in the 37 patients who did not have the ICP monitored. This difference was not statistically significant but did suggest that the ICP monitoring influenced outcome, although the two groups were treated by different physicians and other differences in therapy may have been present in addition to the presence or absence of ICP monitoring.

Miller et al. published a series of 225 patients with severe head injuries treated aggressively using ICP monitoring data. Fifty-six percent of the patients had GR or MD outcomes and only 34% died.[26] They identified 158 patients who were clinically compatible with the IDB groups and found a lower mortality rate (40%) in their patients than that in the IDB group (49%). Miller et al. believed that a real, although modest, reduction in mortality after severe head injury had been obtained by their treatment protocol and that ICP is "an important variable to measure in the head injured patient."[26]

Certainly, there are problems comparing series from one center to another or even in a single center at two different times. Differences in the number of surgical lesions, especially acute subdural hematomas, mean ages or age distributions, Glasgow Coma scores or distributions, or timing of the arrival of the patient to a definitive neurologic center all may alter mortality rates.

In 1982, Saul and Ducker[32] published a report in which the problems of comparison were minimized. They compared two series of patients who were from the same catchment area, had the same prehospital care, and were treated at the same center with the same protocol. The series differed in that series I was treated *without* a strict ICP management protocol; series II was treated using a specific management protocol based on the level of ICP. In series I, ICP was treated at various levels between 20 and 40 mmHg with varying therapies being used. In series II, all patients were giving mannitol and furosemide and hyperventilated as soon as the ICP was 16 mmHg or higher for 10 minutes while the patient was at rest. Cerebrospinal fluid (CSF) drainage was also used. If the patient's ICP went above 25 mmHg, he was randomized into an intravenous barbiturate protocol. Series I and series II had nearly identical numbers of patients, average age and age distributions, incidence of life-threatening associated injuries, the incidence of intracranial surgical mass lesions, and similar distributions of Glasgow Coma scores.

In series II (the early aggressive treatment group), only 25% of the 106 patients had ICP greater than 25 mmHg. More importantly, the overall mortality rate decreased from 46% in series I to 33% in series II. These investigators concluded that early aggressive monitoring and treatment of intracranial hypertension lowers the incidence of life-threatening levels of

ICP and reduces mortality without increasing the number of severely disabled or vegetative patients.

MONITORING TECHNIQUES

ICP monitoring by ventriculostomy was first described by Lundberg[19] and remains a popular and reliable method. An intraventricular catheter (IVC) is inserted into the frontal horn of the lateral ventricle and is connected to an external transducer. The IVC technique provides an accurate, direct ventricular fluid pressure reading and allows CSF drainage to treat ICP elevations. An IVC poses some risk of central nervous system (CNS) infection and of intracerebral hemorrhage, since the catheter penetrates brain tissue to enter the ventricle.[41,43] To reduce the infection risk, a fastidious sterile technique of catheter placement must be followed. We usually place the IVC into the right frontal horn, but occasionally into the left frontal horn if that ventricle seems more accessible. We shave the head bicoronally and also shave the remainder of the right hemicranium (Fig. 8–1) to assure adequate scalp exposure for the purposes of "tunneling" the catheter under the scalp with an exit point 5 to 6 cm away from its entry into the skull (Fig. 8–1). This decreases the chance of intracranial infections. The catheter is then attached to a three-way stopcock. We use a microtransducer for pressure readings (Fig. 8–2); the small transducer is attached to one of the ports of the stopcock and a sterile cap is attached to the other port of the stopcock. Sterile dressings are applied to the incisions. The stopcock/transducer apparatus is wrapped in a dry sterile sponge and then taped to the side of the head, which ensures that the transducer is level with the lateral ventricle regardless of the position of the patient's head or the head of the bed. The stopcock transducer apparatus should be manipulated only with strict sterile technique, such as when connecting the third port of the stopcock to a drainage bag. We have achieved low infection rates using this technique.

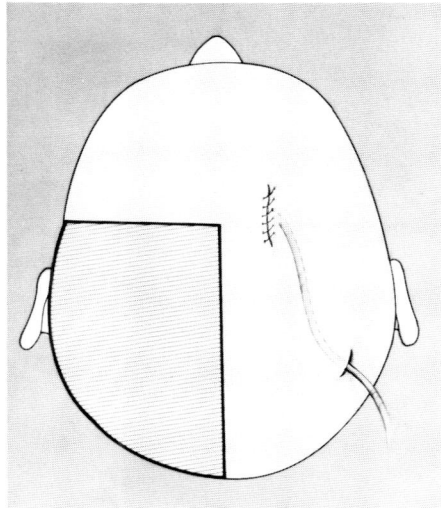

Figure 8–1. Diagram shows technique for insertion of an intraventricular catheter. Note the area of shaving (hatched area is remaining hair) and the "tunneling" of the catheter away from the skull entry.

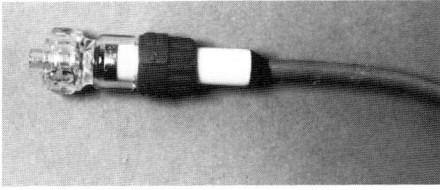

Figure 8–2.   Microtransducer used for ICP monitoring (Statham-Gould P-50).

As ICP monitoring became more popular, new techniques were developed. Vries et al.[41] developed the subarachnoid bolt. This device is a hollow bolt that is implanted via a burr hole into the subdural or subarachnoid space. It functions as a hydrostatic coupler from the intracranial subarachnoid space to an external transducer. The screw can be inserted in the emergency room, operating room, or intensive care unit, using a twist-drill and wrench to screw the bolt into the skull. The external end of the screw is a standard Leur lock that can fit a three-way stopcock, which then is attached to an external transducer for graphic and numerical recordings. The advantages of the subarachnoid screw apparatus are that there may be a lower CNS infection rate and that these devices can be used when the ventricles are collapsed and inaccessible to a ventricular catheter. However, one cannot drain CSF to treat ICP elevations, and the device may become occluded at high pressures because of brain herniating into the lumen of the screw. Figure 8–3 is a diagram of the insertion location of the subarachnoid screw. Once again, sterility should be maintained as with the intraventricular catheter. An important technical point with respect to insertion of a subarachnoid screw is shown in Figure 8–4. If the dura is not adequately coagulated so that it retracts backward, a dural flap may occlude the lumen of the screw and prevent accurate ICP determination.

Wilkinson[43] developed a rectangular-shaped flat catheter with a lumen that opens via a side port or cup opening at the end. The catheter can be placed subdurally through a burr hole at the edge of the bone flap during the closure of a craniotomy. It also is tunneled under the skin and exits a distance from its insertion into the skull (Fig. 8–5). The microtransducer shown in Figure 8–2 can be used for either the subarachnoid screw or the cup catheter. An advantage of the cup catheter is that another insertion technique is not required after a craniotomy is completed.

Figure 8–6 is a diagramatic representation showing a coronal section of the brain with an intraventricular catheter placed in one side and a subarachnoid screw on the other. This

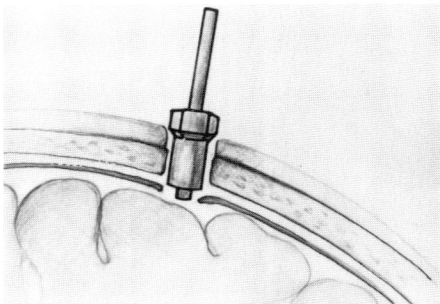

Figure 8–3.   Diagram depicts the placement of ICP bolt in the subdural/subarachnoid compartment.

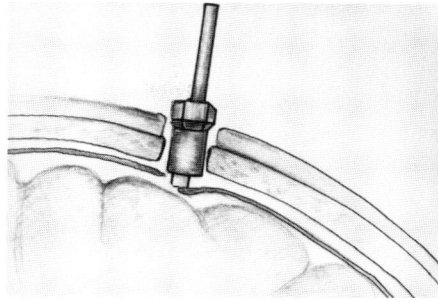

Figure 8–4. Diagram depicts dural flap "occluding" the lumen of bolt, causing malfunction.

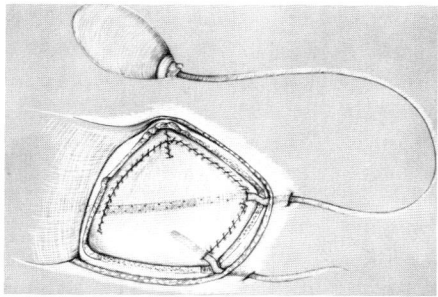

Figure 8–5. Diagram depicts placement of subdural cup catheter (lower exiting tube) at the closure of a craniotomy.

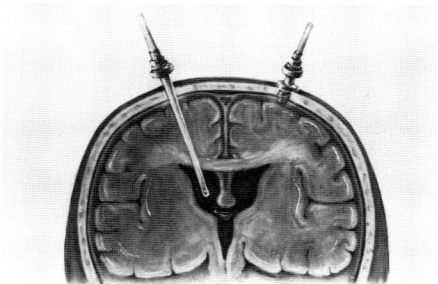

Figure 8–6. Diagram of coronal section of brain depicts monitoring in the ventricle (on left) and in the subdural/subarachnoid compartment (on right).

gives the reader a visual image of the various compartments from which ICP can be monitored.

There are also epidural monitors available, including a fiberoptic epidural probe[18] and an epidural bolt that functions the same way as the subarachnoid bolt.[5] These devices have extremely low CNS infection risks but the reliability of the epidural monitor readings has been questioned.[9,45]

In 1987, Ostrup and colleagues[29] reported their experience of continuous ICP monitoring with a miniaturized fiberoptic device. This device consisted of a 4 F fiberoptic probe with a transducer in the tip. It was initially developed for intravascular pressure recordings but adapted for use intracranially. This device can be placed into the ventricular system, the brain parenchyma, or the subdural space.

When this new monitor device was compared with concurrently functioning IVC monitors or subarachnoid monitors in 15 adult and 5 pediatric patients, the brain parenchyma pressure was within 2 to 5 mmHg of the pressures obtained by the standard monitors. It subsequently was used in adult and pediatric patients for variable lengths of times, occasionally as long as 2 weeks without infections or hemorrhages in 120 patients.[38] The catheter is easy to insert, can monitor ICP from any intracranial compartment, has an extremely low infection rate, and provides reliable readings. I believe that with simple and reliable devices such as this, ICP monitoring will become even more widespread than it already is.

ICP monitoring is not free from complication. Lundberg et al.[20] concluded that "there was no excessive risk in IVC monitoring" but they did not look closely at complications. Rosner and Becker[31] in 1976 reported an infection rate of 4.7% in a combined series of intraventricular catheters and bolts. Winn et al.[44] reported on 650 patients monitored with subarachnoid bolts with an incidence of 0.7% CNS infection; 1.4% superficial skin infection; and an 8% failure rate of the subarachnoid bolt. Finally, Narayan et al.[28] reported on more than 200 monitored patients, 91% having intraventricular catheter and the other 9% having a subarachnoid bolt. The infection rate was 6.3% and there was an intracerebral hemorrhage rate of 1.4% attributed to passing the catheter through the brain. One must weigh the risk of these complications from ICP monitoring against the possible benefits.

PATIENT SELECTION

It is generally agreed that any head-injured patient who can be aroused and who follows commands probably does not require ICP monitoring. Conversely, a patient who is comatose and does not localize to a painful stimulus probably needs ICP monitoring. In one series, patients admitted with severe head injury (less than 8 on the Glasgow Coma Scale) who had abnormal admission computed tomography (CT) scans, were found to be at high risk for developing elevated ICP. Therefore routine ICP monitoring in such patients is justified. Patients with normal CT scans on admission infrequently had elevated ICP. However, the following factors increased the possibility of elevated ICP even in patients with normal CT scans: systolic blood pressure less than 90 mmHg; unilateral or bilateral motor posturing; and age over 40 years.[28] Because of these findings, we generally monitor any comatose trauma patient who exhibits a flexion-withdrawal motor response or worse. If the patient localizes to a painful stimulus, this clinical finding can be used as a "clinical monitor." If the motor response deteriorates and the patient has flexor or extensor posturing, an immediate CT scan is obtained and an ICP monitor is inserted. Occasionally a septic patient will deteriorate neurologically without increase in ICP.[12] If one does not monitor comatose patients with normal CT scans, one should obtain a follow-up CT scan within 24 to 48 hours to rule out delayed intracranial abnormality that could alter the ICP dynamics.

If a patient is to be treated aggressively to decrease intracranial hypertension, ICP monitoring can guide the physician in starting and stopping treatment and indicate whether or not the treatment is effective. The medical regimens described below are not always benign or without complications. Moreover, the timing of various treatment modalities may be important in getting "the most" out of each modality; this can also be guided by continuous ICP measurements.

It is not entirely clear at what level ICP should be treated. Normal ICP is generally accepted as less than 15 mmHg. Pressures greater than 25 mmHg are more difficult to reduce than ICP levels less than 20 mmHg.[17] Over the years, the level of ICP at which specific treatment is instituted has been lowered. We begin treatment when the ICP level is consistently higher than 16 mmHg.[1] Others accept levels up to 20 mmHg before instituting some of the therapies described next. The level at which to begin treating ICP must be decided by the physician and then a well-defined protocol initiated when this level is reached.

MEDICAL TREATMENT

The medical management of ICP can be viewed as "balanced therapy." This concept divides the therapeutic endeavors into general measures and specific measures. General measures are those techniques and medications instituted at all levels of ICP to maintain optimal brain homeostasis discussed in Chapter 7. Specific measures are those aimed at returning elevated ICP to acceptable levels.

Intracranial Hypertension

When ICP exceeds acceptable levels (variously chosen as 15, 20, or 25 mmHg), several treatments are usually effective in reducing intracranial hypertension. This armamentarium is most effective if it is used in an organized fashion. No one therapy is always successful in lowering ICP: rather, a balanced treatment is used in which drugs are alternated and the time of administration of an individual drug is important to derive the maximum benefit. Treatment may include sedation, paralysis, hyperventilation, hyperosmolar agents (mannitol), loop diuretics (furosemide), CSF drainage, and barbiturates.[34] Before any of these treatments is started, the surgeon should obtain a CT scan to exclude intracranial mass lesions that may require surgical removal.

Sedation, Paralysis, and Analgesia

A struggling patient may require sedation to facilitate ventilation and to diminish adverse responses to noxious external stimuli. A patient may become hypertensive from stimuli such as nursing care, diagnostic tests, and associated injuries. Arterial hypertension greater than 180 mmHg systolic can increase hydrostatic pressure in intracranial capillary beds and may worsen vasogenic edema, which could aggravate the ICP problems. Sedation and analgesia may abort or blunt this detrimental cycle.

Stimulation may cause abnormal extension or flexion (decerebrate or decorticate posturing), which can increase systemic blood pressure. Moreover, the valsalva maneuver that accompanies abnormal posturing can increase intrathoracic pressure, which increases intracranial venous pressure and ICP. Paralytic drugs can prevent the chest, abdominal, and extremity muscle contraction responsible for this increased venous pressure. When frequent assessment of neurologic status is required, short-acting paralytic agents should be used; when infrequent assessments are adequate, prolonged paralysis may be best. ICP monitoring and ready access to CT scanning will allow safe use of these drugs. Commonly used drugs in patients with severe head injury in the ICU include diazepam, fentanyl, morphine, vecuronium, and pancuronium.

Hyperventilation

Hyperventilation usually decreases ICP for several hours or longer for any given new lowered level of arterial carbon dioxide tension ($PaCO_2$). However, since CSF alkalosis returns toward normal over time, a reduction in ICP for a lower $PaCO_2$ often will be only transient, and other treatments listed later should be used along with hyperventilation. If ICP is acceptable (less than 15 to 20 mmHg), minute ventilation can be reduced to return $PaCO_2$ to 28 to 32 mmHg so that further increases in ICP can again be treated with hyperventilation. We recommend continued controlled ventilation or hyperventilation therapy as long as ICP remains abnormal. Arterial blood gases should be obtained every 6 to 8 hours during this active phase of treatment.

Hyperosmolar Agents

Intravenous administration of solutions with a high osmolarity will produce an osmotic gradient between brain tissue and the blood. Water (and subsequently electrolytes) will diffuse from regions of lower (brain) to higher (blood vessels) osmolarity, reducing brain volume and therefore decreasing ICP. Urea and glycerol previously were used to produce this effect but both cross the blood-brain barrier and conceivably could increase brain water after an initial brain dehydration. Mannitol is a sugar that is not transported across the blood-brain barrier and so is excluded from normal brain. Thus, the osmotic gradient produced by mannitol is maintained over prolonged periods with persistent dehydration of normal brain. Mannitol may enter injured brain where the blood-brain barrier is not intact and might increase local edema in those areas. However, the blood-brain barrier is preserved in large volumes of brain even after severe brain injury, and the net effect of mannitol use is a reduction in brain volume and ICP.

Mannitol therapy is not free of risk. Patients requiring frequent administration can become dehydrated and can develop significant electrolyte imbalances. Severe dehydration and shock can threaten cardiovascular and renal function and ultimately limit the drug's use. Dosages of 0.25 to 1 g/kg every 4 to 6 hours are effective in reducing ICP and in improving intracranial compliance.[22] Larger doses have little additional effect on lowering ICP but will cause more dehydration.

Mannitol also may be given as a continuous infusion. When bolus doses are required at progressively shorter intervals to sustain the decrease in ICP, a continuous infusion should be considered. A continuous infusion of 20% mannitol, starting at approximately 30 cc/hour is equivalent to 6 g/hour or 24 g/4 hours. Neither a maximal nor optimal mannitol dose has yet been described.

In nonketotic hyerosmolar diabetic states, serum osmolarities of 320 to 330 mOsm are associated with an altered mental status, so that mannitol probably should not be given when serum osmolarity exceeds 320 mOsm. When a patient's ICP readings are consistently above 16mmHg, we administer 25 g of 20% mannitol every 6 hours to maintain an ICP level less than 16 mmHg. If necessary, the dose frequency is increased to every 4 hours to obtain a sustained decreased ICP. If more frequent boluses are required, a continuous infusion is begun. After 36 to 48 hours of good ICP control, the mannitol doses are tapered over the next 24 to 48 hours. Although a cautious dose regimen may help decrease the problems of hyperosmolar electrolyte disorders, it does not abolish them. Frequent (every 6 hours) electrolyte and osmolarity determinations are advised.

Diuretics

Recently, furosemide has been shown to be effective in decreasing ICP.[7,40] Furosemide is a diuretic and decreases intravascular volume; it also decreases the production of CSF and may have a direct effect on brain edema.[40] At the present time, we do not use furosemide alone to lower ICP in severely head-injured patients, but rather use it alternately with mannitol, perhaps decreasing mannitol requirements and minimizing electrolyte imbalances. For example, 25 g of mannitol can be given every 6 hours and 10 to 20 mg of furosemide intravenously every 6 hours between the mannitol doses; the effectiveness of this regimen has not been demonstrated.

Cerebrospinal Fluid Drainage

If an IVC is used to measure ICP, it can be used to drain CSF. This effectively lowers ICP because of the pressure-volume relationship within the cranium,[37] which can be summarized as follows. Intracranial volume is composed of CSF, brain tissue, and blood. The sum of these volumes determines ICP at any given time. If any of these compartments increases in size (such as brain edema, hyperemia) or if an additional volume is added (such as subdural or epidural hematomas), the ICP will increase if there is not a concomitant, compensatory decrease in one of the other compartments.

Compensatory changes include CSF being displaced through the basal subarachnoid cisterns into the spinal canal through the foramen magnum. CSF also may be absorbed into the venous circulation via arachnoidal villi. This "CSF buffering" allows for the addition of some intracranial volume with little change in ICP. However, after compensation has been exhausted, an additional increase in volume will lead to an increase in ICP. This is the concept of elastance, which is the change in pressure divided by the change in volume. Elastance is the reciprocal of compliance. A low elastance value implies that there is substantial intracranial volume reserve. A high elastance value means that even small changes in volume will cause marked pressure changes (that is, a "tight" brain). Thus, removal of small volumes of CSF at high elastance will lower ICP significantly. Although CSF drainage can be effective in controlling ICP, if intracranial hypertension persists, then ventricular size may decrease to the point that no CSF can be removed.

CSF may be drained in a number of ways. Commercially available systems allow continuous closed drainage with a manometer controlling the ICP level at which CSF is drained. Such systems also allow intermittent drainage.

Barbiturates

In recent years, intravenous barbiturate administration has been shown in some patients to lower high levels of ICP that do not respond to other modalities.[4,24,30,34] Although the mechanism or mechanisms by which barbiturates decrease ICP remain controversial, their efficacy in reducing ICP is not. Approximately 75% of the patients with intracranial hypertension will respond to high-dose intravenous barbiturates with decreases in ICP. The question of the efficacy of barbiturates in reducing morbidity and mortality of severe head injuries has not yet been answered completely. Recently, Eisenberg et al.[8] reported the results of a multicenter, randomized study of the efficacy of using barbiturates in severe head-injured patients. They concluded that high-dose barbiturates are an effective adjunctive therapy in decreasing ICP in selected patients.[8]

Barbiturate therapy should be administered only in an intensive care environment. In my opinion, refractory intracranial hypertension (ICP greater than 25 mmHg despite all attempts to reduce it) is the only criteria for instituting barbiturate therapy. I use barbiturate therapy only if a patient is hemodynamically stable and is not devastated neurologically, that is, has intact brainstem reflexes and at least flexes to painful stimuli.

Most reports have recommended using pentobarbital or less commonly sodium thiopental.[4,23,33]

A specific protocol should be followed. All patients placed in barbiturate coma should have an arterial line inserted for constant recording of arterial pressures. ICP should be monitored continuously. In addition, Swan-Ganz catheters or central venous pressure catheters should be used to assess volume status, cardiac output, and pulmonary status, since barbiturates can have a marked depressive effect on cardiopulmonary function. Such monitoring can detect early changes and help avert deleterious cardiac effects and subsequent further impairment of brain function.

We begin barbiturate therapy with pentobarbital, 10 mg/kg/hour for 4 consecutive hours, followed by a maintenance infusion of 1.5 mg/kg/hour.[21] The first-hour dose is given in four separate intravenous injections, 15 minutes apart. The dose over the next 3 hours is given as a constant rate continuous drip. If these doses produce a systolic arterial pressure less than 90 mmHg, the amount is decreased and inotropic agents are given to maintain mean arterial pressure and cardiac output. One hour after the loading dose (5 hours after starting the treatment), the pentobarbital level is determined. Most patients will have a serum level of 3 to 4.5 mg/dl. Thereafter, serum pentobarbital levels are determined daily.

Serum pentobarbital levels and auditory evoked potentials serve as parameters for guiding barbiturate treatment. Serum levels greater than 5 mg/dl may adversely affect myocardial function and often are associated with deterioration of brainstem-evoked potentials. Since many head-injured patients will have isoelectric electroencephalograms and will lose all clinical signs on examination of brain function, brainstem-evoked potentials may be helpful. Ideally, brainstem auditory evoked responses should be obtained before barbiturate therapy and then used for comparison, but this may not be possible since rapid institution of treatment to lower ICP is essential. If brainstem auditory evoked potentials deteriorate during barbiturate therapy, the pentobarbital dose should be reduced or the drug discontinued.

Any ICP increase in a patient undergoing barbiturate therapy warrants an immediate CT scan after a search for other possible causes such as fluid overload or hypercarbia.

Steroids

The use of steroids in the management of severe head injuries is controversial. There is no proof that steroid therapy decreases morbidity and mortality from severe head injuries. The results of experimental and clinical investigations are contradictory, finding beneficial, or no, or adverse effects of steroid therapy.[2,6,10,13,16,26,33,36,39] Steroids do not reduce intracranial hypertension.[14,33] However, I believe that the effect of steroids may be different for different patient groups.[33] I have seen patients with areas of focal contusion whose neurologic status improved within 24 hours, similar to some patients with primary or metastatic brain tumors.[11,25] Therefore I initiate steroid therapy on all comatose head-injured patients. A loading dose of 1 mg/kg of dexamethasone or 5 mg/kg of methylprednisolene is given in the emergency room. If the CT scan shows a specific focal lesion that could be, or is, producing edema, a maintenance dose is given. The daily maintenance dose is the same as the loading dose but in four equal doses and is continued at this dose for approximately 3 days, then tapered over 3 to 4 days.

MISCELLANEOUS PROBLEMS

Other problems may provoke ICP elevations in brain-injured patients, such as nursing care or use of positive end-expiratory pressure (PEEP).[35] Pulmonary management, including use of PEEP, is addressed in Chapter 7.

Good pulmonary and nursing care is crucial in the management of the severely head-injured patient. Chest physiotherapy and pulmonary toilet include regular percussion, postural drainage, and endotracheal suctioning. These and other nursing activities (such as bathing, catheter care) may cause increased ICP.[27] A variety of techniques and drugs can be used to minimize these ICP increases. We schedule nursing activities to occur separately, that is, not within a single block of time. Chest physiotherapy and suctioning can be performed approximately 20 to 30 minutes after the administration of a mannitol or furosemide dose. Manual hyperventilation with an Ambu bag will decrease ICP and facilitate the performance of these maneuvers. A bolus of thiopental, 1 to 3 mg/kg intravenously given immediately before the treatment, may be helpful. In ventilated patients, transient paralysis with succinyl choline may abort ICP elevations more effectively than barbiturates.[42]

SUMMARY

Elevated ICP plays a major role in the pathophysiology of head injury. Uncontrolled ICP elevations are associated with unacceptable morbidity and mortality in these patients. The best management of elevated ICP requires awareness by everyone who cares for the patient of the importance of ICP and its effect on cerebral perfusion. Skillful intensive care of all patients with severe head injury will help to maintain normal ICP dynamics. When intracranial hypertension occurs, the treatments detailed above can be instituted to return ICP dynamics to normal in many patients. These treatment modalities will be most effective when administered according to a well-organized, balanced protocol that is understood by all members of the intensive care team. Such an approach to the treatment of increased ICP can save lives and favorably alter the outcome of severe head injury.

REFERENCES

1. Bellegarrigue R, Ducker TB: Control of Intracranial Pressure in Severe Head Injury. In Intracranial Pressure, vol. V. Berlin: Springer-Verlag, 1983, pp 567–571.
2. Benson VM, McLaurin RL, Foulkes EC: Traumatic cerebral edema: An experimental model with evaluation of dexamethasone. Arch Neurol 23:179–186, 1970.

3. Bowers SA, Marshall LF: Outcome in 200 consecutive cases of severe head injury treated in San Diego County: A prospective analysis. Neurosurgery 6:237–242, 1980.
4. Bruce DA, Schute L, Bruno LA, et al.: Outcome following severe head injuries in children. J Neurosurg 48:679–688, 1978.
5. Cheek WR, Evans AF, Dennis GC, et al.: Device for extradural monitoring of intracranial pressure. Clinical note. Neurosurgery 5:692–694, 1979.
6. Cooper PR, Moody S, Clark WK, et al.: Dexamethasone and severe head injury. A prospective double-blind study. J Neurosurg 51:307–316, 1979.
7. Cottrell JE, Robustelli A, Post K, et al.: Furosemide- and mannitol-induced changes in intracranial pressure and serum osmolality and electrolytes. Anesthesiology 47:28–30, 1977.
8. Eisenberg HM, Frankowski RF, Contant CF: High dose barbiturate control of elevated intracranial pressure in patients with severe head injury. J Neurosurg 69:15–23, 1988.
9. Esparaza J, Manrique A, Lobato RD, et al.: Simultaneous epidural and intraventricular pressure measurement during the occurrence of supratentorial expanding lesions. In Shulman K, Marmarou A, Miller JD, et al. (eds): Intracranial Pressure, vol 4. Berlin: Springer-Verlag, 1980, pp 377–380.
10. Faupel G, Reulen HJ, Muller D, et al.: Double-blind study on the effects of severe closed head injury. In Pappius HM, Feindel W (eds): Dynamics of Brain Edema. Berlin: Springer-Verlag, 1976, pp 337–343.
11. Galicich JH, French LA: The use of dexamethasone in the treatment of cerebral edema resulting from brain tumors and brain surgery. Am Pract 12:169–174, 1961.
12. Gamache F, Ducker TB: Alterations in neurological function in head-injured patients experiencing major episodes of sepsis. Neurosurgery 10:468–472, 1982.
13. Gobiet W, Bock WJ, Liesegang J, et al.: Treatment of acute cerebral edema with high dose of dexamethasone. In Beks, JW, Bosch DA, Brock M (eds): Intracranial Pressure, vol 3, Berlin: Springer-Verlag, 1976, pp 231–235.
14. Gudeman SK, Miller JD, Becker DP: Failure of high dose steroid therapy to influence intracranial pressure in patients with severe head injury. J Neurosurg 51:301–306, 1979.
15. Jennett B, Teasdale S, et al.: Severe head injuries in three countries. J Neurol Neurosurg Psychiatry 40:291–298, 1977.
16. Kobrine AI, Kempe LG: Studies in head injury. Part II. Effect of dexamethasone traumatic brain swelling. Surg Neurol 1:38–42, 1973.
17. Langfitt TW, Gennarelli TA: Can the outcome from head injury be improved? J Neurosurg 56:19–25, 1982.
18. Levin AB: The use of a fiberoptic intracranial pressure monitor in clinical practice. Neurosurgery 1:266–271, 1977.
19. Lundberg N: Continuous recording and control of ventricular fluid pressure in neurosurgical practice. Acta Psychiatr Neurol Scand 36(Suppl 149):1–193, 1960.
20. Lundberg N, Troupp H, Lorin H: Continuous recording of the ventricular-fluid pressure in patients with severe acute traumatic brain injury. J Neurosurg 22:581–590, 1965.
21. Majerus TC, Saul TG, Ducker TB, Cowley RA: Pharmacokinetics of high dose intravenous pentobarbital therapy. Presented at the 50th Anniversary Meeting of the American Association of Neurological Surgeons, Boston, April 5–9, 1981.
22. Marshall LF, Smith RW, Rauscher LA, Shapiro HM: Mannitol dose requirements in brain-injured patients. J Neurosurg 48:169–172, 1978.
23. Marshall LF, Smith RW, Shapiro HM: The outcome with aggressive treatment in severe head injuires. Part I. J Neurosurg 50:20–25, 1979.
24. Marshall LF, Smith RW, Shapiro HM: The outcome with aggressive treatment in severe head injuries. Part II. J Neurosurg 50:25–30, 1979.
25. Meinig G, Aulich A, Wende S, et al.: The effect of dexamethasone and diuretics on peritumor brain edema: Comparative study of tissue water content and CT. In Pappius HM, Feindel W (eds): Dynamics of Brain Edema. Berlin: Springer-Verlag, 1976, pp 301–305.
26. Miller RD, Butterworth JF, et al.: Further experience in the management of severe head injury. J Neurosurg 54:289–299, 1981.
27. Mitchell PH, Mauss NK, Ofuna S, et al.: Relationship of nurse/patient activity and ICP variation. In Shulman K, Marmarous A, Miller ID, et al. (eds): Intracranial Pressure, vol 4. Berlin: Springer-Verlag, 1980, pp 565–568.
28. Narayan RK, Kishore PRS, Becker DP, et al.: Intracranial pressure: To monitor or not to monitor? Review of our experience with severe head injury. J Neurosurg 56:650–659, 1982.
29. Ostrup RC, Luerssen TG, Marshall LF, et al.: Continuous monitoring of intracranial pressure with a miniaturized fiberoptic device. J Neurosurg 67:206–209, 1987.
30. Rockoff MA, Marshall LF, Shapiro HM: High-dose barbiturate therapy in humans: A clinical review of 60 patients. Ann Neurol 6:194–199, 1979.
31. Rosner MJ, Becker DP: ICP monitoring: Complications and associated factors. Clin Neurosurg 23:494–519, 1976.
32. Saul TG, Ducker TB: Effect of intracranial pressure monitoring and aggressive treatment on mortality in severe head injury. J Neurosurg 56:498–503, 1982.

33.   Saul TG, Ducker TB, Salcman M, et al.: Steroids and severe head injury: A prospective randomized clinical trial. J Neurosurg 54:596–600, 1981.
34.   Shapiro HM: Intracranial hypertension. Therapeutic and anesthetic considerations. Anesthesiology 43:445–471, 1975.
35.   Shapiro JM, Marshall LF: Intracranial pressure responses to PEEP in head-injured patients. J Trauma 18:254–256, 1978.
36.   Sparacio RR, Linn TH, Cook AW: Methylprednisolone sodium succinate in acute cranio-cerebral trauma. Surg Gynecol Obstet 121:513–516, 1965.
37.   Sullivan HG, Miller JD, Becker DP, et al.: The physiological basis of intracranial pressure change with progressive epidural brain compression, an experimental evaluation in cats. J Neurosurg 47:532–550, 1977.
38.   Sundbarg G, Nordstrom CH, Messeter K: A comparison of intraparenchymatous and intraventricular pressure. Recording in clinical practice. J Neurosurg 67:841–845, 1987.
39.   Tornheim PA, McLaurin RL: Effect of dexamethasone on cerebral edema from cranial impact in the cat. J Neurosurg 48:220–227, 1978.
40.   Tornheim PA, McLaurin RL, Sawaya R: Effect of furosemide on experimental traumatic cerebral edema. Neurosurgery 4:48–51, 1979.
41.   Vries JK, Becker DP, Young HF: A subarachnoid screw for monitoring intracranial pressure. Technical note. J Neurosurg 39:416–419, 1973.
42.   White PF, Schlobohm RM, Pitts LH, Lindauer JM: A Randomized study of drugs for preventing increases in intracranial pressure during endotracheal suctioning. Anesthesiology 57:242–244, 1982.
43.   Wilkinson HA: The intracranial pressure monitoring cup catheter. Technical note. Neurosurgery 1:139–141, 1977.
44.   Winn HR, Dacey RG, Jane JA: Intracranial subarachnoid pressure recordings: Experience with 650 patients. Surg Neurol 8:41–47, 1977.
45.   Zierski J: Extradural, ventricular and subdural pressure recording comparative clinical study. In Shulman K, Marmarou A, Miller JD, et al. (eds): Intracranial Pressure, vol 4, Berlin: Springer-Verlag, 1980, pp 371–376.

9

Post-Traumatic Sequelae

BRIAN T. ANDREWS

In the past, many studies have concentrated on the pathophysiology, management, and outcome after severe head injury. Outcome evaluation of severely head-injured patients most often has focused on degrees of major motor deficit or levels of independence, while not evaluating in detail subtle abnormalities of cognition and intellectual function.[10,23] Only recently has increased attention been paid to patients who have sustained mild or moderate head injury.[2,21,36] This group represents the vast majority of head-injured patients, accounting for approximately 400,000 to 600,000 persons each year.[13,36] In addition, there has been increasing recognition that persistent clinical symptoms and subtle neurologic, cognitive, and psychologic deficits may follow all grades of head injury and result in a significant and long-lasting disability, even among those patients having no residual sensorimotor deficits.[2,21,36] Significant psychosocial sequelae of head injury may become a major problem for families, and a therapeutic challenge for the clinician.

This chapter will outline some of the symptoms and sequelae that may persist after head injury, and discuss their management. The incidence and treatment of post-traumatic seizures will be described. In addition, the cognitive, behavioral, and psychosocial impact of head injury will be reviewed, as well as some of the recent methods that have been developed to diagnose and treat these disabilities.

POST-TRAUMATIC SYMPTOMS: THE "POSTCONCUSSION SYNDROME"

Persistent physical complaints may occur in patients who have had trauma, ranging from a minor head injury with brief loss of consciousness to a severe head injury with a significant fixed neurologic deficit. These symptoms are usually grouped under the term "postconcussion syndrome" and include headache, dizziness, nausea and vomiting, and alcohol intolerance.[13,21,26,30,36,38] These are often intertwined with additional complaints, such as anxiety, irritability, changes in personality, and difficulties with concentration and memory, symptoms that will be further detailed in subsequent sections of this chapter.

Persistent headache is a frequent complaint, being present in up to 93% of those with mild to moderate head injury[21,30,36] at 3 months postinjury. The headaches are variable in

110

character and duration but are typically diffuse and may be aggravated by movement, position, anxiety, or stress. They are frequently associated with dizziness, nausea, vomiting, and insomnia.[21,26,30,36,38]

Postconcussion dizziness may initially be described as a pronounced vertigo that is exacerbated by movement or changes in position and is frequently associated with nausea. Typically, this resolves weeks after the injury, but may be followed by intermittent unsteadiness, which may be positional or made worse by movement.[38]

There is some evidence that the persistence and severity of postconcussive symptoms are directly related to the severity of the head injury. Among 145 patients with minor head injury, persistence of postconcussive symptoms occurred more frequently among patients having early complaints of diplopia, anosmia, or post-traumatic amnesia for longer than 15 minutes.[39] Patients with persistent symptoms more often have initial abnormalities of smell, vision, hearing, or an intracranial hematoma than those who recover completely.[26] There is also a direct correlation between the incidence of persistent headaches and the severity of the initial head injury: at 3-month follow-up in one study, they were present in 78% of patients with mild head injury and in 93% of patients with moderately severe initial head injury.[21]

The actual cause of postconcussive symptoms is unknown. Although attention had been paid to the roles of psychologic disturbance,[2] compensation, litigation, and malingering,[26] recent evidence indicates that the cause is structural. About half of patients with postconcussive dizziness have abnormalities on electronystagnogram testing and prolonged latencies on brainstem auditory evoked responses, suggesting structural abnormalities of the brainstem.[38] After even minor head injury, subtle evidence of structural injury to the brain has been recognized in human autopsy specimens, including neuronal loss[36] and microscopic lesions in the pyramidal tracts of the medulla oblongata and pons.[2,21] Recently, magnetic resonance imaging (MRI) has shown a variety of structural abnormalities of the frontal and temporal regions among patients with normal computed tomography (CT) scans after mild and moderate head injuries.[28] It is probable that with mild head injury there may be subarachnoid bleeding, which could lead to meningeal irritation, or subsequent abnormalities of cerebrospinal fluid (CSF) flow and intracranial pressure. In addition, stretching and tearing of vascular or dural attachments of the brain such as occurs during basal skull fracture may provide an origin for painful sequelae. Pain from scalp injury or neuralgia from the supraorbital or occipital nerves may also be a cause of postconcussive headaches.[26]

POST-TRAUMATIC EPILEPSY

Post-traumatic epilepsy occurs in a significant number of patients after head injury. Seizures within the first 7 days after injury have been called "early epilepsy," and are seen in approximately 5% of patients after blunt trauma.[25] Early epilepsy is more common after head injury associated with depressed skull fracture, prolonged post-traumatic amnesia, focal neurologic deficit, and intracranial hematoma. It is also more frequent in young children.[25] Early seizures are common after penetrating brain injuries and are seen in as many as 42% of patients not treated with anticonvulsant therapy[4] and in as many as 10% even when anticonvulsants are used routinely.[41]

Delayed post-traumatic epilepsy, defined as seizures that occur longer than 7 days postinjury, is seen in about 5% of patients after closed head trauma.[8,12,24] Among adults with early epilepsy, approximately 25% will develop persistent seizures. Patients with a depressed skull fracture have a 15% incidence of late seizures, and those with an intracranial hematoma have an incidence of 35%.[12] The combination of prolonged post-traumatic amnesia and depressed skull fracture with a focal brain injury increases the risk of delayed epilepsy to as high as 70%. The greatest predictor of persistent epilepsy, however, is the occurrence of a seizure more than 7 days after injury. In this case the risk of additional seizures is at least 75%.[12] Post-traumatic epilepsy is of the grand mal type 70% of the time, although partial seizures without loss of consciousness occur in 10% and complex partial seizures occur in 20%.[24]

More than half of delayed post-traumatic seizures occur within the first year after injury. Among 481 patients with delayed epilepsy reviewed in one study, 27% had an initial seizure within the first 3 months, and 56% within the first year. There was then a progressive decrease in frequency with each subsequent year. However, the first seizure may occurs years later; in 25% of cases the onset was delayed 4 years or more.[24]

Once delayed epilepsy occurs, patients remain at risk for persistent seizures for years. Temporary remissions even as long as 2 years can be followed by recurrent seizures.[5,24] Therefore it may be unwise to discontinue anticonvulsant therapy in patients who have proved to have delayed post-traumatic epilepsy, even years after remaining seizure-free.

COGNITIVE SEQUELAE AFTER MILD TO MODERATE HEAD INJURY

After mild or moderate head injury, patients initially have significant abnormalities of attention, cognitive processing, and memory.[2,21,26,30,36,37] In a multicenter evaluation of outcome after mild head injury (defined as a history of unconsciousness of less than 20 minutes and an initial Glasgow Coma Score [GCS] of 13 to 15) within 7 days of injury, patients had significant deficits of attention, verbal and visual memory, information processing, and hand-eye coordination. By 1 month postinjury in two of the three centers studied, there was significant recovery in these functions, with little difference between the injured groups and control subjects. In contrast, at one center persistent cognitive deficits were detected.[30] Others have similarly shown recovery of cognitive function on most tests within 4 to 6 weeks after minor head injury,[14] although subjective complaints often persisted up to 3 months after injury.[30] In one study 3 months after mild head injury, 59% of patients complained of a deterioration in memory and 14% had difficulties with activities of daily living due to poor attention and cognitive function. One third of such patients had not returned to work; however, the major predictors of unemployment were not the severity of injury, but rather premorbid characteristics (age, education, and socioeconomic status).[36] On neuropsychologic testing, such patients had diffuse but generally mild deficits, although 31% of the patients had the persistence of a severe cognitive deficit.[2,21] In contrast, in the multicenter study, by 3 months postinjury, the cognitive deficits detected earlier had generally resolved.[30] Thus, it appears that despite persistent subjective complaints of attention, memory deficits, and cognitive problems after minor closed head injury, demonstrable deficits on neuropsychologic testing become mild or resolve completely by 1 to 3 months postinjury.

Among patients with an initially moderate injury (GCS 9 to 12), 90% complain of a memory deficit and 87% had difficulties with activities of daily living due to cognitive disorders at the 3-month follow-up. On neuropsychologic testing, significant deficits were detected in all areas, including abnormalities of memory, spatial and temporal orientation, and information processing.[37,44] Two thirds of such patients who were previously employed were unable to return to work, with later unemployment being related to the severity of the injury (length of coma, abnormalities on CT scan, GCS at the time of discharge).[21]

It is probable that the cause for persistent cognitive sequelae after mild and moderate head injury is related to shear-strain involving the brain at multiple levels, including the gray and white matter junction of the cortex, the midbrain, and lower parts of the brainstem. This results in axonal stretching and disruption and secondary neural degeneration.[2,34] Evidence of structural abnormalities in humans after mild head injury includes electrophysiologic abnormalities; as many as 64% of patients with mild head injury have abnormal brainstem auditory evoked potentials.[21,38] After minor experimental head injuries, diffuse axonal degeneration in the brainstem and in the corpus callosum have been demonstrated, and with moderate injury there is diffuse degeneration of axons in the subcortical white matter.[21] Similar abnormalities are seen in human autopsy specimens after head injury.[35] Recently, MRI of patients with mild and moderate head injuries have shown that 85% have multiple abnormalities involving the frontal and temporal regions, which are not apparent on CT scanning. They have also shown that the neuropsychologic deficits seen after head injury are related to the size and distribution of these lesions and that recovery of these deficits are paralleled by improvement in these MRI abnormalities.[28]

COGNITIVE OUTCOME AFTER SEVERE HEAD INJURY

Numerous studies have documented the profound cognitive sequelae that follow severe head injury.[11,26,29,44] Awake patients with severe head injuries had globally impaired memory and intellectual functions soon after injury, whether or not surgery became necessary. Patients with lesions localized to the dominant hemisphere had greater impairment in verbal IQ, and those with lesions of the nondominant hemisphere had greater impairment of performance IQ.[44] By 1 year after injury, patients had improved, but still had significant cognitive deficits, specifically of language and memory. Cognitive outcome was predicted by the patient's age, initial GCS, and the time after injury until the patient could follow simple two-step commands.[44] Some severely head-injured patients had persistent deficits of memory, language, and social adjustment, which generally corresponded to their overall outcome.[29] Although those patients having a good overall outcome had mild cognitive deficits, those having a moderately disabled outcome had significant deficits, primarily of performance IQ and memory; patients with severe disability had profound global intellectual impairment and were the only group to have persistent anomia and dysphasia. Although repetition led to progressive gains in memory among those patients having a good outcome, less improvement occurred among those with a moderately severe deficit, and those patients with severe disability had little improvement. Interestingly, initial abnormalities of the oculocephalic reflexes were predictive of prolonged cognitive and neuropsychologic impairment.[27,29]

Like patients with lesser degrees of head injury, the mechanism for initial and persisting cognitive deficits among the severely head injured is related to diffuse and focal structural damage to the brain. In addition to the damage caused by shear-strain injuries,[2,21,34] there may be diffuse brain injury at the cellular level due to hypotension or hypoxia,[32] increased intracranial pressure,[33] and by focal injuries such as contusions,[7] intracranial hematomas,[43] and brainstem compression due to transtentorial herniation.[1] The location of focal brain injuries can determine the specific types of resulting cognitive deficits. Patients with traumatic lesions involving the left temporal lobe or with diffuse or bilateral lesions have more severe initial deficits of verbal memory than those with focal lesions in other areas. However, patients with left temporal lesions also show a greater degree of recovery in verbal memory function than patients with diffuse injury; recovery may involve increased participation of the nondominant hemisphere.[11] Recent evidence suggests that there is right hemispheric cerebral dominance in spatial attention bilaterally,[46] so that injury to the right hemisphere may lead to bilateral cognitive deficits regarding spatial relationships and performance tasks.

Abnormalities on CT scanning are predictive of neuropsychologic impairment and recovery after severe head injury. Memory and learning ability were best among patients who had evidence of only diffuse swelling on their initial CT scans. Patients with evidence of diffuse axonal injury (midline hemorrhages and small hemorrhages at the gray-white junction) had greater initial impairment, but had more improvement than the other groups. Patients with unilateral intracerebral hemorrhages and contusions on the initial CT scan showed the greatest disability and least improvement of recall and learning.[45] Recently, MRI scanning has demonstrated focal and diffuse white matter and brainstem abnormalities among severely head-injured patients, which are not apparent on CT scanning.[27,47] It is probable that lesions as demonstrated by MRI will correlate with specific cognitive deficits among severely head-injured patients, such as has already been the case among patients with mild and moderately severe head injuries.[28]

PSYCHOSOCIAL IMPACT OF HEAD INJURY

There is an important and often clinically predominant psychosocial and behavioral impact of head trauma. Patients often have depression, withdrawal, and anxiety.[2,9,30,36] Affective symptoms can include increased aggressiveness and hostility[29] and can be as severe as full-blown mania[42] or psychosis.[29] Among patients with mild head injury who had previously been employed, 34% remained unemployed 3 months after injury despite minimal residual cognitive deficits. Emotional stress caused by residual somatic symptoms, such as head-ache, was an important factor relating to persistent disability;[36] 32% of mildly head-injured patients had abnormalities on the Minnesota Multiphasic Personality Inventory. Behavioral dysfunction was only partially related to the severity of cognitive deficits; in some patients there were severe behavioral sequelae but little cognitive impairment.[2] Affective symptoms (anxiety, depression, and sleep disturbance) among patients with mild head injury intensified over the first month, before showing an improvement by 3 months postinjury.[30] Several investigators have noted that emotional distress and affective disorders are more prevalent among patients with greater somatic complaints and cognitive deficits.[2,9,27,30,36]

Patients recovering from more severe degrees of head trauma may also have anxiety and depression, but their behavior is more influenced by residual cognitive disturbance. They often fail to appreciate the severity of their cognitive deficit. Increased irritability, indifference, confabulations, delusions, and aggressiveness have been described.[27] There is also a marked tendency for such patients to become socially isolated. Rarely, such patients may have frankly psychotic symptoms requiring hospitalization.[29] Interviews with the relatives of severely head-injured patients indicate that the behavioral sequelae of the head injury are often more difficult to cope with than the residual cognitive or focal neurologic deficits, and that these difficulties do not diminish by 1 year after injury.[27] These poorly controlled behavioral abnormalities frequently complicate long-term management and rehabilitation of patients after severe head injury.

TREATMENT OF POST-TRAUMATIC SYMPTOMS

Treatment of headache, nausea and vomiting, dizziness, unsteadiness, and insomnia related to the postconcussive syndrome is primarily symptomatic. For the headache, we initially use acetaminophen with 30 mg codeine. This is usually begun during hospitalization or after the initial evaluation and continued for approximately 1 to 2 weeks. Alternative weak narcotic analgesics such as propoxyphene (Darvon) 32 to 65 mg every 3 to 6 hours, may also be used; although this drug is often less effective than codeine, its addictive potential is also less.[19] We then try to begin a nonopiate compound, such as acetaminophen alone 650 mg every 4 to 6 hours, ibuprofen 400 to 800 mg three times a day or another nonsteroidal anti-inflammatory analgesic. Additional medications that we have found to be useful for improving pain tolerance include L-tryptophan 500 to 1000 mg four times daily, which may decrease opiate tolerance.

Nausea and vomiting should be treated only after being sure that these symptoms are not due to increased intracranial pressure, caused by a delayed complication of head injury such as a delayed intracerebral hemorrhage or an enlarging chronic subdural hematoma. This is particularly true if these symptoms are associated with increasing headache or their onset is delayed after injury. Several medications may be effective. Antihistamines such as diphenhydramine (Benadryl) 25 to 50 mg four times daily suppress nausea centrally and may prove to be adequate. The phenothiazine prochlorperazine (Compazine) 25 mg suppository twice daily is a potent centrally acting antiemetic but is known to lower the seizure threshold and therefore may be contraindicated in patients at risk for post-traumatic seizures. As well, the phenothiazines can increase mental dullness, which may be particularly disturbing in the head-injured patient with neuropsychologic sequelae.

Post-traumatic dizziness, if it appears to be vertiginous in nature, may respond to vestibular suppressants. We have used the antihistamine meclizine (Antivert) 25 to 50 mg four times daily as needed, with good results; diphenhydramine 25 to 50 mg four times daily may also be used. Known side effects of this class of compounds are somnolence and mental dullness.

Sleep disturbance after head injury may be treated with a variety of agents. We initially prescribe diphenhydramine 25 to 50 mg, which has sedation as a side effect. The benzodiazepine compound flurazepam (Dalmane) 15 to 30 mg is an effective hypnotic but has significant side effects, including excessive morning drowsiness, vertigo, and ataxia,[20] which may make it inappropriate for head-injured patients who are unsteady or have focal neurologic deficits. Recently, the shorter acting benzodiazepines temazepam (Restoril) 15 to 30 mg and triazolam (Halcion) 0.125 to 0.25 mg have been used as night-time sedatives. These drugs have less residual morning drowsiness, but otherwise have similar side effects to other benzodiazepines. As well, it is generally recommended that the benzodiazepines not be used for longer than approximately 3 weeks,[20] although they may be useful for longer periods in some patients.

TREATMENT OF POST-TRAUMATIC SEIZURES

We begin prophylactic treatment of post-traumatic seizures at the time of admission for patients with particular risk for the development of post-traumatic seizures[8] (Table 9–1). This includes patients with subdural or intraparenchymal hematomas, significant parenchymal contusions, depressed skull fractures,[12] or any penetrating dural injury with cortical laceration.[4,41] Others have recommended initial anticonvulsant therapy for any patient with a severe head injury regardless of the degree of obvious cortical injury.[12] In addition, any head-injured patient in whom a seizure has occurred, except an infant with an early seizure, warrants anticonvulsant therapy. The most frequently used drug for seizure prophylaxis and treatment is phenytoin (Dilantin), which is given first as a loading dosage of 15 mg/kg intravenously. Care must be taken not to infuse intravenous phenytoin more rapidly than 50 mg/minute, because faster administration can lead to myocardial suppression and resulting systemic hypotension; an even slower rate should be used for elderly patients.[49] An initial daily oral or intravenous dosage of 3 to 4 mg/kg is then used, and serum levels are checked to achieve an optimal therapeutic level of 10 to 20 μg/ml. Side effects of phenytoin include nystagmus, ataxia, behavioral changes, hirsutism, coarsening of facial features, gingival hyperplasia, gastrointestinal symptoms, and rash.[8,49] Alternative anticonvulsants include phenobarbitol and carbamazepine, both of which are effective for generalized seizures.[31] These drugs can also cause central nervous system depression and therefore may not be well tolerated by head-injured patients.

Anticonvulsant prophylaxis should be maintained in patients who have a 15% or greater risk of persistent seizures.[39] This would include patients with the occurrence of early or delayed post-traumatic seizures, depressed skull fractures, subdural or intraparenchymal hematomas, and penetrating injury with dural and cortical lacerations.[8] The duration of therapy is somewhat controversial. We maintain patients with minimal cortical injury and those with pure subdural hematomas, but no history of post-traumatic seizures, on prophylaxis for a period of 9 to 12 months. For patients who have had a delayed post-traumatic seizure, and those at high risk for persistent seizures, such as patients with penetrating cortical trauma, gunshot wounds, and significant cortical injury, I recommend maintenance on anticonvulsant therapy indefinitely. Others have suggested that discontinuation of anticonvulsant drugs may be considered among patients in these higher risk groups if they have had no seizures for 1 to 2 years and have no paroxysmal abnormalities on electroencephalogram.[12]

A major concern among patients having a good recovery after head injury is that of being allowed to continue to drive. All patients in whom therapy is discontinued should be advised to not drive for a period of 6 to 12 months.[12,22] It should be realized that even a remission of seizures off of therapy for up to a year may not completely rule out the possibility of a later recurrence.[24] It has been recommended that patients with a sustained

Table 9–1 Risk Factors for Delayed Post-Traumatic Epilepsy

1. Subdural or intraparenchymal hematomas
2. Parenchymal contusions
3. Depressed skull fractures
4. Penetrating dural injury with cortical lacerations

high risk of seizures, including those with penetrating cortical injury,[4] gunshot wounds,[41] and previous seizures while on anticonvulsant therapy give up driving indefinitely.[22]

COGNITIVE AND PSYCHOSOCIAL REHABILITATION

One of the major challenges in the rehabilitation of head-injured patients is to improve neuropsychologic deficits. Recent effort has been focused on rehabilitation programs for patients with minor head injury. Four critical elements of this process include: (1) reassuring the patient that their deficits will improve; (2) education regarding the recovery process and practical techniques of stress management and relaxation; (3) support in cognitive and psychosocial tasks; and (4) regular monitoring of cognitive recovery. This is performed as an outpatient, in conjunction with treatment of postconcussion symptoms and job reintegration. Patients who have an improved understanding of their injury are better able to cope during the recovery process.[17]

Another area of current interest is reintegration of brain-injured children and adolescents into the educational system. Moderately and severely injured patients are generally unable to return to their previous school setting successfully because of significant cognitive and behavioral deficits. With the enacting of the Federal Education for all Handicapped Children's Act of 1975, attention has been paid to developing specialized academic and adaptive-behavioral strategies and vocational-rehabilitation counseling within the school system. Similar efforts have been made regarding postsecondary or vocational education for head-injured adults.[40] Application of one intensive outpatient program emphasizing cognitive, behavioral, and vocational rehabilitation resulted in successful employability or productivity of 84% of previously unemployable head-injured adults.[3]

Attempts have been made at specific rehabilitation of more profound cognitive deficits among the severely head injured, such as attention and memory. Positive reinforcement (reward) to reinforce attention-to-task can result in significant improvement in attentive behavior.[48] Electronic and computerized training methods also have been used to improve deficits of focusing and sustaining attention and have resulted in improvement in psychometric testing and functional skills.[16] The rehabilitation of memory deficits has included the use of mnemonics such as visual imagery, verbal and procedural strategies for storing and retrieving information. These have met with little or mixed success among the severely head injured because of the mental effort required for their use; however, they may benefit moderately impaired patients.[15] Other methods have included the use of external aids, such as notebooks, lists, calculators, computers, cueing devices such as alarm clocks, and structured environments that reduce memory load. However, there has been little systematic evaluation of their efficacy outside of the acute rehabilitation setting.[18]

Finally, social reintegration of head-injured patients requires an evaluation of the family and community setting into which the head-injured patient is placed after inpatient rehabilitation is completed. Difficulties that the family may face in dealing with the behavioral changes and dependency of the patient must be identified, and guidance given to the patient and family to aid the patient in reestablishing a realistic place within the family and community.[6]

It is clear that rehabilitation efforts aimed at the specific cognitive deficits and psychosocial problems seen in head injury are only now being explored. It is crucial that such efforts be directed to patients in all categories of injury severity, including the vast majority with mild but potentially debilitating deficits. Rehabilitation must be extended to the outpatient setting, with a major attempt being to reintegrate the patient into the community. We anticipate improving cognitive recovery and psychosocial and vocational capabilities as these methods become more refined and available.

REFERENCES

1. Andrews BT, Pitts LH, Lovely MP, Bartkowski H: Is CT scanning necessary in patients with tentorial herniation: Results of immediate surgical exploration without CT scanning in 100 patients. Neurosurgery 19: 408–413, 1986.
2. Barth JT, Macciocchi SN, Giordani B, et al.: Neuropsychological sequelae of minor head injury. Neurosurgery 13:529–533, 1983.
3. Ben-Yishay Y, Silver SM, Piasetsky E, Rattok J: Relationship between employability and vocational outcome after intensive holistic cognitive rehabilitation. J Head Trauma Rehabil 2:35–48, 1987.
4. Caveness WF, Liss HR: Incidence of post-traumatic epilepsy. Epilepsia 2:123–129, 1961.
5. Caveness WF: Onset and cessation of fits following craniocerebral trauma. J Neurosurg 20:570–583, 1963
6. Condeluci A, Gretz-Lasky S: Social role valorization: A model for community reentry. J Head Trauma Rehabil 2:49–56, 1987.
7. Cooper PR: Post-traumatic intercranial mass lesions. In Cooper PR (ed): Head Injury. Baltimore: Williams & Wilkins, 1987, pp 238–284.
8. Deutschmann CS, Haines SJ: Anticonvulsant prophylaxis in neurological surgery. Neurosurgery 17:510–517, 1985
9. Dikmen S, Reitan R: Emotional sequelae of head injury. Ann Neurol 2:492–494, 1977.
10. Eisenberg HM: Outcome after head injury: General considerations and neurobehavioral recovery. Part 1: General considerations. In Becker DP, Povlishock JT (eds): Central Nervous System Trauma Status Report. Bethesda, MD: National Institutes of Health, 1985, pp 271–280.
11. Eisenberg HM, Levin HS, Papanicolaou AC: Recovery of memory after head injury. In Dacey RG, Winn HR, Rimel RW, Jane JA (ed): Trauma of the Central Nervous System. New York: Raven Press, 1985 pp 35–47
12. Epstein FM, Ward JD, Becker DP: Medical complications of head injury. In Cooper PR (ed): Head Trauma. Baltimore: Williams & Wilkins, 1987 pp 390–421
13. Feldman WS: Post-concussive syndrome: What a Headache. Leg Aspects Med Pract. 16:4–6, July, 1986.
14. Gentilini M, Nichelli P, Schoenhuber R, et al.: Neuropsychological evaluation of mild head injury. J Neurol Neurosurg Psychiatry 48:137–140, 1985.
15. Gilsky EL, Schacter DL: Remediation of organic memory disorders: Current status and future prospects. J Head Trauma Rehabil 1:54–63, 1986.
16. Grafman J: Memory assessment and remediation in brain-injured patients. In Edelstein B, Couture EC (eds): Behavior Assessment and Treatment of the Traumatically Brain Damaged. New York: Plenum Press, 1983.
17. Gronwall D: Rehabilitation programs for patients with mild head injury: Components, problems and evaluation. J Head Trauma Rehabil 1:53–62, 1986
18. Harris J: Methods of improving memory. In Wilson BA, Moffat N (eds): Clinical Management of Memory Problems. Rockville, MD: Aspen Publishers, 1984.
19. Harvey SC: Hypnotics and sedatives. In Goodman LS, Gilman A (ed): The Pharmacologic Basis of Therapeutics. New York: Macmillan, 1975, pp 124–136.
20. Jaffe JH, Martin WR: Narcotic analgesics and antagonists. In Goodman LS, Gilman A (ed): The Pharmacologic Basis of Therapeutics. New York: Macmillan, 1975, pp 245–283.
21. Jane JA, Rimel RW, Alves WM, et al.: Minor and moderate head injury: Model systems. In Dacey RG, Winn HR, Rimel RW, Jane JA (ed): Trauma of the Central Nervous System. New York: Raven Press, 1985 pp 27–33.
22. Jennett B: Anticonvulsant drugs and advice about driving after head injury and intracranial surgery. Br J Med 286:627–628, 1983
23. Jennett B, Snoek J, Bond MR, Brooks N: Disability after severe head injury: Observations on the use of the Glasgow Outcome Scale. J Neurol Neurosurg Psychiatry 44:285–293, 1981
24. Jennett B, Teasdale G: Neurophysical sequelae. In Jennett B, Teasdale G: Management of Head Injuries. Philadelphia: FA Davis, 1981 pp 271–288.
25. Jennett B, Teasdale G: Management of head injuries in the acute stage. In Jennett B, Teasdale G: Management of Head Injuries. Philadelphia: FA Davis, 1981 pp 211–252.
26. Jennett B, Teasdale G: Recovery after head injury. In Jennett B, Teasdale G: Management of Head Injuries. Philadelphia: FA Davis, 1981 pp 253–269.
27. Levin HS: Neurobehavioral sequelae of head injury. In Cooper PR (ed): Head Trauma. Baltimore: Williams & Wilkins, 1987 pp 442–463.

28. Levin HS, Amparo E, Eisenberg HM, et al.: Magnetic resonance imaging and computerized tomography in relation to the neurobehavioral sequelae of mild and moderate head injuries. J Neurosurg 66:706–713, 1987.
29. Levin HS, Grossman RG, Rose JE, Teasdale G: Long-term neuropsychological outcome of closed head injury. J Neurosurg 50:412–422, 1979
30. Levin HS, Mattis S, Ruff RM, et al.: Neurobehavioral outcome following minor head injury. J Neurosurg 66: 234–243, 1987.
31. Mattson RH, Cramer JA, Collins JF, et al.: Comparison of cabamazepine, phenobarbitol, phenytoin and primidone in partial and secondarily generalized tonic-clonic seizures. N Engl J Med 313:145–151, 1985.
32. Miller JD, Sweet RC, Narayan R, Becker DP: Early insults to the injured brain. JAMA 240:439–442, 1978.
33. Narayan RK, Kishore PR, Becker DP, et al.: Intracranial pressure: To monitor or not to monitor? A review of our experience with severe head injury. J Neurosurg 56:650–659, 1982.
34. Ommaya AK, Gennarelli TA: Cerebral concussion and traumatic unconsciousness: Correlation of experimental and clinical observations on blunt head injuries. Brain 97:633–654, 1974.
35. Oppenheimer DR: Microscopic lesions in the brain following head injury. J Neurol Neurosurg Psychiatry 31: 229–306, 1968.
36. Rimel RW, Giordani B, Barth JT, et al.: Disability caused by minor head injury. Neurosurgery 9:221–228, 1981.
37. Rimel RW, Giordani B, Barth JT, Jane JA: Moderate head injury: Completing the clinical spectrum of brain trauma. Neurosurgery 11:344–351, 1982.
38. Rowe MJ, Carlson C: Brainstem auditory evoked potentials in postconcussion dizziness. Arch Neurol 37: 679–683, 1980.
39. Rutherford WH, Merrett JD, McDonald JR: Sequelae of concussion caused by minor head injury. Lancet 1:1–4, 1977.
40. Savage RC: Educational issues for the head-injured adolescent and young adult. J Head Trauma Rehabil 2:1–10, 1987.
41. Sherman WD, Apuzzo MLJ, Heiden JS: Gunshot wounds to the brain—a civilian experience. West J Med 123:99–105. 1980.
42. Starkstein SE, Pearlson GD, Boston J, Robinson RG: Mania after brain injury: A controlled study of causative factors. Arch Neurol 44:1069–1073, 1987.
43. Stone JL, Rifai MHS, Sugar O, et al.: Subdural hematomas 1: Acute subdural hematomas: Progress in definition, clinical pathology and therapy. Surg Neurol 19:216–231, 1983.
44. Tabaddor K, Mattis S, Zazula T: Cognitive recovery after moderate and severe head injury. In Dacey RG, Winn HR, Rimel RW, Jane JA (ed): Trauma of the Central Nervous System. New York: Raven Press, 1985 pp 49–63
45. Uzzell BP, Dolinskas CA, Wiser RF, Langfitt TW: Influence of lesions detected by computerized tomography on outcome and neuropsychological recovery after severe head injury. Neurosurgery 20:396–402, 1987.
46. Weintraub S, Mesilam MM: Right cerebral dominance in spatial attention: Further evidence based on ipsilateral neglect. Arch Neurol 44:621–625, 1987.
47. Wilberger JE, Deeb Z, Rothfus W: Magnetic resonance imaging in cases of severe head injury. Neurosurgery 20:571–576, 1987.
48. Wood RL: Rehabilitation of patients with disorders of attention. J Head Trauma Rehabil 1:43–53, 1986.
49. Woodbury DM, Fingl E: Drugs effective in the therapy of epilepsies. In Goodman LS, Gilman A (eds): The Pharmacologic Basis of Therapeutics. New York: Macmillan, 1975, pp 201–226.

10

Prediction and Assessment of Outcome Following Closed Head Injury

DENNIS G. VOLLMER AND RALPH G. DACEY

The outcome after closed head injury is the end result of a complex series of interactions begun at the moment of impact (Fig. 10–1). Although the biomechanical forces applied at impact are major determinants of the degree of brain damage and consequently the ultimate functional state of the individual, many other factors play a role in outcome determination.

Preinjury factors such as age, prior psychosocial status, or preexisting physical impairments can significantly affect the probability of survival and can also influence the eventual functional state. Similarly, a number of processes occurring postinjury (such as hypoxia, intracranial hypertension, or infection) can result in secondary brain injuries and alter the outcome. There is also substantial evidence for plasticity within the traumatized nervous system; these reparative processes can affect functional recovery. In addition, extracranial injuries may interact with neurologic deficits, further changing outcome.

The multiple factors and events involved in the pathophysiology of head injury make accurate outcome prediction in individual patients difficult. However, it is desirable to predict outcome after head injury for a number of reasons. First, the patient's family and other physicians caring for the patient need to know the patient's neurologic prognosis so that they can make intelligent decisions regarding medical care options. For example, a complex ankle fracture might be managed without surgery in a patient who is apneic and flaccid after sustaining a severe diffuse axonal injury. Second, a growing number of professionals and laymen are coming to believe that expensive societal resources should not be spent to provide terminal care for severely head-injured patients in whom it is possible to predict accurately that they are destined to die or survive in a persistent vegetative state.[42,46]

Third, as a part of efforts to develop more effective treatment for severe head injury, a number of investigators have developed methods of stratifying patients according to injury severity. The Glasgow Coma Scale (GCS) is the most widely used of these methods. By collecting data on outcome in many patients with consistently defined injuries of known

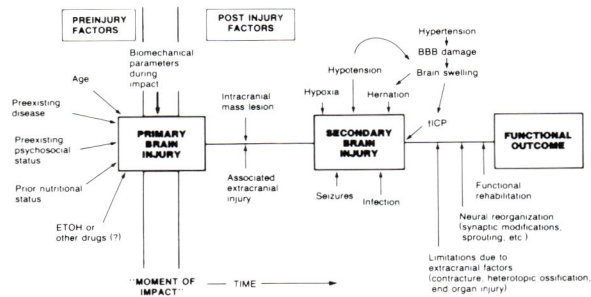

Figure 10–1. Schematic representation of the factors and events that influence outcome after head injury. ETOH: alcohol; BBB: blood-brain barrier.

severity, it has been possible to predict (albeit imperfectly) outcome and to compare outcomes in large groups of patients treated by different methods.

Outcome prediction therefore is useful in the care of head-injured patients for management decisions, triage, and research purposes.

To become more skilled at making correct prognoses, the clinician must be familiar with outcome assessment. In doing so, he begins to understand head injury in terms of eventual functional disabilities. Furthermore, as one examines patients serially over time, the course of recovery is better appreciated. Careful assessment of outcome allows the clinician to evaluate and compare treatment results better, and to recognize factors and events that may have significance in prognostication.

An understanding of functional deficits aids in planning rehabilitation and in counseling patients and families. Understanding the course of recovery allows rehabilitation or other therapy to be maintained as long as they are of benefit or to be discontinued when they are of no further use. Carefully determining patient outcome helps to define the extent of the public health problem, aiding health care planners and government agencies. Finally, by accurately recognizing deficits in individual patients, the physician can assist the patient in obtaining various benefits or social services to which he may be entitled.

In this chapter we will discuss these two aspects of head injury management: outcome assessment and the prediction of outcome, that is, prognosis. We will first consider the nature of functional deficits produced by head injury and how they may be categorized. We will then review means of assessing outcome after head trauma and discuss the time course of recovery. Lastly, we will deal with the problem of prognosis in head injury and the means by which outcome can be predicted. In addressing this latter subject, we will review various factors that have significance for the determination of prognosis, and we will describe methods currently used to predict outcome in individual patients.

FUNCTIONAL DEFICITS FOLLOWING HEAD INJURY

The degree of functional impairment in survivors of closed head injury is, in large part, proportional to injury severity, that is, to the mechanical forces applied to the brain. As already noted, however, this relatively straightforward relationship may be influenced by a number of other factors. The premorbid level of function may influence the final functional level achieved, particularly in mild or moderate degrees of head injury.[13,57,64,76] For example, patients with evidence of premorbid emotional instability appear to be at greater risk for psychiatric consequences after injury.[57] Furthermore, patients with higher levels of education, higher income, or professional occupations are more likely to return to work, at least after mild head injury, and will thus be judged to have had a better outcome.[76]

Secondary brain injuries are events occurring after brain impact, which may alter outcome. They are often generalized insults that diffusely affect the entire brain to some degree, such as hypoxia, hypotension, anemia, increased intracranial pressure (ICP) and metabolic derangements. These secondary insults are not rare. Of 225 severely injured patients studied at admission, 37% were found to be hypoxic, 16% were hypertensive, and 10% were anemic.[58] Hypoxia and hypotension were associated with significantly higher mortality. In this same series, increased ICP was found in 53% of patients monitored with a clear relationship of increasing mortality with ICP elevated above normal. Similar findings have been reported from a number of other series as well.[25,51,61,62] The degree to which such events influence functional status in survivors, however, has been difficult to study and is presently a matter of conjecture.

The types of deficit produced by head injury may be loosely categorized into three main groups: Neurophysical (neurologic); mental (psychologic); and physical (non-neurologic) (Table 10–1). Neurophysical deficits include hemiparesis, cranial nerve injuries, visual field abnormalities, post-traumatic epilepsy, aphasia, and other relatively focal abnormalities. Most deficits of this sort are identifiable with a standard history and physical examination. Neuropsychologic or mental deficits refer to abnormalities of memory, attention, reaction time, and rate of information processing. Psychologic disturbances, changes in personality, and other emotional sequelae, may also be included in this category. Often the deficits within this group are less apparent or underestimated on routine history, physical and neurologic examination. Careful neuropsychologic testing is usually required for full characterization of these deficits. Physical, non-neurological deficits may result from head injury, including contractures or heterotopic ossification, which can produce significant functional problems even in the absence of major ongoing neurologic problems.

Deficits within these three categories may act alone or together to produce various

Table 10–1   A Categorization of Deficits After Head Injury

Neurophysical
  Cortical motor or sensory deficit
  Cranial nerve injury
  Post-traumatic epilepsy
  Post-traumatic movement disorder
  Spasticity
Neuropsychologic
  Memory deficit
  Personality disorder
  Attention and concentration disorder
  Slowed reaction time
  Slowed rate of information processing
Physical, non-neurologic
  Contracture
  Heterotopic ossification
  Other musculoskeletal injury
  Peripheral nerve injury

functional disabilities. It is useful to distinguish between the concepts of deficit and disability: while a deficit may be fixed and permanent, such as a right hemiparesis, the patient may overcome the related disability, for example, by learning to write using the left hand. Disability need not be grossly apparent; a patient who appears normal to a cursory neurologic examination may have a major degree of disability related to neuropsychologic impairments.

Although clinicians treating head-injured patients often focus on neurologic deficits, such as hemiparesis, post-traumatic epilepsy, or cranial nerve palsy, it has been repeatedly shown that patients tend to overcome physical handicaps more readily than mental ones.[14,45,60,90] Consequently, mental sequelae emerge as being more important in determining outcome. Jennett et al.[45] found in a study of 150 severely head-injured patients that neuropsychologic and thinking disorders were the most significant contributors to disability in more than 70% of patients in all outcome groups. Neuropsychologic evaluations of mildly or moderately head-injured patients (GCS 9 to 15) also have demonstrated abnormalities in the majority.[70,76,77] Conversely, neurologic deficits or physical non-neurologic deficits become much less frequent as the severity of head trauma decreases. In one series of 424 minor head injuries, only 2% had neurologic abnormalities.[76]

NEUROPATHOLOGIC CORRELATES OF FUNCTIONAL DEFICIT

In light of our current understanding of head injury neuropathology, it is not surprising that neuropsychologic sequelae predominate. Since Lindenberg et al.[56] and Strich[87,88] called attention to axonal lesions following severe brain trauma, there has been greater awareness of this dimension of brain injury. Adams et al.[1] have further defined the structural abnormalities in white matter after head injury and have clarified their sites of predilection. Similar axonal lesions have also been demonstrated in various primate models of severe[1,28] and minor[41] head injury, a head injury model in cats,[73] and in human head injury.[67,69]

These axonal injuries may not be the result of shearing at the moment of impact, as first suggested by Strich.[88] Povlishock et al.[73] have closely followed the axonal injury after experimental head trauma and noted that the classically described retraction balls developed in a progressive and delayed fashion after impact. Although shearing may have occurred at time of trauma and their myelin stains may not demonstrate the retraction balls immediately, these results raise the theoretical possibility that such axonal events may be preventable or treatable after injury.

These studies emphasize the importance of diffuse white matter injury in the neuropathology of traumatic brain injury and provide a structural basis for the clinical observation of neuropsychologic disturbance after injuries of varying severity. The diffuse nature of these structural and functional aspects underscores the relative insensitivity of assessment methods directed primarily at detecting focal problems, such as computed tomography (CT) scan and neurologic examinations. It is clear that head injury outcome assessment must also be focused on determining loss of more diffusely represented functions.

The neuropathologic correlates for focal neurologic deficit in head injury are primarily cortical contusion, intracranial hemorrhage, and focal injury secondary to increased ICP.[1] These focal injuries, contusions in particular, occur predominantly in the orbital surfaces of the frontal lobe, frontal poles, temporal poles, and inferolateral temporal lobes.[1,2] Other areas may be involved with lesser frequency, particularly under sites of skull fracture. Many of these areas represent relatively "silent" cortex, which accounts for the paucity of focal neurologic findings in many patients with contusions. Although some correlation between focal lesions and subsequent neurologic sequelae has been shown,[95] it is difficult to separate deficits due to focal insult from those due to superimposed diffuse injury.

Hypoxic or ischemic brain damage is common in patients who die after head injury.[31,32] It is largely due to intracranial hypertension with compromise of cerebral perfusion, either focally as with posterior cerebral artery occlusion with tentorial herniation, or in a "watershed" or boundary zone at the margins of territories of the major cerebral arteries. Diffuse hypoxic damage can be found. All of these insults would contribute to the diffuse nature of the hypoxic-ischemic insult.

METHODS OF OUTCOME ASSESSMENT IN HEAD INJURY

Head injury outcome may be assessed in various ways, depending on the purposes of the examiner. The most certain assessment is that of death versus survival, although one must distinguish death due to the head injury from that due to other causes. The study of mortality, though useful, grossly underestimates the overall problem. Head-injured patients are generally young and if they survive the immediate effects of the trauma, are likely to live a near normal life span. Many of these patients survive with considerable deficits and disabilities. The importance of outcome assessment in survivors is obvious.

Outcome in patients surviving head injury may be characterized by specific deficits (neurologic, mental or physical), assessed in terms of functional disabilities (alterations in activities of daily living) or determined by evaluating the patient's subjective symptoms and their severity. The patient's family also should be consulted for their assessment of functional status and quality of life,[18] since the patient may not appreciate or may minimize his problems.

Neuropsychologic tests are probably the most sensitive means of documenting post-traumatic mental sequelae. A discussion of the many testing modalities is beyond the scope of this chapter. The reader is directed to a review by Boll[12] as well as texts on the subject by Levin et al.[52] and Hartlage et al.[34] Some of the more common neuropsychologic tests are listed in Table 10–2.

These tests often require a long time to administer; a complete battery of tests may take as long as 6 hours. Also, the patient must be attentive; this limits the evaluation to patients with the least deficits. The tests require experienced personnel to administer them and to interpret the results,[63] and so can be expensive. However, such testing can document abnormalities that are relatively inapparent by other clinical evaluation. These tests are repeatable and allow follow-up of recovery. By giving a more precise characterization of specific deficits, they also enable rehabilitative efforts to be more specifically directed. Simpler orientation tests also are available[55] but necessarily provide less complete data.

Outcome scales also have been proposed for the quantitation of head injury outcome.[39,43,64,75,78,86] Ideally, the scales standardize outcome information and allow comparisons between individual patients and between different series of patients. To be useful, however, such scales must be reliable, with minimal inter- and intraobserver variability. They must use information that is readily available, and they must make use of unambiguous definitions for assignment of categories. They should be relatively linear without a signifi-

**Table 10–2   Neuropsychologic Tests Commonly Used
in Head Injury Outcome Assessment**

I.   General neuropsychological batteries
    A. Halstead-Reitan Neuropsychological Battery[34]
    B. Luria-Nebraska Neuropsychological Battery (LNNB)[63]
II. Specific neuropsychological tests

Modality Assessed*	Appropriate Tests
1. Resolution of post-traumatic amnesia and retrograde amnesia	Galveston Orientation and Amnesia Test (GOAT)[55]
2. Memory and learning	Benton Visual Retention Test
	Rey Auditory Verbal Learning Test
	Rey-Osterreith Complex Design Test—Recall Mode
	Tactual Performance Test—Memory and Localization
	WAIS-R[†] Digit Span
	Wechsler Memory Scale
3. Language ability	Aphasia Screening Tests
	WAIS-R
	Information Subtest
	Comprehension Subtest
	Similarities Subtest
	Vocabulary Subtest
	Speech Sounds Perception Test
4. Attention and Concentration	Paced Auditory Serial Addition Test (PASAT)[33]
	WAIS-R
	Arithmetic Subtest
	Digit Symbol Subtest
	Trail Making (Parts A & B)[‡]
	Seashore Rhythm[‡]
	Minnesota Multiphasic Personality Inventory (MMPI)
5. Motor skill	Grooved Pegboard Test
	Finger Tapping[‡]
	Grip Strength[‡]
6. Visuospatial and constructional performance	WAIS-R
	Block Design
	Object Assembly
	Picture Arrangement
	Picture Completion
	Tactual Performance Test[‡]
	Rey-Osterreith Complex Figure Test
7. Reasoning and problem solving	Categories Test[‡]
	Wisconsin Card Sort Test

*Many of these tests assay multiple modalities. For detailed discussion see references 12, 33, 34, 52, 55, 63.
†Wechsler Adult Intelligence Scale-Revised.
‡Subset of Halstead-Reitan Neuropsychological Battery.

cant "floor" or "ceiling" effect where numerous categories are crowded into one extreme or the other of the overall spectrum of recovery.

When outcome scales are used to follow individual patients over time, the number of categories must be large enough to allow documentation of small changes.

The neurosurgical unit in Glasgow has developed two scales for classifying head-injured patients: the GCS, which describes injury severity and which will be discussed later in this chapter, and the Glasgow Outcome Scale (GOS). The latter, which has proved to be extremely useful in categorizing the outcome following coma of traumatic or other etiology, will be described briefly. An alternative, the Disability Rating Scale (DRS), which can be more useful for tracking hospitalized patients and which probably can be applied to lesser degrees of head injury, is also described.

Glasgow Outcome Scale

The GOS was devised as a means of categorizing the functional status of patients after traumatic or nontraumatic coma[7,43] and has emerged as the method most often used for this purpose.

The outcome categories are defined in functional terms; they can be applied similarly to patients exhibiting a focal and specific deficit, such as hemiparesis or aphasia, or to patients with impairments resulting from more diffuse central nervous system (CNS) damage, such as memory deficits or behavioral or personality changes. With its functional bias, the GOS focuses on the "bottom line" of outcome after closed head injury, that is, the degree to which the patient is reintegrated into normal levels of activity and social interaction. Assessment of the functional status of a patient does not require extensive neurologic or neuropsychologic testing. Frequently, a discussion with the patient, his family, and others familiar with the patient on a day to day basis can allow appropriate assignment to one of the GOS categories.

Head-injured survivors are placed into one of four GOS categories (Table 10–3). The most severely impaired category has been termed persistent vegetative state (PVS) which, as first used by Jennett and Plum,[44] describes a return of wakefulness that is dissociated from cognitive functioning. The patient may exhibit normal periods of sleep and apparent wakefulness. There is stability of reflex and autonomic function as manifested by stable temperature and blood pressure, normal respiratory control, and stereotyped reflex activity. There is, however, no evidence of any meaningful contact with the environment. As implied by the modifier "persistent," a patient probably should not be placed into this category before 3 months after the head injury. In most series of severe head-injured patients, the outcome category of PVS comprises between 5 and 10% of patients overall.

Severe disability (SD) describes a patient who is conscious but dependent on other persons for some activities on a daily basis. Although many of these patients have severe physical impairments such as marked spastic paresis of the extremities or focal neurologic deficits such as aphasia, others may have relatively limited motor or sensory findings but are severely affected neuropsychologically. These latter patients, although not requiring skilled nursing care, may nonetheless be in need of continuous supervision.

Table 10–3   The Glasgow Outcome Scale*

Dead (D)	
Persistent vegetative state (PVS)	Wakefulness without awareness
Severe disability (SD)	Conscious but dependent
Moderate disability (MD)	Independent but disabled
Good recovery (GR)	Reintegrated (may have nondisabling sequelae)

*Adapted from Jennett and Bond.[43]

The term "moderate disability" (MD) describes patients who are independent but carry some residual disabilities, which though they may be severe, such as memory deficit, hemiparesis, post-traumatic epilepsy, do not preclude an independent life style. In a practical sense, a patient would be in a MD category if he could live alone for a weekend or longer. Patients who can participate in a normal social life in an independent fashion and who can return to work without disability are judged to have attained a good recovery (GR).

Although the GOS has been widely used to categorize outcome in large numbers of patients, with its few categories it is relatively insensitive to small changes in functional status that might occur in a patient over time. In addition, it is difficult to use it before discharge from the hospital or rehabilitation unit where true level of independence is difficult to assess. Thus, the GOS serves primarily (as was intended) as a research tool with little utility for tracking the clinical progress of patients.

Disability Rating Scale

The DRS has been recently proposed by Rappaport et al.[75] as an alternative method of categorizing head injury outcome (Tables 10–4, 10–5). It is a 30-point scale that ranges from 0 (full recovery without gross functional impairment) to 30 (death). It has been validated and has been shown to be a sensitive and reliable means of monitoring patients during and after recovery.[30,35]

The DRS examines the patient's status according to four categories: arousability awareness and responsivity, cognitive ability for self-care, dependence on others, and psychosocial adaptability.

Advantages to the use of the DRS include its incorporation of the GCS, allowing the DRS to be used early after injury. Also, the greater number of points allows for easier tracking of slight improvements in outcome during recovery. Although the DRS has largely been used by rehabilitation specialists, it is easily learned and applied and may be of use to neurosurgeons for following quantitatively the course of severe head injury during and after hospitalization.

Like the GOS, the DRS does not make use of detailed clinical or neuropsychologic data and can therefore be rapidly utilized, although it is more cumbersome than the GOS. Further study of the DRS and broader usage are required before its utility can be fully evaluated.

Timing of Outcome Assessment

To obtain a true picture of outcome after head injury, the assessment must be performed at a time when a steady-state condition has been achieved. Assessments made too early will overestimate morbidity in survivors if recovery is continuing, or underestimate mortality if patients are continuing to die of causes related to the head injury.

In practice, mortality after head injury is rarely underestimated, since more than 50% of patients who will die do so within 48 hours, and a large part of the remainder will die within the first week.[96] However, morbidity is easily overestimated in the early postinjury period.

Our lack of understanding of recovery mechanisms and their time course makes it difficult for us to determine when maximal recovery has been achieved. Bond and Brooks[14]

Table 10–4   Disability Rating Scale—Component Scores*

	SCORE
1. Arousability, awareness, and responsivity (modified GCS)	
Eye opening	
Spontaneous	0
To speech	1
To pain	2
None	3
Best verbal response	
Oriented	0
Confused	1
Inappropriate	2
Incomprehensible	3
None	4
Best motor response	
Obeys	0
Localizes	1
Withdraws	2
Flexor	3
Extensor	4
None	5
2. Cognitive ability for self care (feeding, toileting, grooming); ignore motor disability (maximum 3 points for each task)	
Complete	0
Partial	1
Minimal	2
None	3
3. Level of functioning	
Completely independent	0
Independent in special environment	1
Mildly dependent	2
Moderately dependent	3
Markedly dependent	4
Totally dependent	5
4. Employability	
Not restricted	0
Selected jobs competitive	1
Sheltered workship—noncompetitive	2
Not employable	3

*Adapted from Rappaport et al.[75]

have studied the rate of recovery in relation to GOS status and have found that most patients with PVS or SD outcomes reached a steady state by 3 months. Sixty-eight percent of good recoveries had reached this status by 3 months and 90% were there by 6 months. Two thirds of patients destined for moderate disability were at their final functional status by 3 months and 95% were there by 6 months. Similar findings for recovery rates were noted by Heiden et al.[37] Figure 10–2 is a diagrammatic representation of recovery curves for various ultimate GOS categories. Despite the relative uniformity of recovery rates within the first year observed in terms of GOS category, specific functional modalities may recover at different rates[11,13,45] (Table 10–6).

Table 10–5 Disability Rating Scale; Disability Categories*

TOTAL SCORE	LEVEL OF DISABILITY
0	None
1	Mild
2–3	Partial
4–6	Moderate
7–11	Moderately severe
12–16	Severe
17–21	Extremely severe
22–24	Vegetative state
25–29	Extreme vegetative state
30	Death

*Adapted from Rappaport et al.[75]

OUTCOME PREDICTION IN HEAD INJURY

In this section, we will discuss prognosis and prognostic indicants. Most work on this subject has pertained to severe closed head injury. Consequently, we have generally limited our discussion to severe craniocerebral trauma.

Description of Injury Severity After Head Injury

Several scales have been developed to describe the severity of head injury in the individual patient. The use of these scales facilitates communication between physicians, nurses, and other health care providers and aids in prediction of outcome by allowing patients to be objectively categorized. Four commonly used scales are outlined in Table 10–7.

The most commonly used scale is the GCS, which was developed and validated by Jennett and Teasdale in the mid-1970s[48,91,92] and which describes level of consciousness in terms of three aspects of neurologic function: eye opening, motor response, and verbal performance. The patient's best response in each of these areas is used for scoring purposes.

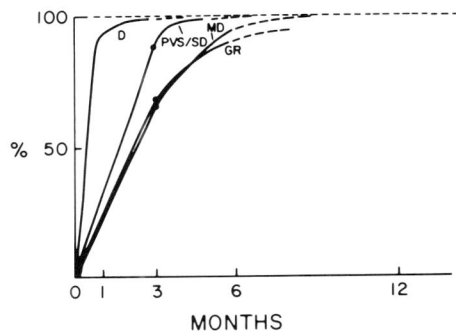

Figure 10–2. Approximate percentage of patients reaching final functional status over time. Note that for all GOS categories 90% of patients will have reached this final status by 6 months; patients who die generally do so in the first month. Adapted from Bond and Brooks,[14] Heiden et al.[37] and Vollmer et al.[96]

**Table 10–6   Cognitive Deficits Associated
with Head Injury and Appropriate Time for Recovery
Following Mild to Moderate Head Injury**

Motor skill and speed	0–3 months
Language skill	3–6 months
Attention/concentration	6–12 months
Memory/learning	6–12 months
Complex problem solving	6–24 months
Mental stamina	6–24 months

From Boll.[11] Reprinted with permission.

There is little interobserver variability among physicians, nurses, and paramedical personnel in patient assessment with the GCS.[93] As a result, the GCS has been used in almost all head injury studies since 1977. The GCS does have some potential weaknesses, however. Assessment of eye opening may be impossible when orbitofacial injury causes lid swelling and speech cannot be assessed in patients with endotracheal tubes in place. Also, the scale does not make use of clinical data, which may independently affect outcome, such as pupillary reactivity or oculovestibular reflexes. It is important to note the interval between injury and the time at which the GCS score is determined, since as many a quarter of patients will improve after resuscitation and treatment of extracranial injuries.[48] Some studies have used the score at 6 hours after injury to decrease the effect of this methodologic problem.

Factors Determining Outcome After Severe Head Injury

Injury Severity

Severe head injury is often defined arbitrarily as that which results in a GCS score of 8 or less. The mortality in recent series of severely head-injured patients varies over a remarkably narrow range from 34 to 50%. In the three-center International Data Bank[48] for which initial GCS was assessed at more than 6 hours after injury, mortality ranged from 48 to 50%. In subsequently reported International Data Bank compatible series, mortality rates have been somewhat lower, around 40%.[27,50,51,61] A relatively small percentage of cases, about 2 to 6%, survive in a vegetative state.[27,50,51,61] The majority of conscious survivors make a good recovery (12 to 48% of all patients). The rest who survive are moderately or severely disabled, accounting for about 5 to 15%.[27,50,51,61] These figures, derived from various neurosurgical centers in Europe and North America, quite consistently describe the outcome of all patients with severe head injury. The variability among centers may be due to several factors, including different proportions of low GCS score patients, differences in mean patient age, frequency of intracranial hematomas, variability in application of GOS, and different mechanisms of injury.

There is a consistent relationship between GCS and mortality among severely head injured patients.[15,16,27] About 12 to 27% of patients with GCS of 7 will die, whereas mortality for patients with GCS of 4 ranges between 51 and 80%.[15,16] The GCS score at the time of entry into a study therefore is a useful predictor of outcome.

Table 10–7 Level of Consciousness: Classification and Grading Systems*†

BECKER ET AL.[9]	RANSOHOFF AND FLEISCHER[74]	GRADY COMA SCALE[6]	GLASGOW COMA SCALE[92]	
I Transient loss of consciousness; now alert and oriented without neurologic deficit; may have headache, nausea, or vomiting	I Alert; responds immediately to questions; may be disoriented and confused; follows complex commands	1 Drowsy, lethargic indifferent, uninterested/belligerent, and uncooperative; does not lapse into sleep when left undisturbed	Eye opening	*E*
			Spontaneous	4
			To speech	3
			To pain	2
			Nil	1
II Impaired consciousness but able to follow at least a simple command; may be alert, but with a focal neurologic deficit	II Drowsy, confused, uninterested, does not lapse into sleep when undisturbed; follows simple commands only	2 Stuporous; will lapse into sleep when not disturbed; may be disoriented to time, place, and person	Best motor response	*M*
			Obeys	6
			Localizes	5
III Unable to follow even a single simple command because of disordered level of consciousness; may use words, but inappropriately; motor response varies from localizing pain to posturing or nil	III Stuporous; sleeps when not disturbed; responds briskly and appropriately to mildly noxious stimuli	3 Deep stupor, requires strong pain to evoke movement	Withdraws	4
			Abnormal flexion	3
		4 Does not respond appropriately to any stimuli; may exhibit decerebrate or decorticate posturing; retains deep tendon reflexes	Extensor response	2
	IV Deep stupor; responds defensively to prolonged noxious stimuli		Nil	1
			Verbal response	*V*
			Oriented	5
IV No evidence of brain function (brain death)	V Coma; no appropriate response to any stimuli, decorticate and decerebrate responses included	5 Does not respond appropriately to any stimuli; flaccid, no deep tendon reflexes	Confused conversation	4
			Inappropriate words	3
			Incomprehensible sounds	2
	VI Deep coma; flaccidity; no response to any stimuli		Nil	1
			Coma score	
			(E + M + V = 3 to 15)	

*Categories are based on initial presentation and provide a simple system for triage of patients into a management system appropriate to the degree of their brain injury.

†From Dacey and Dikmen.[24] Reprinted with permission.

Patient Age

Age has a substantial effect on outcome after head injury. Younger patients have better outcomes after severe head injury.[10,19,65] Patients more than 60 years of age have mortality rates between 70 and 90%,[51,65,72] whereas those for patients between 40 and 60 years are significantly lower. In the International Data Bank series a continuous relationship was found between age and outcome.[94] Other studies have suggested that there may be inflections in the age—outcome curve (at 20, 40, and 60 years of age).[16,38]

The reason for the effect of age on outcome is not understood. Extracranial injuries and illnesses have been blamed for the increase in mortality associated with aging.[8,21] Intracranial factors (such as the degree of brain atrophy) may also be important, however, in affecting the response of the brain to impact and secondary injuries. Underlying brain atrophy or an alteration in the viscoelastic properties of brain or bridging veins may contribute to the higher incidence of acute subdural hematoma seen in the elderly. In addition, the epidemiology of head injury changes with age. Falls, which seem to have a propensity for producing intracranial hematomas, increase, whereas vehicular accidents decline. The high mortality associated with acute subdural hematoma is well known.

Pediatric patients have better outcomes after head injury than older patients. Bruce et al.[19] reported that only 6% of a group of children with a mean age of 7 years died. Berger et al.[10] noted a mortality of 33% in their series of pediatric head injuries. Although patients less than 5 years recovered less well than those 5 to 19 years in the International Data Bank series, overall recovery from prolonged or deep coma is better in patients younger than 20 years of age.[21,38,94] Despite the preponderance of evidence that children have lower mortality rates after closed head injury, children may not uniformly fare better when other aspects of recovery are examined. Levin et al.[53,54] studied the recovery of memory in a group of children, adolescents, and adults after severe head injury. Their results demonstrated less cognitive recovery in the head-injured children than in a similarly injured group of adolescents.

Impact and Prehospital Factors

Outcome after head injury is significantly affected by a variety of factors at the time of impact and in the prehospital phase. The mechanism of injury is important. Vehicular accidents involving either passengers or pedestrians occur at relatively high velocities and tend to produce diffuse brain injury.[15,48] In contrast, falls produce a higher incidence of hematomas.[15,25,47] Vehicular trauma tends to involve young adults, falls most commonly affect the elderly and the very young. Gunshot wounds are associated with a very high mortality rate of 85%.[49] However, with the exception of gunshot wounds, Jennett et al.[48] found that mechanism of injury was one of a number of factors that had little independent effect on outcome.

Extracranial injury and prehospital systemic physiologic abnormalities affect outcome, Miller et al.[62] demonstrated that patients admitted to the emergency room with either shock or hypoxia have worse outcomes than those who do not. Eisenberg et al.[25] considered shock and hypoxia separately and found that they adversely affected outcome in the Traumatic Coma Data Bank. Hypotension in the prehospital period is associated with a higher incidence of increased ICP, which can adversely affect outcome.[66]

Extracranial injuries (such as hand or long bone fractures) may affect outcome (as determined by the GOS) by affecting the patient's ability to work after injury independent of neurologic injury.[22]

Pupillary Size and Reactivity

Absence of the pupillary light reflex in the head-injured patient is usually a grave prognostic sign. Ninety-five percent of patients with nonreactive pupils in the International Data Bank series progressed to poor outcomes (dead, vegetative, severe disability); nonreactive pupils are even more ominous in patients older than 50 years, for 95% of such patients died compared with 82% of those younger than 50 years.[47] Braakman et al.[16] reported mortality rates of 29, 54, and 90% with both pupils reacting, one nonreacting, or both pupils nonreacting, respectively. Narayan et al.[65] reported a somewhat lower mortality of 61% in patients with bilaterally impaired pupillary reactivity. Eighty-six percent of patients with bilaterally absent pupillary responses died.[51]

Oculocephalic or Oculovestibular Response

Pathways mediating eye movements in response to vestibular stimulation span a relatively large portion of the brainstem. Not surprisingly, impaired oculocephalic or oculovestibular responses usually correlate with a poor prognosis. In the International Data Bank series,[47] 90% of those with absent or impaired eye movements died or were left vegetative. Ninety-five percent of patients with absent oculovestibular responses died, as reported by Braakman et al.[16] Levati et al.[51] and Narayan et al.[65] reported somewhat lower mortalities of 73 and 51%, respectively, in patients with impaired or absent oculocephalic responses.

Motor Response

Flaccidity or decerebrate posturing is usually associated with a poor neurologic outcome after head injury.[20] In the International Data Bank series, 83% of patients having extensor posturing had poor outcomes. Decorticate posturing (abnormal flexion) was found by Bricolo et al.[17] to correlate with a mortality rate of 57%, whereas decerebrate posturing was associated with a mortality of 85%. Levati et al.[51] reported a significant correlation between best motor response and mortality in a series of head-injured patients: localize or withdrawal—25% mortality; abnormal flexion—44%; abnormal extension—60%. Narayan et al.[65] found that patients were twice as likely to die after severe head injury if motor posturing was present. Patients who are flaccid on admission have a high mortality rate (76%) and a high incidence of elevated and uncontrollable ICP.[28]

Computed Tomography and Magnetic Resonance Imaging: Effect on Outcome

When information from the CT scan is added to clinical data, the ability to predict outcome is significantly enhanced.[65,100] In general, the presence of a mass lesion on the CT indicates a worse prognosis. Narayan et al.[65] found mortalities of 10% with normal CT scan versus 46% with high-density lesions. When operative hematomas were considered separately, a mortality of 40% was found. Acute subdural hematoma is the lesion consistently associated with higher mortality, ranging from 60% to 80%. Some have speculated that severe associated cerebral parenchymal injury accounts for this high mortality. The finding that early removal of acute subdural hematoma improves outcome, however, suggests that the mass lesion itself is a major determinant of mortality.[83]

Gennarelli et al.[27] examined outcome in a group of patients and found a hierarchical relationship between combined CT and clinical findings and outcome. By combining length of coma and motor response with type of CT lesion (subdural or epidural hematoma or other focal lesion), a rank-outcome list could be determined (Fig. 10–3). This ranking of outcome by lesion type was independent of injury severity as measured by GCS score. An independent, adverse effect of mass lesions on outcome can be inferred from experience with those patients who "talk and deteriorate."[59,79,80] The fact that outcome can be poor in patients whose impact damage is not severe enough to render them comatose from the outset, but who later develop intracranial hematomas, confirms an independent effect.

Magnetic resonance imaging in severely head-injured patients with normal CT scans may reveal lesions indicative of diffuse white matter shearing injury. Wilberger, et al.[98] found a correlation between poor outcome and widespread rostral brainstem injury seen on magnetic resonance imaging.

Intracranial Pressure

Intracranial hypertension is generally associated with a poor outcome, although it has been difficult to quantitate the effect of episodes of increased ICP in terms of their duration, frequency, and amplitude. Saul et al.[82] described a lowering of head injury mortality in two consecutive series in which treatment for elevations of ICP was begun at 15 mmHg compared with 25 mmHg. Narayan et al.[65] subsequently reported a mortality of 51% when ICP was elevated above 20 mmHg compared with a 16% mortality when ICP remained normal. It is unclear whether elevated ICP has an effect on outcome that is independent of injury severity. Some studies have failed to demonstrate that treatment of elevated ICP affects outcome.[84,89] Eisenberg et al.,[25] however, showed that ICP elevations of greater than 30 mmHg were associated with a significantly poorer outcome even when patients were stratified into three groups based on initial GCS (Fig. 10–4).

Evoked Potentials

Impairment of somatosensory, visual or auditory evoked potentials predicts a poor outcome after severe head injury. Combined data from multimodality evoked potentials (MMEP) are the most accurate single prognostic indicators, with 91% correct outcome predictions.[65] Patients with either normal or "focal" abnormalities on MMEP had good outcomes (GR,

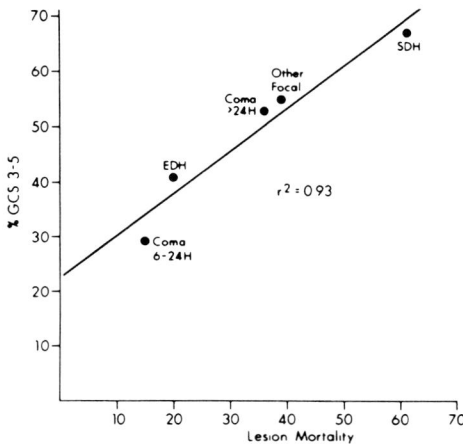

Figure 10–3. The relationship between lesion severity, as determined by percent of patients with GCS score of 3 to 5, and percent mortality. Note strong positive correlation, that is, lesions that have more patients with GCS scores 3 to 5 have a higher mortality rate. SDH: subdural hematoma; EDH: extradural hematoma. (From Gennarelli et al.[27] Reprinted with permission.)

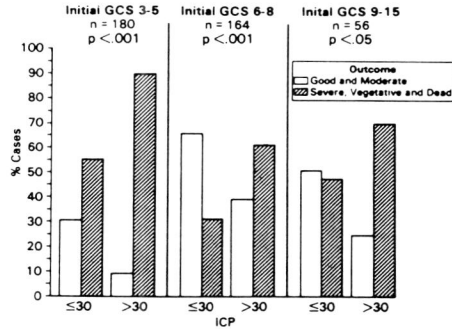

Figure 10–4. The relationship between ICP and outcome at three levels of GCS (GCS = 3–5: χ^2 = 17.5, df = 1), (GCS = 6–8: χ^2 = 11.55, df = 1), (GCS = 9–15: χ^2 = 4.69, df = 1). (From Eisenberg et al.[25] Reprinted with permission.)

MD) in 79% of cases, whereas those with disseminated deficits had good outcomes in only 3% and death in 82%.[65] Walser et al.[97] found a close correlation between degree of impairment of somatosensory evoked potentials, neurologic outcome, and extent of neuropathologic evidence of injury. Since the cerebral hemispheres are more vulnerable than the brainstem to the effects of head injury, brainstem auditory evoked responses (BAERs) are not always impaired in patients who have poor outcomes.[71] When they are impaired in severe head injury, they usually indicate that the head-injured patient will die.[71] It is of interest, however, that BAERs may also be abnormal in a significant number of patients with mild injuries (GCS 13 to 15), but these abnormalities do not necessarily correlate with post-traumatic deficits or symptoms.[68,81] Thus, BAERs taken independently are of limited value in outcome prediction.

Blood and Cerebrospinal Fluid

A number of markers found in cerebrospinal fluid (CSF) have been reported to have prognostic significance after severe head injury. Elevation of CSF creatine kinase BB isoenzyme (CK BB) concentrations almost exclusively indicates brain injury[3] despite the potential for CSF contamination by blood. CK BB activity in CSF is inversely proportional GCS score and outcome after head injury (Fig. 10–5).[4] Lactate dehydrogenase is also elevated in CSF after brain injury but contamination from systemic sources is more of a problem.[4] CSF cyclic adenosine monophosphate levels are significantly related to severity of injury (and presumably to outcome) in traumatic coma.[26] Circulating catecholamine levels reflect the severity of brain injury. Plasma concentration of norepinephrine correlates with GCS score and length of ventilation and hospitalization.[36,99]

Prediction of Outcome Based on Multiple Indicants of Prognosis

There are two common approaches to using statistical models for prediction of outcome after head injury: Bayesian statistics and linear logistic regression.

Jennett et al.[47] analyzed outcome in the International Coma Data Bank series using a Bayesian method for prediction. Calculations are made using the probabilities of a particular outcome given the presence of a prognostic indicant, such as whether or not the pupils react to light. The probabilities of a poor outcome using this method of prediction as noted by Giannotta et al.[29] are shown in Table 10–8.

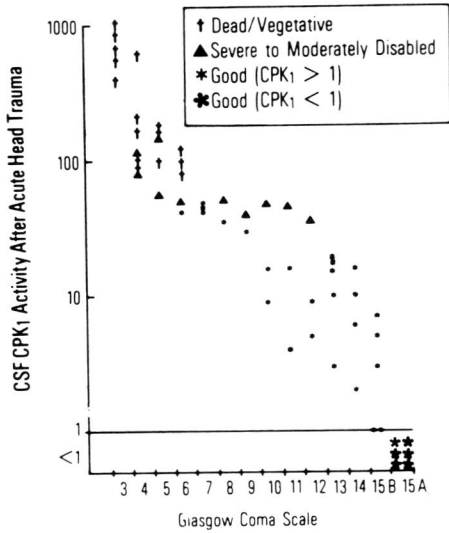

Figure 10–5. Correlation of Glasgow Coma Scale score, creatine phosphokinase (CPK), levels in the CSF (CPK_1 = CPK BB), and outcome from head injury. (From Bakay and Ward.[4] Reprinted with permission.)

Stablein et al.[85] developed an alternative method for predicting outcome after head injury using the linear logistic regression model to analyze data that are collectable within an hour of admission after head injury. This approach may be better than the Bayesian model because it is not based on the assumption that prognostic indicants (such as the age of a patient and occurrence of acute subdural hematoma) vary independently of one another. In the linear logistic calculations each indicant is assigned a weighting that represents its statistical importance and the degree to which it is dependently associated with other indicants. The most important variables in the study by Stablein et al. were (in rank order): requirement for surgical decompression, age, physiologic status on admission (presence of hypoxia, hypercapnia, hypotension, low hematocrit), motor response, and pupillary response. Using this predictive model, 91% of predictions were correct, with 69% of predictions being at the 0.90 level. This accuracy is impressive given that the data used were collected within 1 hour of the patient's admission.

Clinicians surveyed by Barlow and Teasdale[5] have shown interest in using computer

Table 10–8 Probabilities of Poor Outcome Related to Three Clinical Variables: Age, Pupillary Response, and Motor Response*

| | AGE (YR)* | | | | | |
| | ≤20 | | 20–59 | | ≥ 60 | |
MOTOR RESPONSE	N[†]	R[†]	N	R	N	R
Obeys/localizes	0.6812	0.1175	0.8179	0.2191	0.9638	0.6373
Withdrawal/flexor	0.8489	0.2593	0.9223	0.4241	0.9874	0.8231
Extensor/nil	0.9662	0.6254	0.9837	0.7779	0.9972	0.9579

*Data derived from Jennett et al.[48] From Gianotta et al.[29] Reprinted with permission.
[†]N: nonreactive pupils; R: reactive pupils.

modeling methods for outcome prediction when making clinical decisions about care of patients with severe head injury.

CONCLUSIONS

In this chapter, we have conducted a brief review of head injury outcome in terms of the functional deficits that may be produced, the time course of recovery, and some of the common methods of assessment. We have attempted to provide an overview of outcome prediction, discussing the various factors known to influence survival or eventual recovery. At present, much information is lacking regarding the functional consequences that affect patients in the GOS categories of good recovery and moderate disability. Until recently, most of the interest in head injury research was directed at severely injured patients. However, there is now a greater appreciation for the functional consequences of moderate and perhaps even mild degrees of brain trauma. It is hoped that further work in these areas will soon be forthcoming.

Recently, two controversial studies have failed to show significant differences in the mortality rates of severely head-injured patients, whether treated in an aggressive fashion using extensive monitoring or with significantly less intensity and intervention.[23,40] Reports such as these imply that an aggressive attitude regarding severe head injury management is of little benefit in reducing mortality, particularly in patients who have sustained injuries from which recovery is impossible. Before such a conclusion can be reached, survivors must also be examined before the true effects of treatments can be assayed. In answering questions regarding effects of treatment or comparing therapies, the value of outcome assessment is apparent.

REFERENCES

1. Adams JH, Graham DI, Gennarelli TA: Head injury in man and experimental animals. Neuropathol Acta Neurochir [Suppl] 32:15–30, 1983.
2. Adams JH, Graham DI, Scott G, Parker LS, Doyle D: Brain damage in fatal non-missile head injury. J Clin Pathol 33:1132–1145, 1980.
3. Bakay RAE, Sweeney KM, Wood JH: Pathophysiology of cerebrospinal fluid in head injury: Part 2. Neurosurgery 18:376–382, 1986.
4. Bakay RAE, Ward AA: Enzymatic changes in serum and CSF in neurological injury. J Neurosurg 58:27–37, 1983.
5. Barlow P, Teasdale G: Prediction of outcome and the management of severe head injuries: The attitudes of neurosurgeons. Neurosurgery 1986; 19:989–991.
6. Barrow D. Wood J: Cerebral Rescusitation. In Chernow B, Lake CR (eds): The Pharmacological Approach to the Critically Ill Patient. Baltimore: Williams & Wilkins, 1983.
7. Bates D, Caronna JJ, Cartlidge NFF, Knill-Jones RP, Levy DE, Shaw MB, Plum F: A prospective study of nontraumatic coma: Methods and results in 310 patients. Ann Neurol 2:211–220, 1977.
8. Becker DP, Miller JD, Ward JD, Greenberg RP, Young HF, Sakalas R: The outcome from severe head injury with early diagnosis and intensive management. J Neurosurg 47:491–502, 1977.
9. Becker DP, Miller JD, Young HF, Selhorst JB, Kishore PRS, Greenberg RP, Rosner MJ, Ward JD: Diagnosis and treatment of head injury in adults. In Youmans JR (ed): Neurological Surgery, vol 4, ed 2. Philadelphia: WB Saunders, 1982, p 1938.
10. Berger MS, Pitts LH, Lovely M, et al.: Outcome from severe head injury in children and adolescents. J Neurosurg 62:194–199, 1985.
11. Boll TJ: Behavioral sequelae of head injury. In Cooper PR (ed): Head Injury. Baltimore: Williams & Wilkins, 1982, pp 363–375.

12. Boll TJ: Diagnosing brain impairment. In Wolman BB (ed): Clinical Diagnosis of Mental Disorders. New York: Plenum Press, 1978, pp 601–675

13. Bond MR: Assessment of the psychosocial outcome of severe head injury. Acta Neurochir (Wien) 34:57–70, 1976.

14. Bond MR, Brooks DN: Understanding the process of recovery as a basis for the investigation of rehabilitation for the brain injured. Scand J Rehabil Med 8:127–133, 1976.

15. Bowers SA, Marshall LF: Outcome in 200 consecutive cases of severe head injury treated in San Diego county: A prospective analysis. Neurosurgery 6:237–242, 1980

16. Braakman R, Gelpke GJ, Habbema JDF, Maas AIR, Minderhoud JM: Systematic selection of prognostic features in patients with severe head injury. Neurosurgery 6:362–370, 1980.

17. Bricolo A, Turazzi S, Alexandre A, Ruzzuto N: Decerebrate rigidity in acute head injury. J Neurosurg 47:680–698, 1977.

18. Brooks DN, McKinlay WW: Personality and behavioral change after severe blunt head injury—a relative's view. J Neurol Neurosurg Psychiatry 46:336–344, 1983.

19. Bruce DA, Schut L, Bruno LA, Wood JH, Sutton LN: Outcome following severe head injuries in children. J Neurosurg 48:679–688, 1978.

20. Butterworth JF, Selhorst JB, Greenberg RP, Miller JD, Gudeman SK: Flaccidity after head injury: Diagnosis, management, and outcome. Neurosurgery 9:242–248, 1981.

21. Carlson C, Von Essen C, Lofgren J: Factors affecting the clinical course of patients with severe head injuries. J Neurosurg 29:242–251, 1968.

22. Colohan ART, Alves WM, Jane JA, et al.: Factors affecting social outcome following mild head injury. Presented at the Congress of Neurological Surgeons Meeting, Hawaii, September, 1985.

23. Colohan ART, Alves W, Tandon PN, et al.: Mortality following serious head injury: Comparison of two series with radically different treatment protocols. Presented at the American Association of Neurological Surgeons, Atlanta, April, 1985.

24. Dacey RG, Dikmen SS: Mild head injury. In Cooper PR (ed): Head Injury, 2nd ed. Baltimore: Williams & Wilkins, 1982, pp 125–140.

25. Eisenberg H, Cayard C, Papanicolau A, Weiner R, Franklin D, Jane J, Grossman R, Tabaddor K, Becker DP, Marshall LF, Kunitz S: The effects of three potentially preventable complications on outcome after severe closed head injury. In Ishii S, Nagai H, Brock M (eds): Intracranial Pressure, vol V. New York: Springer-Verlag, 1983, pp 549–553.

26. Fleischer AS: Prognostic value of cyclic AMP in ventricular cerebrospinal fluid of patients following severe head injury. In Popp AJ, Bourke RS, Nelson LR, Kimelberg HK (eds): Neural Trauma. New York: Raven Press, 1979, pp 245–252.

27. Gennarelli TA, Spielman GM, Langfitt TW, Gildenberg PL, Harrington T, Jane JA, Marshall LF, Miller JD, Pitts LH: Influence of the type of intracranial lesion on outcome from severe head injury. J Neurosurg 56:26–32, 1982.

28. Gennarelli TA, Thibault LE, Adams JH, Graham DI, Thompson CJ, Marcincin RP: Diffuse axonal injury and traumatic coma in the primate. In Dacey RG, Winn HR, Rimel RW, Jane JA (eds): Trauma of the central Nervous System. New York: Raven Press, 1985, pp 169–193.

29. Giannotta SL, Weiner JM, Cereverha BB: Prognosis and outcome in severe head injury. In Cooper PR (ed): Head Injury. Baltimore: Williams & Wilkins, 1982, pp 377–406.

30. Gouvier D, Blanton PD, LaPorte KK, Nepomunceno C: Reliability and validity of the disability rating scale and the levels of cognitive functioning scale in monitoring recovery from severe head injury. Arch Phys Med Rehabil 68:94–97, 1987.

31. Graham DI, Adams JH: Ischaemic brain damage in fatal head injuries. Lancet 1:265–266, 1975.

32. Graham DI, Adams JH, Doyle D: Ischaemic brain damage in fatal non-missle head injuries. J Neurol Sci 39:213–234, 1978.

33. Gronwall D, Wrightson P: Delayed recovery of intellectual function after minor head injury. Lancet 2:605–609, 1974.

34. Hartlage LC, Asken MJ, Hornsby JL: Essentials of Neuropsychological Assessment. New York: Springer, 1987.

35. Hall K, Cope DN, Rappaport M: Glasgow Outcome Scale and Disability Rating Scale: Comparative usefulness in following recovery in traumatic head injury. Arch Phys Med Rehabil 66:35–37, 1985.

36. Hamill RW, Woolf PD, McDonald JV, Lee LA, Kelly M: Catecholamines predict outcome in traumatic brain injury. Ann Neurol 21:438–443, 1987.

37. Heiden JS, Small R, Caton W, Weiss M, Kurze T: Severe head injury; clinical assessment and outcome. Phys Ther 63:1946–1951, 1983.

38. Heiskanen O, Sipponen P: Prognosis of severe brain injury. Acta Neurol Scand 46:343–348, 1970.

39. Imes C: Rehabilitation of the head injury patient. Cognit Rehab 1:11–19, 1983.

40. Jane JA, Rimel RW, Pobereskin LH, et al.: Outcome and pathology of head injury. In Grossman RG, Gildenberg PI (eds): Head Injury: Basic and Clinical Aspects, New York: Raven Press, 1982.

41. Jane JA, Steward O, Gennarelli T: Axonal degeneration induced by experimental noninvasive minor head injury. J Neurosurg 62:96–100, 1985.
42. Jennett B: Resource allocation for the severely brain damaged. (Editorial). Arch Neurol 33:595–597, 1976.
43. Jennett B, Bond M: Assessment of outcome after severe brain damage; a practical scale. Lancet 1:480–484, 1975.
44. Jennett B, Plum F: Persistent vegetative state after brain damage; a syndrome in search of a name. Lancet 1: 734–737, 1972.
45. Jennett B, Snoek J, Bond MR, Brooks N: Disability after severe head injury: Observations on the use of the Glasgow Outcome Scale. J Neurol Neurosurg Psychiatry 44:285–293, 1981.
46. Jennett B, Teasdale G: Management of Head Injuries. Philadelphia: FA Davis, 1981.
47. Jennett B, Teasdale G, Braakman R, Minderhoud J, Heiden J, Kurze T: Prognosis of patients with severe head injury. Neurosurgery 4:283–289, 1979.
48. Jennett B, Teasdale G, Galbraith S, et al.: Severe head injuries in three countries. J Neurol Neurosurg Psychiatry 40:291–298, 1977.
49. Kaufman HH, Loyola WP, Makela ME, et al.: Civilian gunshot wounds: The limits of salvageability. Acta Neurochir (Wien) 67:115–125, 1983.
50. Langfitt TW, Gennarelli TA: Can the outcome from head injury be improved? J Neurosurgery 56:19–25, 1982.
51. Levati A, Farina ML, Vecchi G, Rossanda M, Marrubini MB: Prognosis of severe head injuries. J Neurosurg 57:779–783, 1982.
52. Levin HS, Benton AL, Grossman RG: Neurobehavioral Consequences of Closed Head Injury. Central Nervous Trauma Status Report—1985. New York: Oxford University Press, 1982.
53. Levin HS, Eisenberg HM: Neuropsychological outcome of closed head injury in children and adolescents. Childs Brain 5:281–292, 1979.
54. Levin HS, Eisenberg HM, Wigg NR, Kobayashi K: Memory and intellectual ability after head injury in children and adolescents. Neurosurgery 11:668–673, 1982.
55. Levin HS, O'Donnell VM, Grossman RG: The Galveston orientation and amnesia test: A practical scale to assess cognition after head injury. J Nerv Ment Dis 167:675–684, 1979.
56. Lindenberg R, Fisher R, Durlacher SH, Lovitt WV, Freytag E: Lesions of the corpus callosum following blunt mechanical trauma to the head. Am J Pathol 31:297–317, 1955.
57. Lishman WA: The psychiatric sequelae of head injury: A review. Psychol Med 3:304, 1973.
58. Lutz HA, Becker DP, Miller JD, Ward JD: Monitoring, management, and the analysis of outcome. In Grossman RG, Gildenberg PL (eds): Head Injury: Basic and Clinical Aspects. New York: Raven Press, 1982, pp 221–228.
59. Marshall LF, Toole BM, Bowers SA: The National Traumatic Coma Data Bank: Part 2. Patients who talk and deteriorate: Implications for treatment. J Neurosurg 59:285–288, 1983.
60. McLean A Jr, Dikmen S, Temkin N, Wyler AR, Gale JL: Psychosocial functioning at one month after head injury. Neurosurgery 14:393–399, 1984.
61. Miller JD, Butterworth JF, Gudeman SK, Faulkner JE, Choi SC, Selhorst JB, Harbison JW, Lutz HA, Young HF, Becker DP: Further experience in the management of severe head injury. J Neurosurg 54:289–299, 1981.
62. Miller JD, Sweet RC, Narayan RK, Becker DP: Early insults to the injured brain. JAMA 240:439–442, 1978.
63. Moses JA Jr, Golden CJ, Ariel R, Gustavson JL: Interpretation of the Luria-Nebraska Battery, Vol 1. New York: Grune & Stratton, 1983.
64. Najenson T, Mendelson L, Schecter I, David C, Mintz N, Groswasser Z: Rehabilitation after severe head injury. Scand J Rehabil Med 6:5–14, 1974.
65. Narayan RK, Greenberg RP, Miller JD, Enas GG, Choi SC, Kishore PRS, Selhorst JB, Lutz HA, Becker DP: Improved confidence of outcome prediction in severe head injury. A comparative analysis of the clinical examination, multimodality evoked potentials, CT scanning, and intracranial pressure. J Neurosurg 54: 751–762, 1981.
66. Narayan RK, Kishore PRS, Becker DP, Ward JD, Eras GG, Greenberg RP, Dasilva AD, Lipper MH, Choi SC, Mayhall CG, Lutz HA, Young HF: Intracranial pressure: To monitor or not to monitor? J Neurosurg 56: 650–659, 1982.
67. Nevin NC: Neuropathological changes in the white matter following head injury. J Neuropathol Exp Neurol 26:77–84, 1967.
68. Noseworthy JH, Miller J, Murray TJ: Auditory brainstem responses in postconcussion syndrome. Arch Neurol 38:275–278, 1981.
69. Oppenheimer DR: Microscope lesions in the brain following head injury. J Neurol Neurosurg Psychiatry 31: 299–306, 1968.
70. O'Shaughnessy EJ, Fowler RS Jr, Reid V: Sequelae of mild closed head injuries. J Fam Pract 18:391–394, 1984.

71. Papanicolaou AC, Loring DW, Eisenberg HM, Raz N, Contreras FL: Auditory brain stem evoked responses in comatose head-injured patients. Neurosurgery 18:173–175, 1986.

72. Pazzaglia P, Frank G, Frank F, Gaist G: Clinical course and prognosis of acute post-traumatic coma. J Neurol Neurosurg Psychiatry 38:149–154, 1975.

73. Povlishock JT, Becker DP, Cheng CLY, Vaughn GA: Axonal change in minor head injury. J Neuropathol Exp Neurol 42:225–242, 1983.

74. Ransohoff J, Fleischer A: Head Injuries. JAMA 234:861–864, 1975.

75. Rappaport M, Hall KM, Hopkins K, Belleza T: Disability rating scale for severe head trauma: Coma to community. Arch Phys Med Rehabil 63:118–123, 1983.

76. Rimel RW, Giordani B, Barth JT, Boll TJ, Jane JA: Disability caused by minor head injury. Neurosurgery 9: 221–228, 1981.

77. Rimel RW, Giordani B, Barth JT, Jane JA: Moderate head injury: Completing the clinical spectrum of brain trauma. Neurosurgery 11:344–351, 1982.

78. Roberts AH: Long term prognosis of severe accidental head injury. Proc R Soc Med 69:137–140, 1976.

79. Rockswold GL, Leonard PR, Nagib MG: Analysis of management in thirty-three closed head injury patients who "talked and deteriorated." Neurosurgery 21:51–55, 1987.

80. Rose J, Valtonen S, Jennett B: Avoidable factors contributing to death after head injury. Br Med J 2:615–618, 1977.

81. Ruth RA, Ringers BB, Vollmer DG, Alves WA, Jane JA: Use of the auditory brainstem response in the assessment of minor head injury. Presented at the Houston Conference on Neurotrauma, Houston, Texas, May, 1984.

82. Saul TG, Ducker TB, Salcman M, Carro E: Steroids in severe head injury. A prospective randomized clinical trial. J Neurosurg 54:596–600, 1981.

83. Seelig JM, Becker DP, Miller JD, et al.: Traumatic acute subdural hematoma. Major mortality reduction in comatose patients within four hours. N Engl J Med 304:1511–1518, 1981.

84. Smith HP, Kelly DL, McWhorter JM, Armstrong D, Johnson R, Transou C, Howard G: Comparison of mannitol regimens in patients with severe head injury undergoing intracranial monitoring. J Neurosurg 65: 820–824, 1986.

85. Stablein DM, Miller JD, Choi SC, Becker DP: Statistical methods for determining prognosis in severe head injury. Neurosurgery 6:243–248, 1980.

86. Stover SL, Zeiger HE Jr: Head injury in children and teenagers: Functional recovery correlated with duration of coma. Arch Phys Med Rehabil 57:201–205, 1976.

87. Strich SJ: Diffuse degeneration of the cerebral white matter in severe dementia following head injury. J Neurol Neurosurg Psychiatry 19:163–185, 1956.

88. Strich SJ: Shearing of nerve fibres as a cause of brain damage due to head injury; a pathological study of twenty cases. Lancet 2:443–448, 1961.

89. Stuart GG, Merry GS, Smith JA, et al.: Severe head injury managed without intracranial pressure monitoring. J Neurosurg 59:601–605, 1983.

90. Tabaddor K, Mattis S, Zazula T: Cognitive sequelae and recovery course after moderate and severe head injury. Neurosurgery 14:701–708, 1984.

91. Teasdale G, Jennett B: Assessment and prognosis of coma after head injury. Acta Neurochir (Wien) 34:45–55, 1976.

92. Teasdale G, Jennett B: Assessment of coma and impaired consciousness. A practical scale. Lancet 2:81–83, 1974.

93. Teasdale G, Knill-Jones R, Van Der Sande J: Observer variability in assessing impaired consciousness and coma. J Neurol Neurosurg Psychiatry 41:603–610, 1978.

94. Teasdale G, Skene A, Parker L, Jennett B: Age and outcome of severe head injury. Acta Neurochir [Suppl] (Wien) 28:140–143, 1979.

95. Uzzell BP, Zimmerman RA, Dolinskas CA, Obrist WD: Lateralized psychological impairment associated with CT lesions in head injured patients. Cortex 15:391–401, 1979.

96. Vollmer DG, Torner JC, Charlebois D, Sadovnic B, Jane JA: Age and outcome following traumatic coma: Why do older patients fare worse? Presented at the Annual Meeting of the American Association of Neurological Surgeons, Dallas, Texas, May 3–7, 1987.

97. Walser H, Emre M, Janzer R: Somatosensory evoked potentials in comatose patients: Correlation with outcome and neuropathological findings. J Neurol 233:34–40, 1986.

98. Wilberger JE, Deeb Z, Rothfus W: Magnetic resonance imaging in cases of severe head injury. Neurosurgery 20:571–576, 1987.

99. Wolf PD, Hamill RW, Louyse LA, Cox C, McDonald JV: The predictive value of catecholamines in assessing outcome in traumatic brain injury. J Neurosurg 66:875–882, 1987.

100. Young B, Rapp RP, Norton JA, Haack D, Tibbs PA, Bean JR: Early prediction of outcome in head-injured patients. J Neurosurg 54:300–303, 1981.

11

Initial Assessment
and Management
of Spinal Injuries

FRANKLIN C. WAGNER, JR.

The potentially grave consequences of a spinal injury have long been known. In the 5000-year-old Edwin Smith papyrus six cases of spinal trauma are described.[2] The author of this document recommends that treatment should not be given in those cases of spinal trauma in which the patient is unconscious of his arms and legs and in which priapism and urinary incontinence are experienced. Although advances in the treatment of spinal injuries and in rehabilitation have made this advice invalid, the cure of the spinal cord injury in such cases remains elusive.

It is estimated that between 40 and 50 patients per million population annually are hospitalized with spinal cord injuries in the United States.[1] The patients are most likely to be adolescent or young adult males. The majority of cases of spinal cord injury are transport related, with motor vehicle collisions being chiefly responsible.[11]

STABILIZATION

After trauma, the presence of a spine or spinal cord injury is usually obvious. When multiple trauma has occurred, however, other injuries may mask the presence of a spine or spinal cord injury. Examples of trauma with which injuries of the spine and spinal cord may be associated include head trauma sufficient to result in unconsciousness, trauma above the clavicles to the head and neck, and any trauma associated with a high-speed motor vehicle accident or a fall from a height roughly three times that of the patient's.

When a spine or spinal cord injury has occurred or is likely to be present, it is important to immobilize the spine. Immobilization requires that the head, thorax, and pelvis be stabilized as a unit.[7] This may be accomplished by applying a semirigid collar to the neck, a short spine board to the head and back if it is necessary to extricate the patient, and, after extrication, applying a long spine board without removing the short spine board. The back of the head should be padded when either the short or the long spine boards are used. Padding the head will prevent extending the cervical spine beyond the neutral position of approximately 12°. The accident patient must be firmly secured to the spine boards. In doing this one should not use the chin as a point of suspension. Only after adequate immobilization has been achieved should the patient be transported.

The airway should be protected during transportation with either a nasal or oral airway and supplemental 100% oxygen provided. Should endotracheal intubation be necessary once the patient has arrived in the emergency room, the neck must be maintained in a neutral position. An assistant standing alongside the patient's chest may do this by stabilizing the head, placing his hands over the patient's ears from in front. As the cervical spine is immobilized in this manner, an endotracheal tube may be inserted orally. The "sniffing position," which is commonly used when placing an oral endotracheal tube but which flexes the cervical spine at C5 and C6 and extends it at C1 and C2, must be avoided.

A midcervical or high cervical spinal cord injury may produce a loss in sympathetic tone resulting in what is referred to as neurogenic shock.[10,12] Clinically, the patient will have hypotension, a slow pulse rate, and a warm, dry skin. The intravascular volume will be normal, but, as a result of the decrease in peripheral vascular tone, the vascular space will be expanded.

Mild cases of neurogenic shock in which the hypotension is not profound and which improves within hours of the patient's hospitalization, of course, do not need treatment. Other cases in which the hypotension persists and is sufficient to threaten adequate perfusion require treatment. In these patients, central venous pressure or pulmonary wedge pressure monitoring will help determine the relative importance of treatment with fluids or vasopressers.

Since it is the peripheral vasculature that is dilated, treatment usually is aimed at reducing the expanded vascular space by administering a vasopressor whose effect is primarily peripheral rather than central. Phenylephrine hydrochloride, which is predominantly a peripheral vasoconstrictor, is the drug of choice. It can be given as a solution of 50 mg in 1000 ml of 5% dextrose in water or a balanced salt solution at the rate of 0.5 to 1.5 ml/min.

SPINAL EXAMINATION

An injury to the vertebrae, intervertebral disks, and ligamentous structures with secondary spasm of the paravertebral muscles will produce local pain. This is described as being a persistent, nonradiating, aching, deep, dull soreness of the neck or back muscles. The pain will vary in intensity with changes in posture.

Inspection may show a deformity of the spine and ecchymoses of the overlying skin. Palpation of the muscles in the area of injury will detect spasm, and local pressure or percussion is likely to produce tenderness.

The number of times a patient with a potential spinal injury is moved should be minimized. The danger of moving a patient with an unstable spinal injury may outweigh the value of inspecting and palpating the injured area. When it is not possible to palpate the spine of a patient lying supine by the examiner gently sliding his hand between the spine and the gurney or board, diagnostic imaging should be relied on to rule in or out the presence of a spinal injury.

NEUROLOGIC EXAMINATION

The neurologic examination of the patient with a spinal cord injury should accurately describe the patient's neurologic deficit and should be reproducible by subsequent examiners. Since a change in the patient's neurologic status during the period of initial evaluation may be subtle, it is helpful to record the results of each examination.

What should be regarded as the level of spinal cord injury has not always been clear. Most investigators now agree that the most caudal spinal cord segment with fully intact sensation and motor power should be considered as the spinal cord level.[9] Utilizing this method avoids confusing partially preserved root function, which may persist for as many as three levels caudal to the injury, with spinal cord function.[6]

Motor power should be assessed in a systematic manner. The muscles tested should be selected on the basis of their functional significance, the ease with which they may be examined, and the spinal cord segments they represent. For example, it is helpful in the upper extremity to examine two muscles each in the arm, the forearm, and the hand. The strength of each muscle tested should be graded according to an accepted method, such as that devised for the Medical Research Council.[8]

Sensation should be judged to be present, present but diminished, or absent. It is also important to remember as the sensory examination is being done that the C5 through C8 dermatomes are fully represented in the upper extremities but have no representation on the trunk and that the T1 dermatome has little representation on the trunk. If only the trunk is examined, the danger exists of giving the patient with a cervical spinal cord injury a fallaciously high or low sensory level, since the C4 dermatome is immediately cephalad to the T2 dermatome.

The fibers conveying the sensation of light touch have the widest distribution in the spinal cord, being located in both the posterior and the lateral columns of the white matter. Consequently, light touch may be the one sensory modality preserved when all other modalities are absent. Therefore the physician should determine whether pin sensation is sharp or felt only as a touch. Posterior column function should be assessed by testing position and vibratory sense.

As the fibers subserving perianal sensation ascend within the spinal cord, they migrate toward the periphery of the spinal cord as other fibers enter more rostally. As a consequence of their more peripheral location in the thoracic and cervical spinal cord, they may escape injury should the central portion of the spinal cord in these two regions be injured. It is important therefore that sensation in the perianal area be tested to determine whether or not "sacral sparing" is present.

After a significant spinal cord injury, the deep tendon reflexes below the level of injury will be absent. They then are likely to reappear and become hyperactive within 3 to 6 weeks of the injury as the period of spinal shock subsides. In contrast to the deep tendon reflexes, the bulbocavernosus and anocutaneous reflexes may reappear as soon as 6 hours after a complete injury to the lumbar spinal cord.[5]

DIAGNOSTIC IMAGING

The lateral spine roentgenogram is the most useful view in determining the presence or absence of a spinal fracture or fracture-dislocation.[4,13] Furthermore, obtaining a lateral roentgenogram of the spine does not require any undue movement of the patient.

Because of its comparative mobility, the lower cervical region, including the cervico-thoracic junction, is a frequent site of injury; thus, it is essential that this region be visualized on the lateral roentgenogram. To avoid the superimposition of the shoulders, it may be necessary to pull the arms downward as this view is being obtained. If this maneuver is unsuccessful, a swimmer's view should be attempted. This can be accomplished by raising the arm above the head on the same side as the x-ray cassette and pulling downward on the opposite arm. If the neck is carefully maintained in a neutral position during the radiographic examination, additional risk of neck movement and new cord injury is minimized.

A systematic review of the lateral roentgenogram of the cervical spine will initially involve detecting any malalignment. Once alignment has been evaluated, damage to the bones, the joints, and the surrounding soft tissue can be assessed. Normally, four lordotic curves formed by the anterior and posterior surfaces of the vertebral bodies, by the bases of the spinous processes, and by the tips of the spinous processes can be appreciated in the cervical spine. Alternatively, the spinal canal within the uninjured cervical spine should form a funnellike figure with a smoothly curved spout. Any disturbance in these curves or outline will indicate an abnormality in alignment. (See Chapter 13 for additional discussion.)

The superimposition of the ribs on the thoracic spine make the interpretation of the lateral roentgenogram of this region difficult. Therefore the standard radiographic examination of the thoracic spine includes the anteroposterior projection as well as the lateral view. The upper portion of the thoracic spine is often obscured by the shoulders. Should this be the case, adequate visualization may be obtained with the swimmer's projection.

The lumbar spine is initially evaluated with anteroposterior and lateral projections. If it is not possible to obtain a satisfactory lateral view with the horizontal beam, one may consider placing the patient in the lateral position, which should be done only with extreme caution.

Computed tomography (CT) has added greatly to the radiologic evaluation of the patient with a spine and spinal cord injury. By demonstrating the spine in cross-section, the size and the shape of the spinal canal and the integrity of the pedicles, laminae, and spinous processes besides the vertebral bodies can be assessed. Reconstruction in the coronal and sagittal planes can also add useful information, particularly in regions where conventional roentgenograms of the spine may be difficult to interpret. When one is reviewing axial views, it is necessary to remember that a fracture or fracture-dislocation occurring in the same plane as the scan may not be evident.

Visualization of the spinal cord and the cauda equina is still not possible with CT alone. To accomplish this CT must be combined with myelography with a water-soluble contrast agent. After the contrast agent has been introduced intrathecally, compression or enlargement of the spinal cord or an obstruction to the flow of the contrast agent may be revealed by CT.

The usefulness of magnetic resonance imaging (MRI) in the evaluation of patients with acute spinal injuries has not yet been determined. Although MRI is unable to image cortical bone, it shows soft tissue within the spinal canal well. Among the reasons this modality has not been more rapidly adopted is the difficulty of obtaining a scan in patients requiring mechanical ventilation, electrical monitoring, or immobilization with ferrous-containing materials. However, because MRI depicts the spinal cord so well, it likely will become an important adjunct in evaluating patients with spinal cord injuries (see Chapter 13).

INITIAL MANAGEMENT

Once the patient with a spine and spinal cord injury has been stabilized and evaluated by diagnostic imaging, further treatment can be carried out. What form this treatment will take will be influenced by whether the patient has an incomplete or a complete spinal cord lesion.[3] Since the patient with an incomplete lesion may regain a significant amount of his lost neurologic function, the objective of treatment will be to correct any condition that might compromise neurologic recovery. In contrast, the patient with a complete lesion is unlikely to recover neurologically to the same degree. Consequently, in patients with complete lesions, treatment will be aimed at preventing any further neurologic damage.

After immobilization, stabilization, neurologic examination, and radiographic evaluation of the patient with a spine and spinal cord injury, decisions regarding additional treatment can be made. If a fracture-dislocation is present, its reduction will improve the malalignment of the spine and may decompress the spinal cord or cauda equina. If the cervical spine is involved, an attempt at closed reduction is justified initially. The forces required to achieve a closed reduction of a fracture-dislocation involving the thoracic and the lumbar spine are much greater. Therefore attempting a closed reduction in these regions is usually not worthwhile.

If it is possible to reduce a cervical fracture-dislocation by closed means, what is done next will be determined by the patient's neurologic status. Continuing observation while maintaining immobilization is indicated in the patient who is improving. Whether or not the patient is placed in a cervical orthosis, such as a halo vest, or undergoes internal stabilization at a later time rests with the judgment of how stable the fracture is. The patient who worsens neurologically or who at first improves and then becomes stable requires further investigation to try to determine a cause for these changes. This can be done with myelography and CT or MRI.

Patients with either an incomplete or complete cervical spinal cord injury in whom it has not been possible to achieve a closed reduction of their fracture-dislocation will require an open reduction, at which time a fusion may also be done. If not already done as a part of their initial evaluation, CT should be carried out before an open reduction so that the physician may better understand the disordered anatomy.

In view of the difficulty achieving a closed reduction of a fracture-dislocation of the thoracic or of the lumbar spine, an open reduction at these levels will probably be necessary. The timing of this procedure, as with patients with cervical injuries, will be determined by the patient's overall condition, by the degree the dislocation may be compressing neural structures, especially in those with incomplete lesions, and by the need to mobilize patients with complete lesions to lessen the chances of respiratory complications developing. Early mobilization might be allowed by internal stabilization.

REFERENCES

1. Bracken M3, Freeman DH, Hellenbrand K: Incidence of acute traumatic hospitalized spinal cord injury in the United States, 1970–1977. Am J Epidemiol 113:615–622, 1981.
2. Breasted JH: The Edwin Smith Surgical Papyrus. In Wilkins RH (ed): Neurosurgical Classics. New York: Johnson Reprint, 1965, pp 1–5.

3. Chehrazi B, Wagner FC, Collins WF, Freeman DH Jr: A scale for evaluation of spinal cord injury. J Neurosurg 54:310–315, 1981.
4. Harris JH: Radiographic evaluation of spinal trauma. Orthop Clin North Am 17:75–86, 1986.
5. Holdsworth F: Fractures, dislocations and fracture-dislocations of the spine. J Bone Joint Surg 52A:1534–1551, 1970.
6. Lucas JT, Ducker TB: Recovery in spinal cord injuries. Adv Neurosurg 7:281–294, 1979.
7. McSwain NE Jr: Patient Assessment and initial management. In McSwain NE Jr, Kerstein MD (eds): Evaluation and Management of Trauma. Norwalk, CT: Appleton-Century-Crofts, 1987, pp 58–59.
8. Medical Research Council of the United Kingdom: Aids to the Examination of the Peripheral Nervous System. Memorandum no. 45. London: His Majesty's Stationery Office, 1943.
9. Michaelis LS: International inquiry on neurological terminology and prognosis in paraplegia and tetraplegia. Paraplegia 7:1–5, 1969.
10. Nelson PB: Fluid and electrolyte physiology, pathophysiology, and management. In Wirth FP, Racheston RA (eds): Neurosurgical Critical Care. Baltimore: Williams & Wilkins, 1987, p 72.
11. Tator CH, Edmonds VE: Acute spinal cord injury: Analysis of epidemiologic factors. Can J Surg 22:575–578, 1979.
12. Watts CC, Pulliam MW: Problems associated with multiple trauma. In Youmans JR (ed): Neurological Surgery, 2nd ed, vol. 4. Philadelphia: WB Saunders, 1982, pp 2509–2510.
13. Williams CF, Bernstein TW, Jelenko C III: Essentiality of the lateral cervical spine radiograph. Ann Emerg Med 10:198–204, 1981.

12

Spinal Trauma Imaging

CAROLE A. MILLER
AND REBECCA P. BRIGHTMAN

Imaging of the traumatized spine and spinal cord has changed dramatically over the past decade. Plain roentgenograms and tomography have been used for many years to evaluate the injured spine. With the advent of myelography, the spinal subarachnoid space could be directly visualized and thus indirect conclusions about associated damage to the spinal cord could be made.

Computed tomography (CT) of the spine revolutionized the evaluation of trauma. The details of a bony injury and the integrity of the spinal canal and thecal sac could, for the first time, be directly assessed. Contrast-enhanced CT scanning has further defined the extent and significance of canal compromise and neural compression.

Most recently, magnetic resonance imaging (MRI) and now three-dimensional CT have been added to our diagnostic tools. The significance of MRI in the evaluation of spine and spinal cord injury is becoming apparent; however, its full impact has yet to be realized. These newer imaging techniques have enabled us to define more accurately the extent of spine and spinal cord injury and thus aid the clinical management of these patients, particularly as it relates to neurosurgical and orthopedic operative procedures.

The purpose of this chapter is to (1) help the trauma physician in his or her initial radiologic evaluation of the spine-injured patient; (2) point out pitfalls and areas where errors in diagnosis can be avoided; and (3) alert physicians to the newer radiologic techniques available.

PLAIN SPINE FILMS

The initial radiographic evaluation of the traumatized spine in the emergency room is with plain radiographs. A cross-table lateral cervical spine film is absolutely essential in any multiple trauma patient, conscious or unconscious. In several large series of trauma patients none of the alert patients without cervical spine pain were found to have any cervical injury.[1,5] Quadriplegia, however, is such a devastating consequence of a missed cervical fracture that obtaining a cervical spine series may be considered in all trauma patients. Most importantly, it is necessary to see clearly all seven cervical vertebrae. Localization of the area of injury should be done initially with plain radiographs. Only after the area of presumed or actual injury is thus identified does one proceed with other more sophisticated neuroimaging techniques. Importantly, up to two thirds of patients with one spinal fracture will have two or more injuries.[1,5] Therefore additional fractures must be aggressively looked for. A note should be made that all trauma patients should be evaluated and assessed for areas of spine pain by palpation of the entire vertebral column. Other indicators of injury besides local pain include gibbus, prevertebral swelling, and reversal of the normal lordotic curve, particularly in the cervical spine.

The cross-table lateral film shows evidence of fracture in approximately 75% of cervical spine injuries.[20,22] Thus, a cross-table lateral view alone is an inadequate screening film because it leaves an unacceptably high frequency of undetected fractures. With completion of the anteroposterior (AP) and open mouth odontoid views, an additional 10% of cervical fractures will be identified.[22] Trauma obliques of the cervical area often are quite helpful in evaluation of the pedicles, laminae, and neural foramina. All of these films, however, offer only a static view of the cervical spine. In patients with persistent neck pain but without signs of bony injury, controlled flexion and extension views of the cervical spine are mandatory to rule out ligamentous injury and instability. In patients with significant paraspinous muscle spasm full flexion and extension films may not be possible. This spasm is an important physical sign because it is a protective mechanism for the patient. In these cases a period of conservative therapy with repeat dynamic views of the spine may be necessary to demonstrate a ligamentous injury (Fig. 12–1 A, B). Flexion injuries with disruption of the posterior ligamentous complex that are unrecognized and untreated may result in late displacement and even occasional deterioration in neurologic status.[24]

The cervicothoracic junction is often difficult to see with plain films due to the superimposed density of the shoulders. The so-called swimmer's view may be helpful in

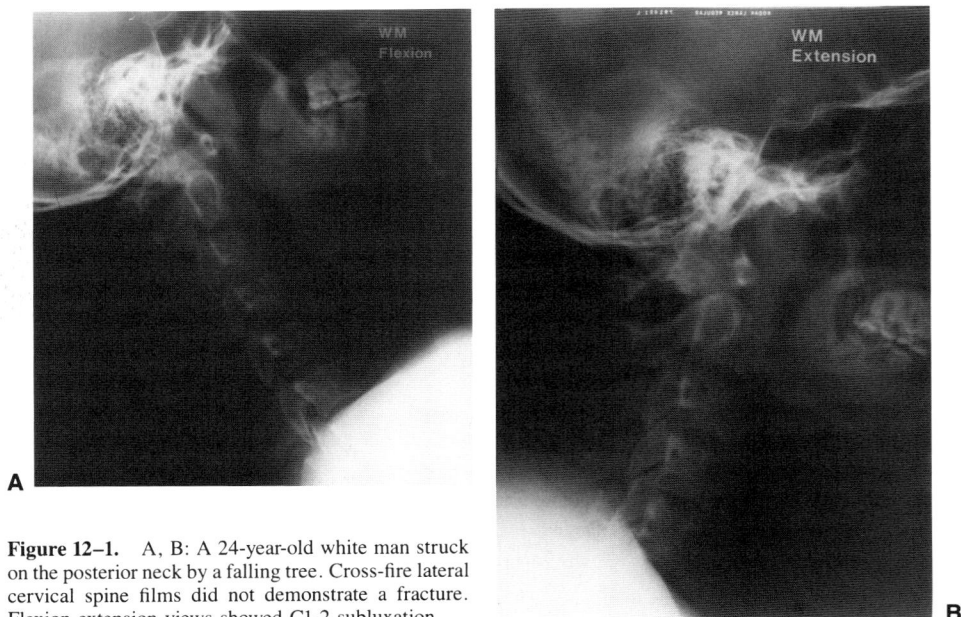

Figure 12–1. A, B: A 24-year-old white man struck on the posterior neck by a falling tree. Cross-fire lateral cervical spine films did not demonstrate a fracture. Flexion-extension views showed C1-2 subluxation.

evaluating this area. In this view, the patient is positioned so that the x-ray beam is directed through one axilla toward the C7-T1 area. Another technique that is especially helpful is to have one person stabilize the patient's head and to have two assistants, one on each arm, pull the patient's arms down. Unless someone is extremely muscular, this will usually provide good visualization of all seven cervical vertebrae. The upper thoracic spine is also notoriously difficult to visualize with plain roentgenograms. In patients with possible thoracic and lumbar spine injuries, cross-table lateral views and AP films must be taken. In the lumbar area, obliques and occasionally flexion and extension films are necessary, as well as spot films of the lumbosacral junction.

Plain films are important in demonstrating the level of spinal injury. However, ligamentous injury is difficult to assess with plain roentgenography alone, and movement x-rays such as flexion-extension may be necessary to demonstrate instability. Also vertebral body fractures with posterior displacement of bony elements into the spinal canal can often be hidden by the pedicle when viewed on a lateral spine film (Fig. 12–2). Posterior neural arch fractures are also difficult to visualize.

TOMOGRAPHY

Multicycloidal tomography has been used as an adjunctive method for evaluation of spinal trauma for many years. Certain areas of the spine, including the cervicomedullary and cervicothoracic junctions and the upper thoracic levels, are often difficult to evaluate by plain spine films. Tomograms of these regions allow visualization of fractures, particularly of the posterior elements, which were previously not well demonstrated.[12] Detail of odontoid fractures is also well seen by tomography (Fig. 12–3 A, B). Tomographic

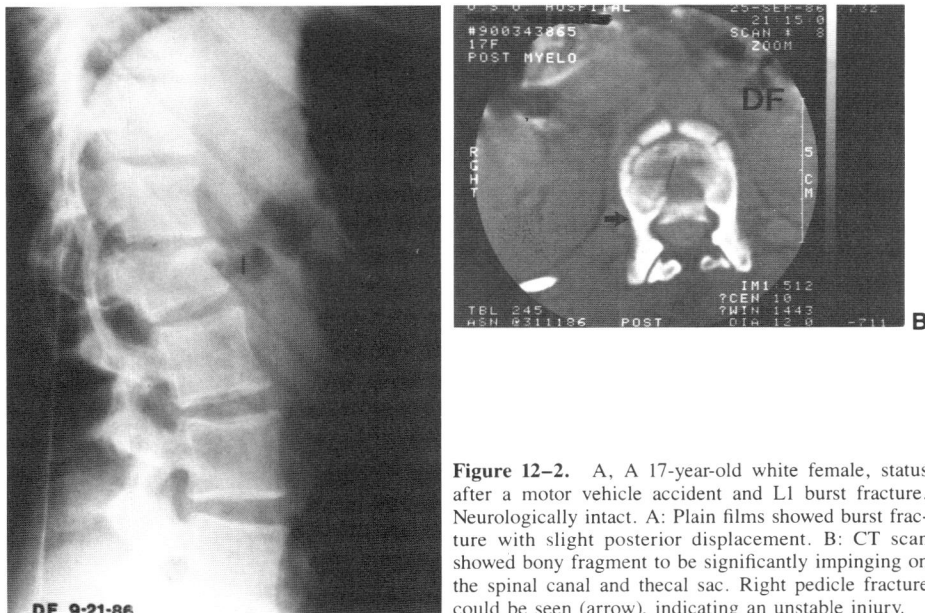

Figure 12–2. A, A 17-year-old white female, status after a motor vehicle accident and L1 burst fracture. Neurologically intact. A: Plain films showed burst fracture with slight posterior displacement. B: CT scan showed bony fragment to be significantly impinging on the spinal canal and thecal sac. Right pedicle fracture could be seen (arrow), indicating an unstable injury.

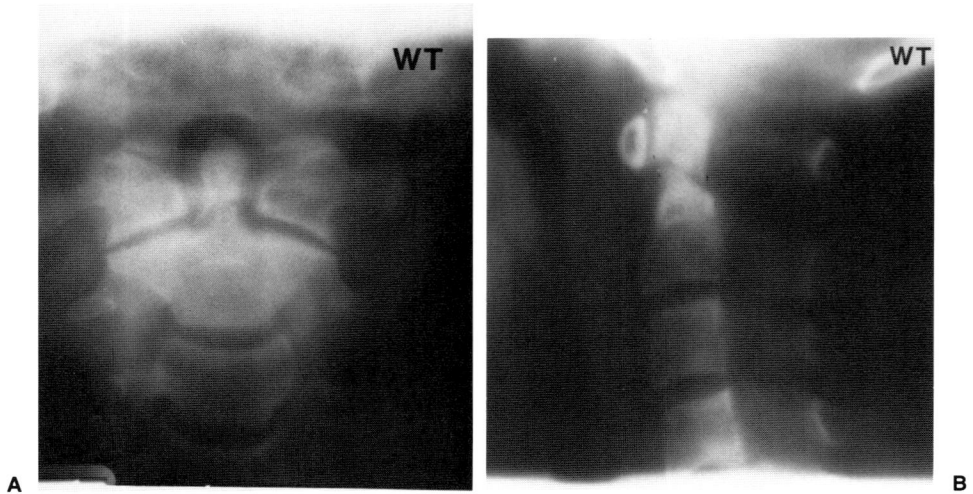

Figure 12–3. A 19-year-old white man, status after a motor vehicle accident with type II odontoid fracture. Anteroposterior (A) and lateral (B) polytomography shows good detail of the fracture and no displacement.

evaluation of the injured spine, however, requires significant manipulation of the patient with the risk of further instability, neural damage, and often severe pain. Importantly, if a position causes pain, the radiologist and other physicians must stop and reevaluate the patient's neurologic status. This increased pain may be heralding a progression in neurologic deficit. Listen to the patient!

Before CT, thin section tomography was extremely useful in revealing additional fractures not seen on plain films. In centers where CT scanning is available, however, it has virtually replaced conventional multidirectional tomography due to its ability to image the patient without significant manipulation.

MYELOGRAPHY

The use of myelography in spinal trauma has primarily been to evaluate the patency of the subarachnoid space. Lateral cervical puncture for myelography in trauma was introduced by Kelly and Alexander.[9] Other investigators have utilized this technique with both Pantopaque and metrizamide injections.[3] With this technique, a C1-2 puncture is performed in a supine patient and the dye is injected into the cervical subarachnoid space. Failure of passage of the dye column past the level of injury indicates block of the subarachnoid space. This, however, is a nonspecific finding. It can be interpreted as due to bony fragments in the canal, epidural hemorrhage, widening of the cord at the level of impingement, or an acutely herniated disk. Differentiation between these various causes of block is occasionally difficult. A lacerated dura can also sometimes be identified by the extravasation of dye during myelography, and root avulsions can be seen.

A recent advance in myelography is the introduction of the water-soluble contrast materials, which are much less likely to produce arachnoiditis than the oil-based materials, such as Pantopaque. Better anatomic detail generally is possible with the water-soluble materials, and there is no danger of depositing a permanent oil-based radiopaque material in the posterior fossa. The water-soluble compounds have caused occasional seizures concentrations have lowed intracranially. The intrathecal ingestion of contrast material is frequently followed by CT. Using this technique of thecal sac opacification, one often gains additional information about the thecal sac and the neural elements.

In centers were MRI is readily available, it may replace myelography in the acute spine-injured patient, since it is less invasive and more informative. However, in an unstable patient with multiple injuries, plain radiographs followed by myelography and CT scanning is a quick and relatively easy way to evaluate the patency of the spinal canal. The introduction and more frequent use of C2 myelography have made this procedure in the trauma patient much safer and more rapid, since it does not require manipulation of the patient in order to evaluate the spinal canal.

COMPUTED TOMOGRAPHY

Computerized axial tomography was introduced commercially in 1972 and was in use clinically soon thereafter. The first CT of the spine was done in 1978.[18] Since then, spinal CT scanning has revolutionized the evaluation of the injured spine. It provides a safe and accurate radiologic technique and is now considered essential in the evaluation and treatment of vertebral fractures.

Standard radiographs can identify areas of injury and correctly assess the amount that a vertebral body has been compressed. However, they do not consistently evaluate damage to the posterior elements or involvement of the neural canal. Keene et al.[8] found that in approximately 20% of their patients with posterior element fractures the extent of the injury could not be determined from standard radiographs. They also found that in 40% of their patients estimates of the amount of compromise of the neural canal using standard radiographs differed by at least 20% from those made from computed axial tomography scans.

Contrast enhancement of the spinal canal with subsequent CT scanning has a limited but important place in the evaluation of the injured spine. Better definition of the thecal sac and any encroachment from bone, blood, or disk can be evaluated best with contrast-enhanced CT scans (Fig. 12–2 B). In addition, dural tears can be identified with extravasation of the dye seen on CT scan.

It has been thought that polytomography demonstrates a greater number of posterior elements than CT scanning. However, experience with improved scanning techniques using scanners capable of providing 2 mm thick axial sections and sagittal and coronal reconstructions has allowed improved detection and definition of fractures.[2] This is especially true of those fractures that occur parallel to the scanning plane. CT scanning is also superior to polytomography for evaluation of the neural canal. Using conventional polytomography, the patency of the neural canal cannot accurately be evaluated if only AP tomograms are available for interpretation. When anterior, posterior, and lateral tomograms are obtained, there is sufficient information to estimate the degree of compromise; however, the estimates obtained in this manner differ by approximately 20% or more from those based on a computerized scan.[8] CT scanning is also preferred because it poses less potential danger to the patient with a spine injury. For lateral tomography, the patient must be placed in the lateral decubitus position. This change in position subjects anyone with an unstable or potentially unstable fracture of the spine to a greater risk of spinal cord or nerve root injury.

Also, combined anterior, posterior, and lateral polytomography exposes the patient to ten times the radiation exposure needed for CT.[8] It should be noted, however, that this comparison of exposure is based solely on the average radiation received at the skin.

Computed axial tomography of the spine in the trauma patient often provides important information regarding paraspinous structures, such as kidney, liver, spleen, and lung as well as paravertebral hematomas. Additionally, it is convenient to combine spinal CT scans with CT of the abdomen, chest, or head without moving the patient.

We, and others, have found the CT scan particularly helpful in the evaluation of fractures of the thoracic and lumbar spine and specifically the thoracolumbar junction.[13] Burst fractures in this area usually involve the superior posterior margin of the vertebral body and the retropulsed fragment is often hidden between the pedicles on lateral spine films. The compromise of the neural canal as seen with plain radiographs is sometimes quite deceptive and the degree of angulation of the spinal column is not necessarily consistent with the degree of retropulsion and compression of the neural elements. Although axial CT has thus become standard in the management of patients with spinal trauma (Fig. 12–2 B), limitations of spinal CT in traumatic injuries exist. Abnormalities that occur in the axial plane may not be evident on CT scan, including horizontal and compression fractures as well as distraction injuries.[7] Subluxations may also be difficult to identify. In these cases, fine quality sagittal reconstructions are crucial.

Medical imaging combined with computer graphics now allows us to generate high-resolution quality three-dimensional images of the skull and vertebral column. Using the GE 3D83 software package in current CT scanners, selected anatomic features can be displayed in a three-dimensional manner to create a realistic picture of the desired spinal unit.[6] Completed reconstructions may be displayed on the computer screen at any angle desired. We have found this new technique to be of benefit in evaluating spinal trauma, since it has the ability to image occult lesions that are often not adequately defined by conventional radiographic means (Fig. 12–4). The ability to construct an accurate 3-dimensional picture of a pathologic area of the spine allows better appreciation by the surgeon of the extent of the injury. This noninvasive method may eventually replace other invasive and less precise imaging techniques. Additionally, a CT scan obtained acutely on the spine-injured patient can later be reconstructed and reformatted into a three-dimensional image.

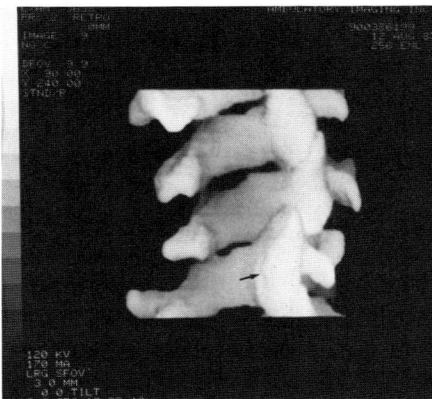

Figure 12–4. A 16-year-old white male, status after a motor vehicle accident with C4 quadriplegia and C4-5 subluxation on plain films. Three-dimensional CT scan shows unilateral jumped facet with fractured superior articular process of C5 (arrow).

MAGNETIC RESONANCE IMAGING

MRI has added a new dimension to the evaluation of the traumatized spinal column and neural elements. Magnetic resonance has been used in analytic chemistry since 1946. It was not until the early 1970s, however, that crude anatomic images were first produced by Lauterbur.[10] Images are created by manipulating the naturally occurring magnetic properties of the nucleus by man-made magnetic fields. The inherent differences in tissue chemistry are reflected by differences in intensity and distribution of the magnetic resonance signal produced.[16] These different signals allow anatomic images to be produced. Tissue contrast can be controlled by the operator through changes in the pulse sequences used.

Early clinical use of MRI in evaluation of trauma to the spinal column and the craniovertebral junction has been very rewarding.[14] With the introduction of surface coils, allowing an increased signal-to-noise ratio, improved images of spinal structures and pathologic conditions can be obtained. The entire length of the spinal cord and cervicomedullary junction, as well as their longitudinal relationship with structures in the posterior fossa, can now for the first time be directly imaged in any plane. Bony artifact is absent. The use of intrathecal contrast materials or ionizing radiation is eliminated. The noninvasive nature of MRI and the lack of known biologic hazards of current magnetic field strength and radiofrequency pulse sequences allow increased patient tolerance.

MRI is clinically useful in spinal trauma for several reasons. First, it gives excellent information concerning spinal cord integrity and edema (Fig. 12–5).[16] Spinal cord parenchyma and its architecture can be directly evaluated with MRI. Axial scans can delineate the butterfly-shaped central gray matter of the normal cord.[4] Recognition of central hemorrhagic necrosis in patients with hyperextension injuries and clinical central cord syndrome is thus possible, since edema and hemorrhage into the cord distorts this architecture. Follow-up examination of patients with cord trauma is also useful because changes in cord edema can readily be diagnosed by MRI. Ascending cord swelling, as in the case of the patient in Figure 12–5, can be directly seen on sagittal images and this knowledge may change the clinical management. Since MRI is superior in the detection of intramedullary pathologic conditions, it is invaluable in the evaluation of patients with progressive deficits after operative intervention. Additionally, it allows us to detect cystic intramedullary abnor-

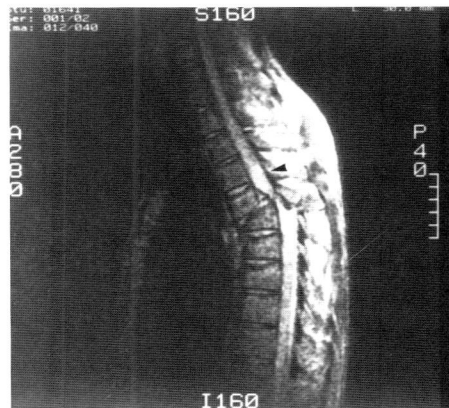

Figure 12–5. A 17-year-old white male, status after a sledding accident with T3-4 fracture, subluxation, and complete paraplegia. Tingling up to C8 dermatome. MRI shows total spinal cord transection with cord edema above level of injury (arrowhead).

malities and differentiate between myelomalacia and syrinx formation in the injured cord.[19] MRI has become the radiologic procedure of choice for evaluation of syringomyelia because it allows for excellent delineation of the cranial and caudal extent of the syrinx.[20]

Soft tissue injuries in the form of ligamentous disruption can also be identified by MRI.[14] Evaluation of the integrity of the anterior and posterior longitudinal ligaments is possible with MRI and is especially important. These ligaments can be seen as signal voids along the border of the vertebral bodies and disks. As they travel over the vertebral bodies, the image blends with the cortex of the bone but can be well seen over the margin of the high signal disk. Disruption of these ligaments has a significant impact on the stability of the spinal column and knowledge of this may alter the clinical and surgical management of the patient (Fig. 12–6) This is particularly true in the thoracolumbar region where McArdle et al.[14] have recently shown MRI to be useful in assessing patients with acute and chronic thoracolumbar injuries. We have found this particularly true in the acute situation when the integrity of the ligaments and stability of the fracture is of utmost importance. Additionally, damage to the ligamentum flavum, interspinous and supraspinous ligaments also can be seen and this knowledge will add to the evaluation of the stability of that spinal segment.

Magnetic resonance also provides more comprehensive information concerning the degree of subarachnoid space narrowing and actual spinal cord compression than does conventional CT. Important data concerning the patency of the epidural and subarachnoid spaces, which have previously been available only through invasive procedures, can be obtained by MRI. Intervertebral disk protrusions or extrusions associated with trauma are best evaluated by MRI in the acute traumatic injury (Fig. 12–7 A, B, C).[23] As previously mentioned, the cause of anterior cord compression after trauma is difficult to determine with myelography alone. Even a CT scan, although more specific, cannot always differentiate between traumatic disk herniation and epidural hemorrhage. The presence and extent of epidural hematomas, which may be responsible for cord compression, are clearly shown with magnetic resonance. Imaging of bony fractures is also possible with MRI, particularly in the thoracolumbar and lumbar spine with its large amount of contrasting epidural fat. In the cervical spine it is at times difficult to visualize directly fractures of the posterior elements because the small bones, and the paucity of fat surrounding the neural arches provide little contrast. For the present, CT scanning provides the most precise method for accurately visualizing all fracture lines.

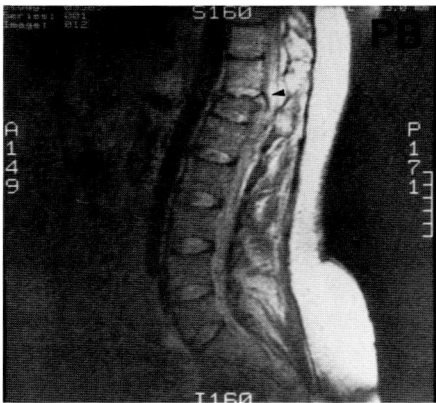

Figure 12–6. A 44-year-old white woman, status after a motor vehicle accident and T12 burst fracture. MRI shows disrupted anterior (arrow) and posterior (arrowhead) longitudinal ligaments. Ligaments appear as signal voids traveling over bony cortex and disk space. Anterolateral operative decompression confirmed that the posterior bony fragment was attached to the torn posterior ligament.

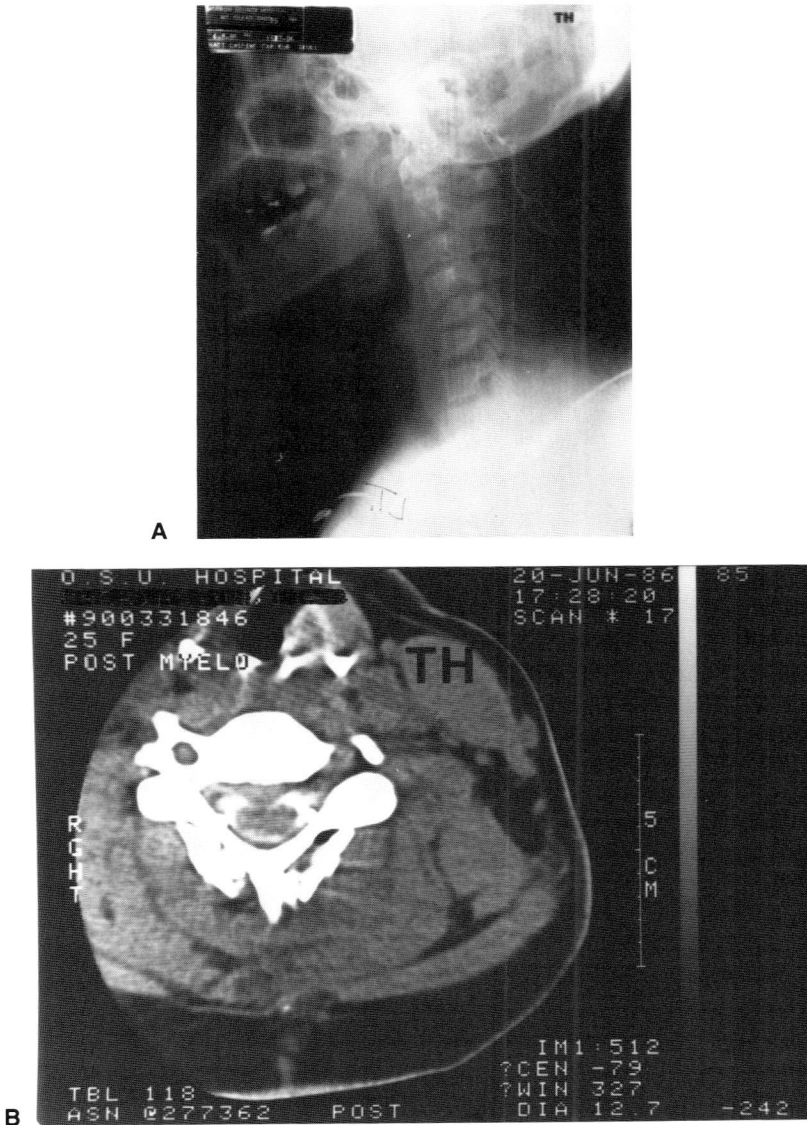

Figure 12–7. A 25-year-old white woman, status after a diving accident with immediate, complete quadriplegia. A: Spine films showed C4-5 subluxation. B: CT scan with intrathecal contrast showed ventral extradural mass. (Figure continued on next page)

The major limitations of MRI in the trauma setting are in the severely injured patient who requires intubation or other mechanical and metal devices in and around his body for support. These life-support devices contain many ferromagnetic materials that cannot remain in the room with the magnet. In many institutions, another limiting factor is simply the location of the MR scanner in relation to the emergency room.

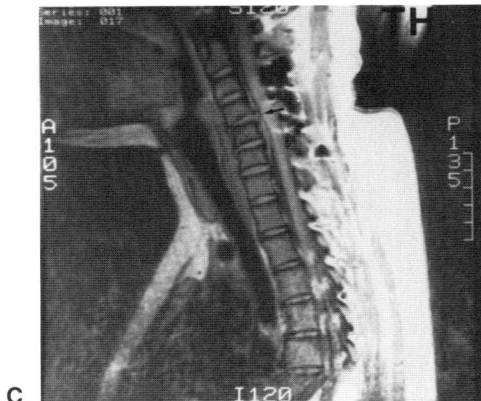

Figure 12–7, cont. C: MRI confirmed traumatic disk rupture (arrow) with epidural hemorrhage. Spinal cord is not significantly encroached on.

Although clinical experience with MRI in trauma is limited at the present time, we believe that it is rapidly establishing itself as one of the primary imaging modalities in the evaluation of pathologic conditions of the injured spine. Unfortunately, most MRI suites are not presently equipped to image patients with multisystem injuries who require complex life-support equipment.

RADIOLOGIC ASSESSMENT

Our recommendations for patients with suspected spinal injuries are that they be assessed in the following manner. An algorithm incorporating these recommendations is outlined in Figure 12–8. First, standard AP and lateral radiographs should be taken to establish whether

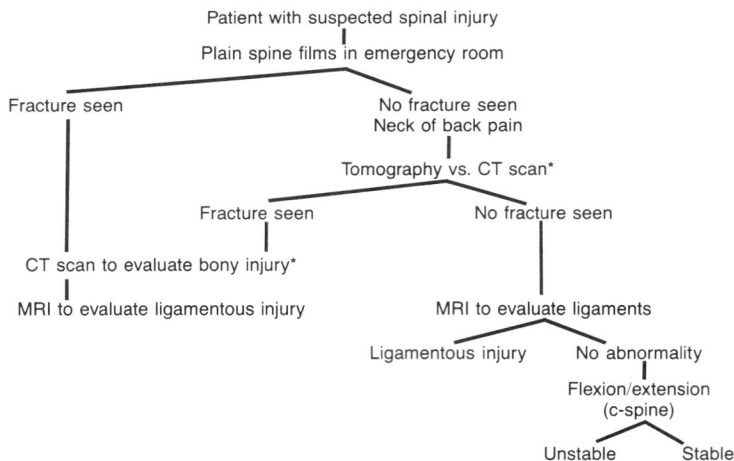

Figure 8. Algorithm for radiographic evaluation of patients with suspected spinal injury. *Three-dimensional CT may aid in presurgical evaluation.

a fracture has occurred. If a vertebral injury is demonstrated, additional plain films, including views of the injured segment or segments, should be taken. We, like others, have found that these supplemental radiographs improve the accuracy of standard radiography. Second, axial CT should be obtained to evaluate further the neural canal and posterior elements. Conventional tomograms may be performed if a CT scanner is not available or if a fracture line in the transverse plane is suspected but not demonstrated on the standard radiographs or CT scans. Water-soluble myelography is a worthwhile addition if the patient's neurologic deficit is not consistent with the level of the vertebral injury seen on the plain radiographs and CT scans. Dural lacerations also can be diagnosed with this technique. Finally, an MR scan should be done in the medically stable patient to evaluate the extent of spinal cord damage and ligamentous injury.

In a patient with persistent spine pain, if no fracture or ligamentous injury is seen with the imaging techniques just mentioned, flexion and extension views should be performed. Repeated clinical and radiographic evaluation should be performed in the symptomatic patient to ensure that no significant spinal injury goes unnoticed.

CONCLUSION

The radiologic evaluation of the spine-injured patient has become quite complex. Plain spine films remain important in initial evaluation but are frequently supplemented by tomography, myelography, and CT scanning. The superior depiction of bony detail with CT allows clear demonstration of fracture lines and is particularly important in the assessment of posterior neural arch lesions. MRI, when available, contributes a great deal of additional information about spinal cord parenchyma and vertebral column ligaments. For the first time, direct evidence of spinal stability is available. MRI is quickly becoming invaluable in the clinical and surgical decision-making process.

With a multitude of new imaging techniques available, the physician must devise his own decision tree to evaluate the spine-injured patient. This should be based on the medical stability of the patient and his neurologic status. The physician's past experience with these techniques as well as the availability of the necessary technology are also essential factors.

REFERENCES

1. Bachulis BL, Long WB, Hynes GD, Johnson MC: Clinical indications for cervical spine radiographs in the traumatized patient. Am J Surg 153:473–478, 1987.
2. Cacayorin ED, Kieffer SA: Applications and limitations of computed tomography of the spine. Radiol Clin North Am 10:185–206, 1982.
3. Carol M, Ducker TB, Byrnes DP: Minimyelogram in cervical spinal cord trauma. Neurosurgery 7:219–224, 1980.
4. Chakeres DW, Flickinger F, Breshnahan JC, Beattie MS, Weiss KL, Miller CA, Stokes BT: MR imaging of acute spinal cord trauma. AJNR 8:5–10, 1987.
5. Fischer RP: Cervical radiographic evaluation of alert patients following blunt trauma. Ann Emerg Med 13: 905–907, 1984
6. Hadley MN, Sonntag VKH, Amos MR, Hodak JA, Lopez LJ: Three-dimensional computed tomography in the diagnosis of vertebral column pathological conditions. Neurosurgery 21:186–192, 1987.
7. Handel SF, Lee Y: Computed tomography of spinal fractures. Radiol Clin North Am 19:69–89, 1981.
8. Keene JS, Goletz TH, Lilleas F, Alter AJ, Sackett JF: Diagnosis of vertebral fractures. A comparison of conventional radiography, conventional tomography and computed axial tomography. J Bone Joint Surg 64A: 586–595, 1982.

9. Kelly DL, Alexander E: Lateral cervical puncture for myelography, Technical note. J Neurosurg 29:106–110, 1968.

10. Lauterbur PC: Image formation by induced local interactions: Examples employing nuclear magnetic resonance. Nature 242:190–191, 1973.

11. Leo JS, Bergeron RT, Kricheff II, Benjamin MV: Metrizamide myelography for cervical spinal cord injuries. Neuroradiology 129:707–711, 1978.

12. Maravilla KR, Cooper PR, Sklar FH: The influence of thin-section tomography on the treatment of cervical spine injuries. Diagn Radiol 127:131–139, 1978.

13. McAfee PC, Yaun HA, Fredrickson BE, Lubicky JP: The value of computed tomography in thoracolumbar fracture. J Bone Joint Surg 65A:461–473, 1983.

14. McArdle CB, Crofford MJ, Mirfakhraee M, Amparo EG, Calhoun JS: Surface coil MR of spinal trauma: Preliminary experience. AJNR 7:885–893, 1986.

15. Miller MD, Gehweiler JA, Martinez S, Charlton OP, Daffner RH: Significant new observations on cervical spine trauma. AJR 130:659–663, 1978.

16. Modic MT, Hardy RW, Weinstein MA, Duchesneau PM, Paushter DM, Boumphrey F: Nuclear magnetic resonance of the spine: Clinical potential and limitation. Neurosurgery 15:583–592, 1984.

17. Norman D, Mills CM, Brant-Zawadzki M, Yeates A, Crooks LE, Kaufman L: Magnetic resonance imaging of the spinal cord and canal: Potentials and limitation. AJNR 5:9–14, 1984.

18. Nykamp PW, Levy JM, Christensen F, Dunn R, Hubbard J: Computed tomography for bursting fracture of the lumbar spine. Report of a case. J Bone Joint Surg 60A:1108–1109, 1978.

19. Quencer RM, Sheldon JJ, Post MJD, Diaz RD, Montaivo BM, Green BA, Eismont FJ: MRI of the chronically injured cervical spinal cord. AJR 147:125–132, 1986.

20. Shaffer MA, Doris PE: Limitation of the cross table lateral view in detecting cervical spine injuries: A retrospective analysis. Ann Emerg Med 10:508–513, 1981.

21. Sherman JL, Barkovich AJ, Citrin CM: The MR appearance of syringomyelia: New observations. AJNR 7: 985–995, 1986.

22. Streitwieser DR, Knopp R, Wales LR, Williams JL, Tonnemacher K: Accuracy of standard radiographic views in detecting cervical spine fractures. Ann Emerg Med 12:538–542, 1983.

23. Tarr RW, Drolshagen LF, Kerner TC, Allen JH, Partain CL, James AE: MR imaging of recent spinal trauma. J Comput Assist Tomogr 11:412–417, 1987.

24. Webb JK, Broughton RBK, McSweeney T, Park WM: Hidden flexion injury of the cervical spine. J Bone Joint Surg 58B:322–327, 1976.

13

Post-Traumatic Spinal Instability

SANFORD J. LARSON

For the vertebral column, stability and immobility are not synonymous, although immobility may become necessary to achieve stability. The normal vertebral column can be flexed, extended, bent laterally, and rotated with different degrees of freedom at different levels. The spinal canal becomes longer in flexion and shorter in extension. The cross-sectional area is reduced during extension because of inward bulging of the anulus fibrosis, the yellow ligaments, and the dura. The spinal cord and roots have a fixed volume, and therefore adapt to changing dimensions of the spinal canal during motion, becoming longer and thinner in flexion and shorter and thicker in extension.[1] If the physiologic limits of motion are exceeded, the spinal cord is at risk, since it may not be able to tolerate an abnormal increase in length, or a decrease in cross-sectional area of the spinal canal.

If a force applied to the spinal column is sufficient to cause structural change, the spinal cord and roots can be injured in either or both of two ways: by transfer of energy at the moment of impact and by deformity that may be persistent. Although little can be done about neural changes secondary to energy transfer, further deformity of the spinal cord can be prevented, and at an appropriate time the deformity can be relieved.

Many patients with injury to the vertebral column have associated injuries that demand prompt treatment and take precedence over the vertebral lesion. If this involves moving and positioning the patient for surgery, it becomes important to know whether or not the spinal column is stable. Identification of instability is also important in determining when the patient can be allowed up with or without an orthosis, and whether surgical treatment is necessary. Post-traumatic spinal instability can be defined as osseous and ligamentous injury sufficient to allow progressive vertebral malalignment under physiologic loads. In most instances, this requires damage to both neural arch and vertebral body or related ligamentous elements.[3] Instability does not necessarily require surgical treatment, but it is an indication for appropriate immobilization to prevent injury to the spinal cord and roots secondary to the development or progression of malalignment.

Patients with stable fractures can be moved and positioned as necessary for a surgical procedure. They may need an orthosis when not recumbent primarily for comfort and secondarily as a precaution. Those with unstable fractures that can be expected to heal with immobilization should be maintained in the neutral position while recumbent and can be up and about in an orthosis. Patients with higly unstable fractures require great care when moved for diagnostic and surgical procedures and need internal fixation as well as external splinting before they can be allowed up.

The deformity produced by a load depends on the direction in which it is applied relative to the vertebral column. A compressive force applied axially is, except at C1, largely absorbed by the vertebral body, which becomes shortened vertically but expanded circumferentially in a relatively symmetrical fashion (Fig. 13–1). If the posterior elements remain

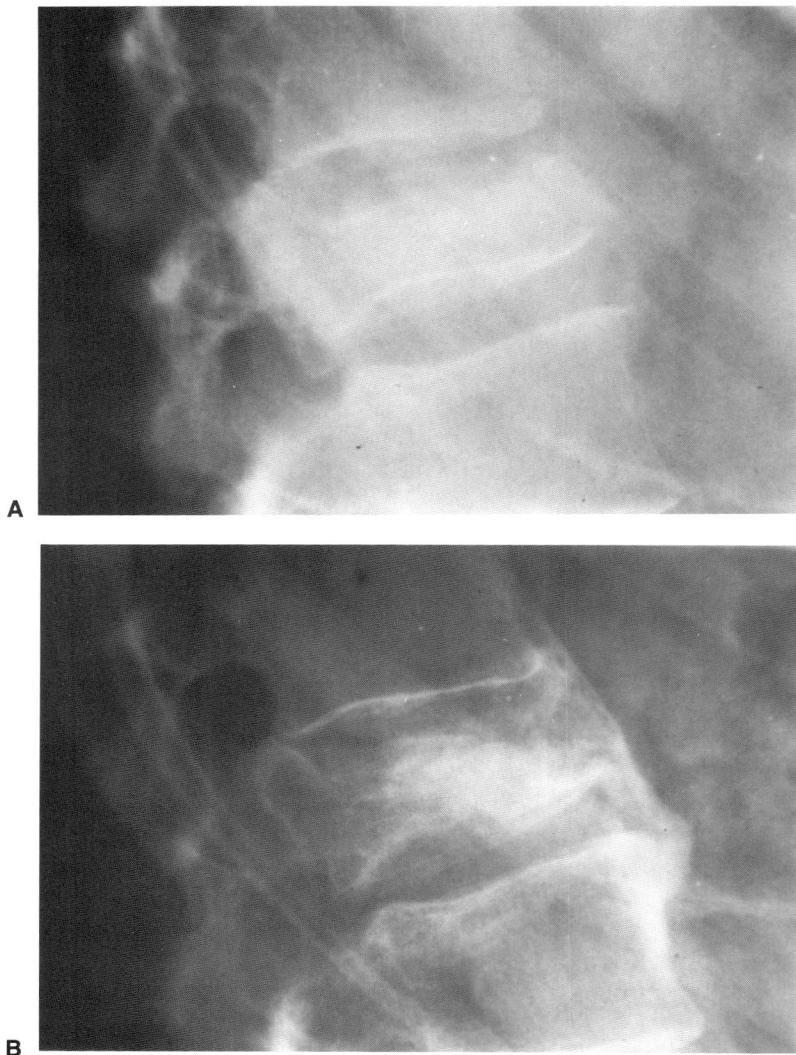

Figure 13–1.   A: The patient with this burst fracture of L1 had a mild neurologic deficit that cleared within a few days. From Larson.[5] (Reprinted with permission.) B: Same patient 3 years later. He was neurologically normal and without symptoms. (From Larson.[5] Reprinted with Permission.)

intact the fracture is stable, and further deformity would not be anticipated unless a load is applied exceeding that which produced the fracture. At C1, because the vertebral body is absent, the load falls on the medially directed, wedge-shaped articular pillars of the atlas and tends to separate them. If fracture occurs, it is through the anterior and posterior portions of the C1 ring with lateral displacement of one or both of the C1 articular pillars (Fig. 13–2). This lateral displacement may cause avulsion or rupture of the transverse atlantal ligament.[4] Since this would permit anterior displacement of C1 on C2, the fracture is unstable. Axial forces applied in distraction pull the vertebrae apart, producing circumferential disruption. These injuries usually occur in pedestrians struck by rapidly moving vehicles. The acceleration of the body relative to the head ordinarily results in atlanto-occipital separation (Fig. 13–3 A), but separation occasionally occurs at a lower level (Fig. 13–3 B). Skeletal traction should not be used; it not only might increase the distraction, but would also oppose the reflex contraction of the muscles, which can effect reduction. Because these lesions are highly unstable, the patient is kept recumbent in an orthosis until fusion can be performed.

In flexion and compression the force is not distributed uniformly, but is concentrated anteriorly, producing anterior wedging of the vertebral body (Fig. 13–4 A). A portion of the vertebral body may be displaced posteriorly into the spinal canal (Fig. 13–4 B). If the posterior elements remain intact (Fig. 13–4 B, C), further deformity should not occur under physiologic loads and the fracture can be considered stable (Fig. 13–4 D). However, if the axis of rotation is located more anteriorly in the vertebral body, there may be distraction posteriorly with disruption of the neural arch (Fig. 13–4 E). If the posterior elements are disrupted (Fig. 13–4 E, F, G), then progressive deformity can be anticipated, since flexion is not adequately opposed.

Pure flexion produces ligamentous injuries[2] without significant changes in bone (Fig. 13–5). Separation of the spinous processes implies rupture of the interspinous ligament, injury to the joint capsules, the posterior longitudinal ligament, and anulus. Even slight separation of the spinous processes and slight subluxation may be significant, especially

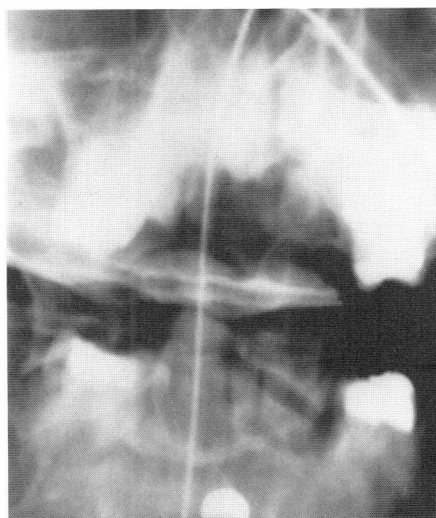

Figure 13–2. Anteroposterior view of a C1 fracture produced by an axial load. The right articular pillar of C1 is displaced laterally.

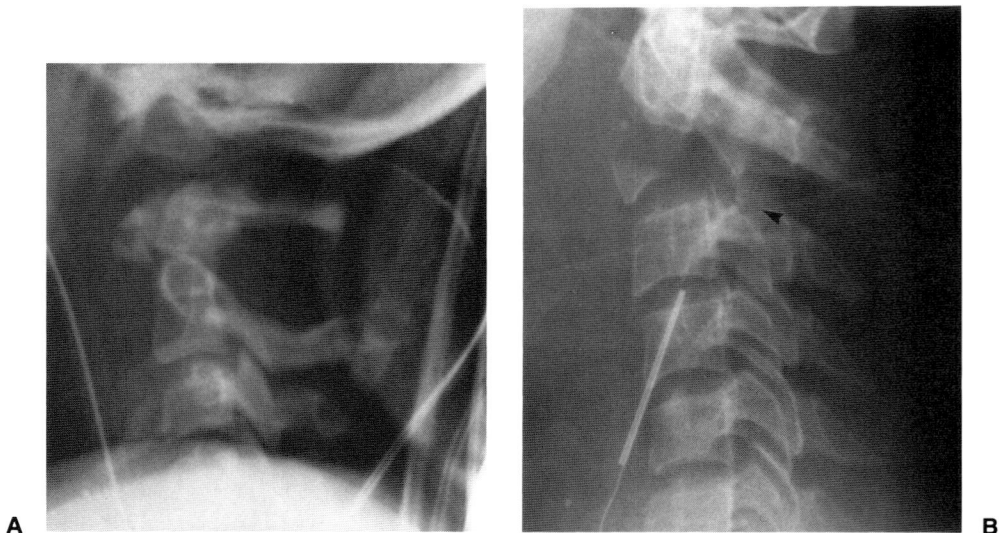

Figure 13–3.   A: Lateral film from a pedestrian struck by a motor vehicle. The occiput is separated from C1, and the anterior portion of C1 is fractured transversely. The spinal cord function was normal. B: Circumferential disruption at C2-C3 in a pedestrian struck by a motor vehicle. The C2-C3 facets are separated (arrow). The patient recovered from an incomplete myelopathy after postural reduction followed by posterior fusion of C2 and C3.

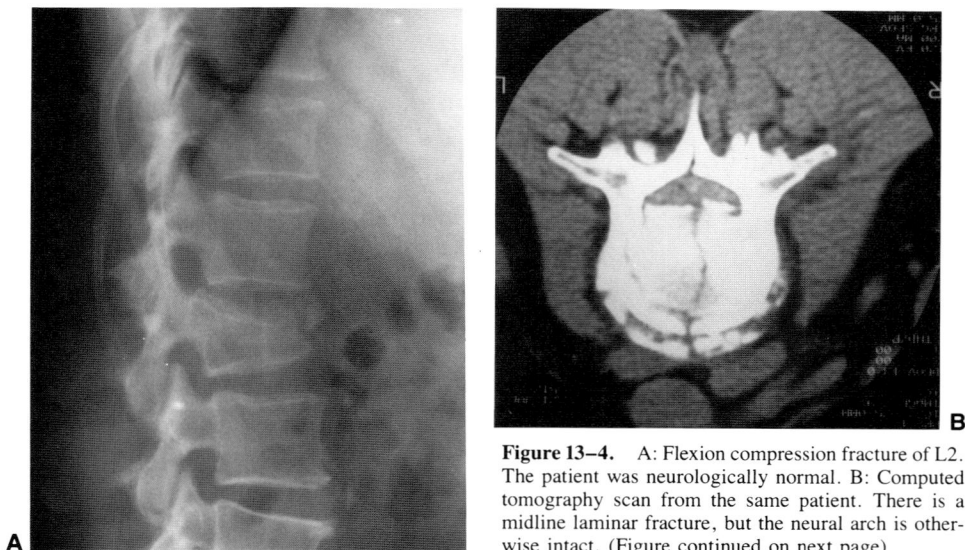

Figure 13–4.   A: Flexion compression fracture of L2. The patient was neurologically normal. B: Computed tomography scan from the same patient. There is a midline laminar fracture, but the neural arch is otherwise intact. (Figure continued on next page)

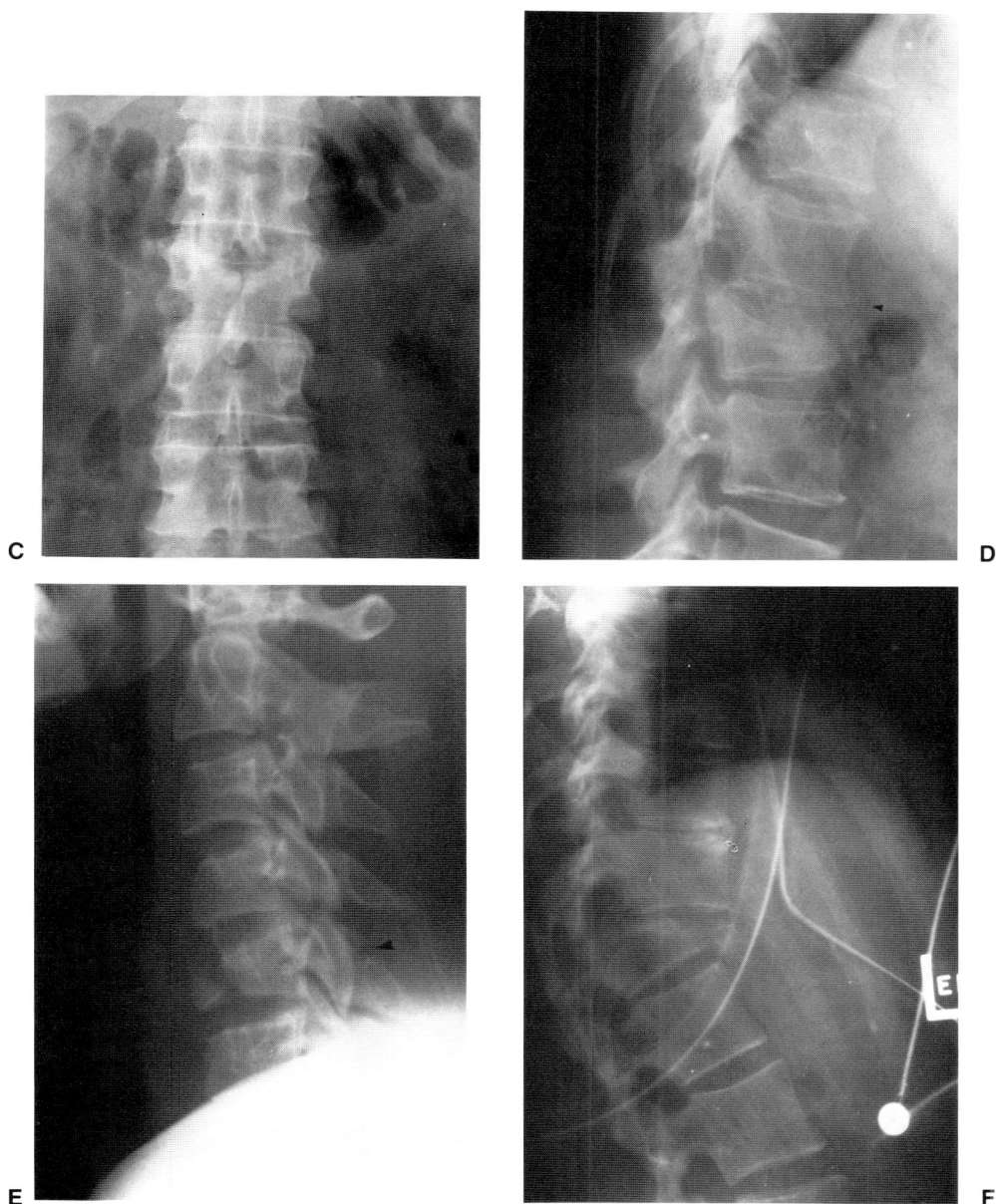

Figure 13–4, cont. C: Anteroposterior view in the same patient demonstrating intact pedicles and normal interspinous process distances. D: Neurologic function remained normal. E: A cervical flexion compression injury with posterior disruption (arrow). F: A thoracic flexion compression injury with an element of shear and anterior and posterior disruption. (Figure continued on next page)

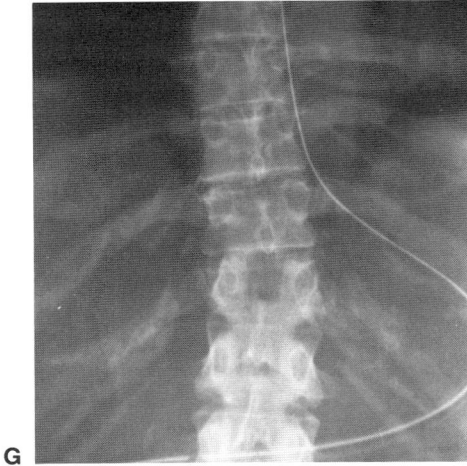

Figure 13–4, cont. G: Same patient as in Figure 4F demonstrating separation of the T11 and T12 spinous processes.

G

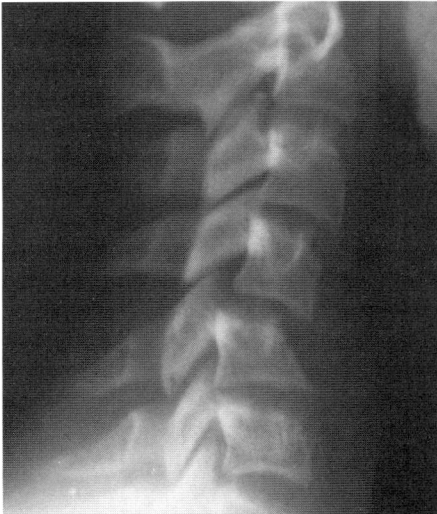

Figure 13–5. Flexion injury with anterior and posterior ligamentous disruption. The spinous processes of C4 and C5 are separated, a space exists between the superior processes of C5 and the posterior inferior surface of the C4 body, and C4 is displaced anteriorly.

when motion of the spinal column is limited by muscle spasm and pain and the actual extent of ligamentous injury cannot be demonstrated by flexion or extension films.[8] The disruption of these posterior ligamentous elements permits progressive flexion deformity (Fig. 13–6 A, B).

Flexion and distraction in the cervical portion of the vertebral column can cause bilateral locked facets (Fig. 13–7). Here the movement of the articular processes allows the anterior and superior edges of the lower facets to clear the posterior and inferior edges of the upper facets. With reflex contraction of the extensor muscles, the inferior facets of the upper vertebra become locked anterior to the superior processes of the lower vertebra. Because of the circumferential disruption of the ligaments and anulus, this is a highly unstable lesion. Only muscle contraction holds the vertebral bodies in apposition, and excessive skeletal

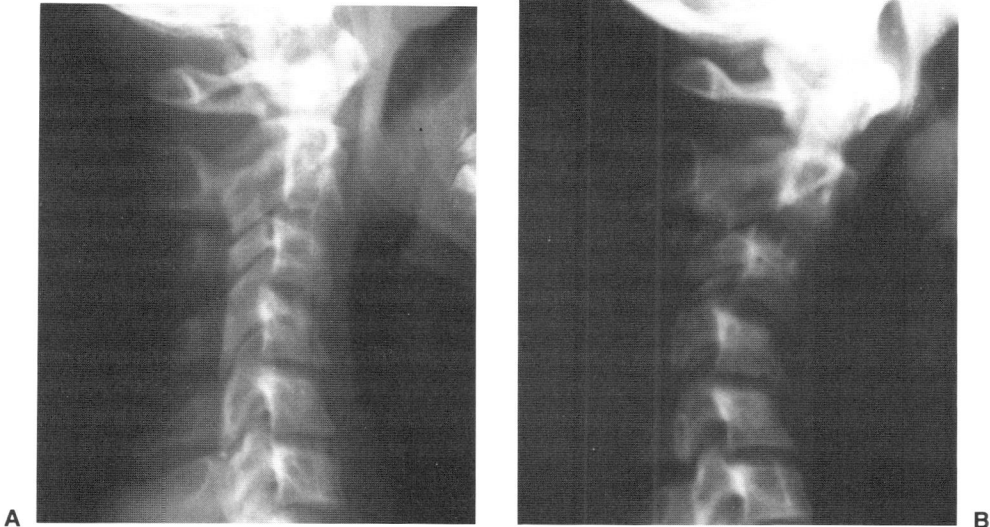

Figure 13–6. A: Films taken shortly after a flexion injury. Very little motion had been demonstrated on flexion-extension films. B: Same patient 3 weeks later.

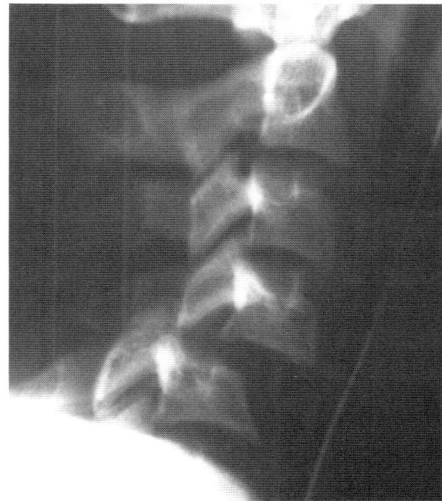

Figure 13–7. Lateral films demonstrating bilaterally locked facets.

traction may result in distraction of the vertebral bodies with increased neurologic deficit.[6] In the thoracolumbar area, flexion-distraction injuries produce the Chance fracture and its variants. The separation begins posteriorly in the spinous process or interspinous ligament and moves anteriorly through the pedicles and vertebral bodies or disk (Fig. 13–8 A, B). The Chance fracture is an unstable lesion, since flexion forces will not be adequately resisted.

In the cervical region, because of the orientation of the facets, rotational movement is coupled with lateral movement. For example, if the head and neck are rotated to the right, the

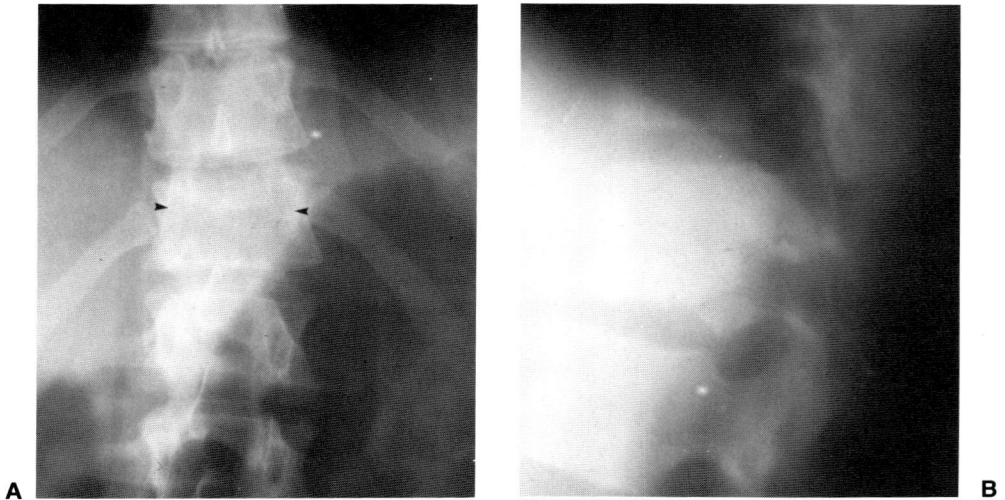

Figure 13–8.   A: Flexion-distraction injury with fractures through the pedicles (arrows). The T12-L1 interpedicular distance is greater than normal. B: Lateral polytomogram demonstrating the fracture through the T12 pedicle and vertebral body.

inferior facets move caudally on the right and rostrally on the left, the vertebral column tilting to the right as it rotates. This combination of movement brings the posterior and inferior edge of a left facet progressively closer to the anterior and superior edge of the subjacent facet, and with sufficient rotation, the upper facet clears the lower and becomes locked anterior to it by reflex muscle contraction (Fig. 13–9 A, B). Because of the associated soft tissue disruption, this is usually considered an unstable lesion. In the thoracolumbar area, rotation produces the slice fracture.[2] This fracture usually occurs in the vicinity of the transitional vertebra, which has a horizontal thoracic type superior articular process and a more vertical lumbar type inferior process. The transitional vertebra is usually either the 11th or the 12th thoracic vertebrae. Rotational movement of the transitional vertebra is blocked by contact between its vertically oriented inferior articular process and the superior facet of the vertebra below it. With sufficient force, a fracture occurs either through the pedicle or sometimes through the vertebral body with displacement of the facet and transverse process of the inferior vertebra laterally.[5] Usually, the superior portion of the inferior vertebra remains attached to the rotating transitional vertebra (Fig. 13–10). Because disruption is circumferential, this is a particularly unstable lesion, even though alignment may appear good while the patient is recumbent.[3]

In the cervical spine, only C2 has a pars interarticularis. With sufficient extension force, the fracture occurs through the pars. This is not a highly unstable lesion, but spondylolisthesis is possible and therefore immobilization is required until healing takes place. However, if the anterior longitudinal ligament and the anulus have been disrupted (Fig. 13–11) by hyperextension, the instability is much greater, and more rigorous immobilization is necessary. In the other cervical vertebrae, extension produces fractures through the pedicle, which can be either unilateral (Fig. 13–12 A, B, C) or bilateral. For this to occur, the neural arches come into apposition and the facets are in full extension. With further

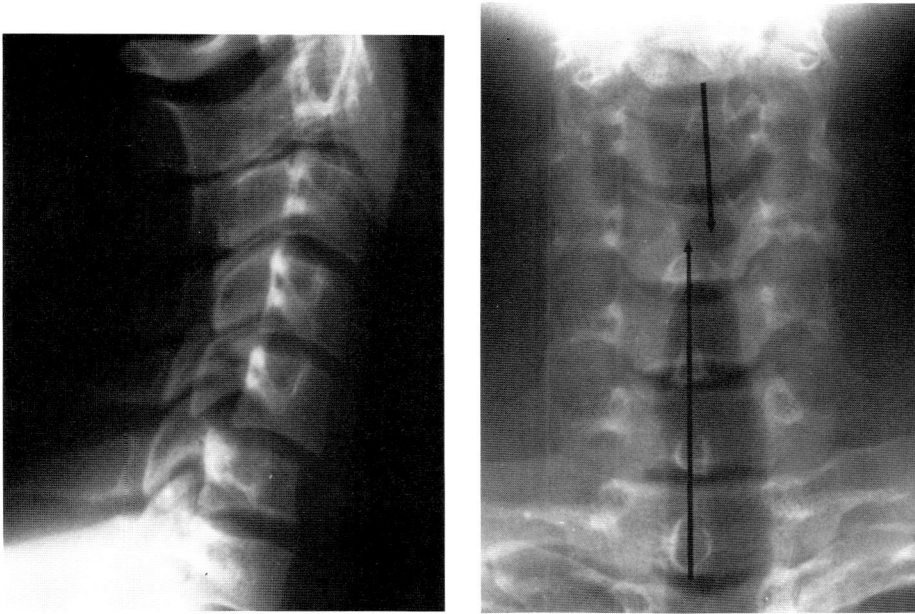

Figure 13–9. A: Unilaterally locked facet at C5-6. B: Same patient showing the typical lateral displacement of the spinous processes above the level of the locked facet.

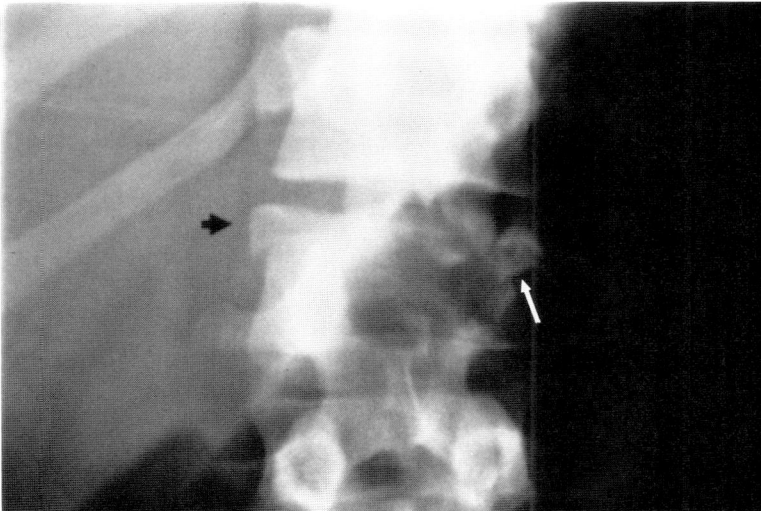

Figure 13–10. Anteroposterior films in a patient with a slice fracture. A portion of the pedicle, superior articular process, and transverse process of L1 have been displaced laterally (white arrow). The superior portion of the body of L1 remains attached to T12 (black arrow).

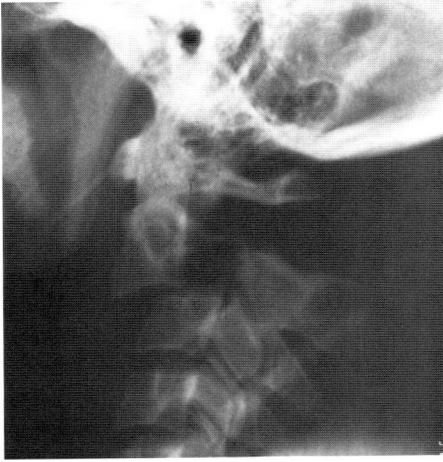

Figure 13–11. Hyperextension injury with fracture of the C2 pars interarticularis and disruption of the longitudinal ligaments and anulus.

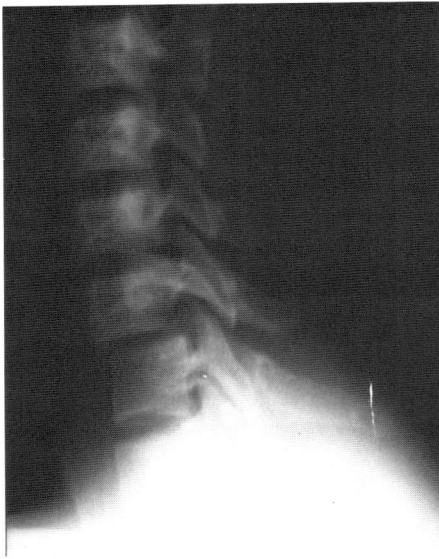

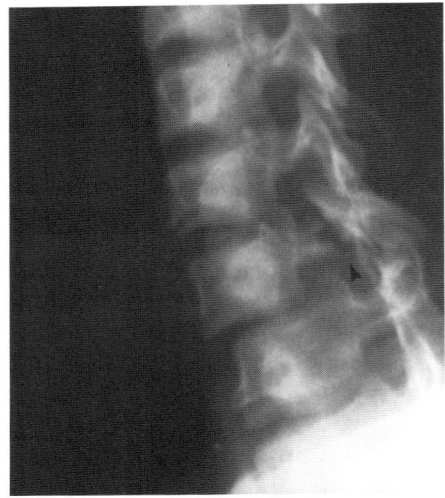

A

B

Figure 13–12. A: Hyperextension injury with anterior displacement of C6 on C7. B: Oblique view demonstrating the pedicle fracture (arrow). The opposite pedicle was intact. (Figure continued on next page)

extension, the anterior longitudinal ligament and the anulus fail, and if the facet joint remains intact, the pedicle fractures. Although the injury occurs in extension, anterolisthesis results. This is an unstable lesion. With extension plus compression, a shear force is added, producing circumferential disruption, severe malalignment (Fig. 13–13), and a highly unstable vertebral column.

The odontoid process can be fractured (Fig. 13–14) by forces applied either anteriorly or posteriorly. If the force is applied from in front, the anterior portion of the atlantal ring

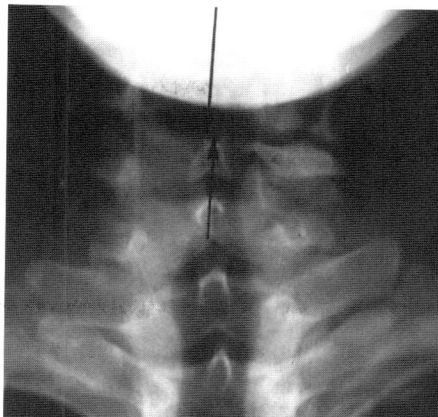

C

Figure 13–12, cont. C: Same patient. Because the pedicle fracture permits unilateral anterior movement without much rotation, lateral displacement of the spinous processes is minimal. With bilateral pedicular fracture, the anterior displacement is bilateral and greater, but the spinous processes are not deviated.

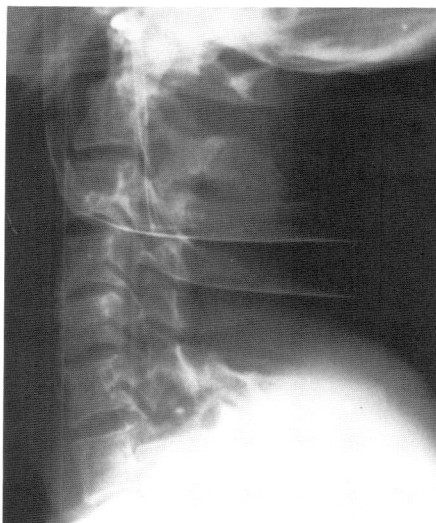

Figure 13–13. Extension-compression injury with severe disruption. The body of C7 lies in front of T1.

fractures the odontoid posteriorly. If the force is applied from behind, the transverse atlantal ligament fractures the odontoid anteriorly. However, the radiographically demonstrated position of the odontoid relative to C2 may not necessarily reflect the direction in which the force was applied, and the extent of displacement is not an indicator of the degree of instability[7] but may rather be a function of head movement subsequent to injury.

SUMMARY

Instability occurs when both the vertebral body and the neural arch or related soft tissue elements are disrupted. Under these conditions, progressive deformity and malalignment

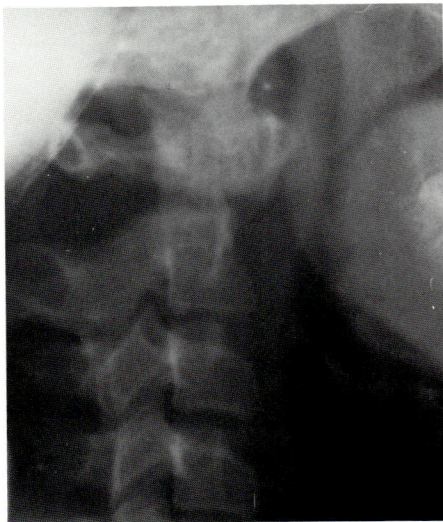

Figure 13–14. Fracture through the base of the odontoid process with anterior displacement of the odontoid.

can be anticipated, with the possibility of neurologic deficit in previously normal patients, or further loss of function in those with incomplete deficit.[5] Consequently, identification of instability is necessary so that the spinal cord can be protected during necessary surgical procedures, such as laparotomy and thoracotomy, and until the vertebral lesion can be treated definitively.

Acknowledgment

This research was supported in part by the Veterans Administration Medical Research Fund.

REFERENCES

1. Breig A: Adverse Mechanical Tension in the Central Nervous System. Stockholm: Almquist & Wiksells, 1978.
2. Green JD, Harle TS, Harris JH Jr: Anterior subluxation of the cervical spine: Hyperflexion sprain. AJNR 2: 243–250, 1981.
3. Holdsworth FW: Fractures, dislocations, and fracture-dislocations of the spine. J Bone Joint Surg 45B:6–20, 1963.
4. Johnson RM, Wolf JW Jr: Stability. In The Cervical Spine. Philadelphia: JB Lippincott 1983, pp 35–53.
5. Larson SJ: The thoracolumbar junction. In Dunsker SB, Kahn A, Schmidek H, Frymoyer J (eds): The Unstable Spine. New York: Grune & Stratton, 1986; pp 127–152.
6. Maiman DJ, Barolot G, Larson SJ: Management of bilateral locked facets of the cervical spine. Neurosurgery 18:542–546, 1986.
7. Southwick WO: Current concepts review: Management of fractures of the dens (odontoid process). J Bone Joint Surg 62A:482–486, 1980.
8. Webb JK, Broughton BK, McSweeney T, Park WM: Hidden flexion injury of the cervical spine. J Bone Joint Surg 58B:322–327, 1976.

14

Stabilization and Management of Cervical Injuries

GEORGE W. SYPERT

Cervical spine injuries are among the most serious traumatic injuries. The vast majority are closed, occurring as a result of indirect forces. Injuries range in consequence from simple myofascial stretch injuries and neck pain (sprains, strains) to quadriplegia and death. Serious injury to the cervical spinal cord is a major health problem, since its sequelae result in severe long-term disability, much individual suffering, and huge financial demands on public resources.

The principal objectives of the physicians responsible for caring for patients with such injuries are to provide an optimal environment for the spinal cord to recover, to correct spinal malalignment, and to reestablish the stability of the cervical spine. Inappropriate management can prevent recovery or result in further loss of neurologic function.[9] Treatment must be designed to prevent complications that may lead to further disability or inhibit spontaneous recovery of function.

About 6000 new cases of spinal cord injury are identified annually, of whom 52% will have a cervical spinal cord injury.[76] The mean age at the time of spinal cord injury is 30 years.[75] Cervical spinal cord injuries are most common in the 15- to 30-year-old age group, and males are more commonly afflicted than females by 4:1.[76] Most spinal cord injuries result from motor vehicle accidents (48%), followed by falls (28%), penetrating injuries (15%), and recreational and sports-related activities (14%), particularly water-related diving.[40,41,76]

FUNCTIONAL ANATOMY OF THE CERVICAL SPINE

The cervical spine consists of seven vertebrae with eight motion segments that anatomically and clinically can be divided into two main segments: the upper cervical spine (occiput-C2) and the lower cervical spine (C3-T1).[34]

The cervical spine encloses the cervical spinal cord, protecting it from injury when the spine is under physiologic loads, while permitting great flexibility of movement of the head in four planes. Given this inherent flexibility and the relative weakness of the spine's osseoligamentous complex, the cervical spine is particularly susceptible to injury because it links the rigidly supported trunk and the relatively heavy, extremely mobile head.

The cervical spine has six degrees of freedom of motion. Major motions include: flexion-extension (sagittal plane), lateral bending (frontal plane), and rotation. Distraction-compression, anterior-posterior translocation, and lateral translocation are fine movements that occur in conjunction with the three major motions of the cervical spine.[27] The combination of a major motion with a fine movement is referred to as "coupling." The greatest flexion-extension of the cervical spine occurs at the occipitoatlanto joint (25°) and at the lower cervical spine between C5 and C6 (21°).[44] Essentially, no rotation or lateral bending occurs at the occipitoatlantal joint, whereas about one half of the normal cervical rotation occurs at the atlantoaxial joint.[42] The lower cervical spine (C3-T1) is responsible for lateral bending and contributes to the remaining rotational function of the cervical spine. The C5-C6 motion segment has the greatest range of flexion-extension motion in the lower cervical spine and is subject to the highest incidence of fracture (C5) and fracture-dislocation (C5-C6) in cervical spine trauma.

The cervical spinal cord is an elongated soft tubular structure continuous with the caudal end of the medulla oblongata at the foramen magnum and the rostral end of the thoracic spinal cord at the level of the T1 vertebra. The diameter of the spinal cord is widest at the cervical spinal cord enlargement (C5-C8), where the nerve roots supplying the upper extremities emerge. There are eight pairs of cervical nerve roots that exit the spinal canal. The first cervical nerve, made up of only ventral root filaments, emerges between the occiput and atlas. The remaining cervical spinal nerve roots (C2-C8) emerge from the neural foramina with the same numbers as the caudal cervical vertebrae (that is, C6 spinal nerve emerges from the neural foramen between C5 and C6 vertebrae).

The spinal cord and nerve roots are enclosed by protective membranes. The outermost is the spinal dura mater, which is composed of dense fibrous connective tissue. The arachnoid membrane is a membrane loosely connected to the dura, which encloses the spinal fluid and neural elements. The innermost membrane is the pia mater, a thin, vascular membrane intimately applied to the surface of the spinal cord. Three spaces related to the meninges are important to an understanding of cervical traumatic pathologic conditions; the epidural space lies between the dura mater and the interior surface of the vertebral canal. The subdural space is a potential space between the dura mater and arachnoid. The subarachnoid space exists between the arachnoid and the neural elements and is filled with cerebrospinal fluid. The subarachnoid space is largest in the upper cervical spine.

BONE AND LIGAMENT INJURIES

Cervical spine injuries usually result from trauma to the head or trunk, or both, with injury forces indirectly transmitted to the cervical spine. Harris et al.[39] have presented a clinically useful cervical spine injury classification in which acute cervical spine osseoligamentous injuries are assumed to be the result of either pure vector forces (flexion, extension, axial loading) or combinations of such forces (flexion-rotation, extension-rotation) and are grouped accordingly. (Table 14–1.) Since the majority of serious cervical spine injuries are caused by being accelerated head first against a nonyielding object, significant axial loading of the cervical spine probably occurs in most injuries classified as flexion and extension

**Table 14–1   Mechanistic Classification
of Cervical Spine Osseomusculoligamentous Injuries***

I.	Flexion
	A. Anterior dislocation (hyperflexion sprain)
	B. Bilateral facet dislocation (locked facets)
	C. Simple wedge compression fracture
	D. Clay-shoveler fracture (spinous process avulsion)
	E. Flexion tear drop fracture
II.	Flexion-rotation
	A. Unilateral facet dislocation
III.	Vertical compression (axial loading)
	A. Jefferson's bursting fracture of atlas
	B. Burst fracture
IV.	Extension
	A. Hyperextension dislocation (hyperextension sprain)
	B. Avulsion fracture of anterior arch of atlas
	C. Extension teardrop fracture of axis
	D. Fracture of posterior arch of axis
	E. Laminar fracture
	F. Hangman's fracture (C2 spondylolisthesis)
	G. Hyperextension fracture-dislocation
V.	Extension-rotation
	A. Lateral mass (pillar) fracture
VI.	Lateral flexion (bending)
	A. Uncinate process fracture
VII.	Unclassified mechanisms
	A. Atlanto-occipital dislocation
	B. Atlantoaxial dislocation
	C. Odontoid fractures

*Modified from Harris et al., Orthop Clin North Am 17:15–30, 1986.

injuries. Different injuries may be caused by a single predominant vector force with a direct relationship between the magnitude of the force or forces and the type of injury.[1,59]

Cervical spine stability has been defined using three parameters: (1) the motion segment will not further displace or deform under physiologic loads; (2) there is not progressive displacement or deformity during the healing process; and (3) there is no progressive compression or injury to the neural elements. In the clinical situation it may be difficult to determine definitely the stability of many cervical spine injuries. As a general rule, it is safest to assume that all cervical spine injuries are unstable and initially to treat them as such until it is determined that the lesion is stable.

White et al.[82] defined biomechanically instability of the lower cervical spine as imminent or existing if there is more than 3.5 mm of horizontal displacement of one vertebra on the adjacent vertebra, or if there is more than 11° of angulation between adjacent vertebra. However, less displacement or angulation in a later lateral cervical spine radiograph does not ensure stability.

Recently, a three column concept of spine instability has been proposed that may be applicable to the cervical spine.[19] The posterior column is formed by the posterior neural arch, spinous process, facet articular processes, and their corresponding posterior ligamentous complex. The middle column consists of the posterior third of the vertebral body and annulus fibrosus and posterior longitudinal ligament. The anterior column is comprised of the anterior longitudinal ligament and the anterior two thirds of the vertebral body and annulus fibrosus. If two or more columns are disrupted, then acute spinal instability probably exists and predicts the possibility of late instability. Injuries that involve a single column generally do not lead to instability.

CLASSIFICATION OF NEUROLOGIC INJURIES

The pathologic extent of trauma to the neural elements depends on the degree to which the forces of injury transmitted to the cervical spine are in turn transmitted to the cervical spinal cord or nerve roots. Severe destruction of the nerual structures may occur without evidence of correspondingly severe osseous or ligamentous disruption and displacement, whereas gross osseoligamentous damage may occasionally be associated with minimal disturbance of neural function. Certain underlying conditions also predispose some patients to the development of a serious spinal cord injury. A small cervical spinal canal (such as congenital, spondylosis, prior trauma) or excessive rigidity of the spine (such as congenital, spondylosis, ankylosing spondylitis) is of great importance.

The classification of neurologic injuries is based on a detailed neurologic examination and notes that a patient: (1) is neurologically normal; (2) has a complete transverse myelopathy; (3) has an incomplete myelopathy; or (4) has a radiculopathy.

The most severe spinal cord injury is the complete transverse myelopathy in which all sensorimotor function below the level of the lesion is lost. Acute complete transverse myelopathy is generally associated with the phenomenon of spinal shock, which may last days or weeks. Spinal shock secondary to a complete cervical spinal cord injury is characterized by total absence of all sensorimotor function, flaccidity, and the absence of deep tendon reflexes. The signs of autonomic dysfunction, hypotension and bradycardia, that may accompany spinal shock are referred to as neurogenic shock.

Three of the more common incomplete spinal cord syndromes are illustrated in Figure 14–1. Most incomplete traumatic myelopathies do not conform strictly to the classic descriptions of those syndromes.

The most common incomplete traumatic myelopathy appears to be the anterior spinal cord syndrome.[64] The clinical picture is one of dysfunction of the anterior two-thirds of the cervical spinal cord in which there is both upper and lower motor neuron paralysis of the upper extremities associated with an upper motor neuron paralysis of the lower extremities. There is bilateral loss of pain and temperature sensation below the level of the lesion, but light touch, joint position, and vibratory sense are preserved distally. Reflex activity is usually absent initially but tends to return rapidly in the lower extremities without substantial return of voluntary motor function. This syndrome is particularly associated with flexion-type injuries, which can cause stretching of the spinal cord over a ventral mass or ischemia of the anterior two thirds of the spinal cord by compromise of the anterior spinal artery.[65]

The second most common incomplete acute traumatic myelopathy is the central spinal cord syndrome. This frequently follows contusions of the spinal cord with the most severe injury in the central gray matter of the cervical spinal cord. Pathologically, there is hemorrhagic necrosis of the central gray matter and variable extension into the surrounding white matter.[66] This injury is frequently produced by hyperextension of the stenotic cervical

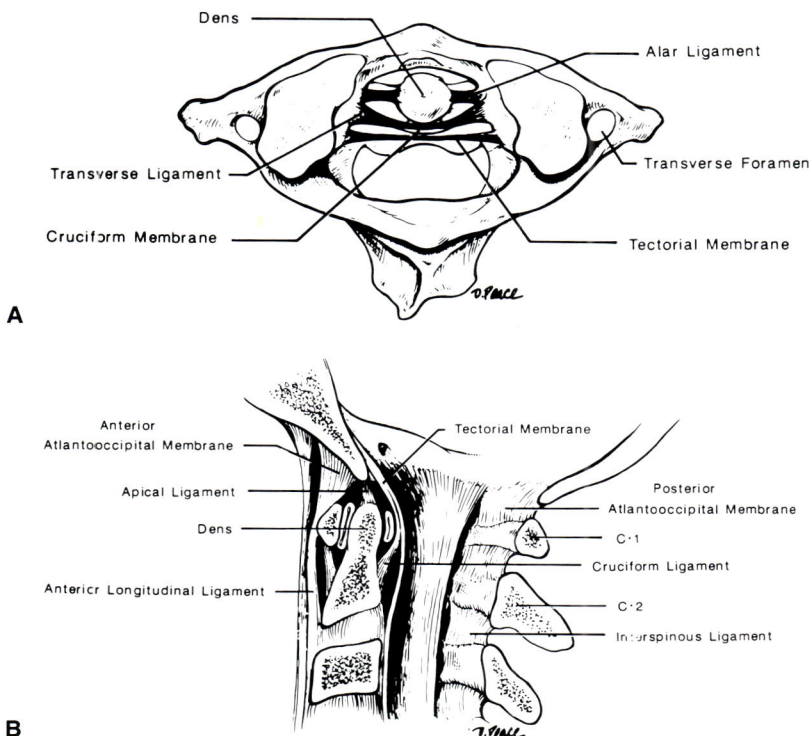

Figure 14–1.   Lateral (A) and anteroposterior (B) schematic of craniovertebral junction.

spinal column in the older patient. Neurologic examination reveals a more severe paresis in the upper extremities than in the lower extremities. Sensory function and bladder and bowel control are variably preserved.

The classic Brown-Sequard syndrome (either anatomic or functional hemisection of the spinal cord) is rare following closed injuries of the spinal cord. However, in incomplete spinal cord traumatic lesions, it is common for one side of the spinal cord to be more severely involved than the other.

Occasionally, the greatest neurologic deficits are found in the functions of the posterior columns after an acute cervical spine injury.[6]

Finally, patients sustaining cervical spine injuries may have an isolated nerve root lesion (traumatic radiculopathy). Although any nerve root in the cervical area may be injured, the fifth or sixth cervical nerve roots are usually involved due to the high incidence of spinal column injuries at these levels.

PROGNOSIS FOR NEUROLOGIC RECOVERY

The most important determinant of long-term functional outcome for the acute cervical spinal cord-injured patient is the initial extent of the spinal cord injury. There is presently no evidence to indicate that any individual or combination therapy enhances outcome for such patients.[20,41,69,80,87] The extent to which persistent compression of the spinal cord by either bone or soft tissue following the initial impact injury impedes neurologic recovery remains to be clarified. In selected patients, delayed surgical decompression and stabilization with reconstruction of the spinal canal can result in neurologic improvement.[8]

INITIAL ASSESSMENT AND MANAGEMENT

As many as one fourth of spinal cord injuries occur after the initial insult, either during prehospital care or early in the course of therapy.[9,58] Therefore, a principal goal in the care of patients who may have sustained cervical spine and spinal cord injuries is to prevent these secondary injuries. This requires immediate prehospital recognition of the possibility of a cervical spine injury with prompt immobilization of the spine.

INITIAL HOSPITAL CARE—EMERGENCY ROOM

When a patient who is suspected of having a cervical spine injury arrives at the emergency room, he or she must be promptly resuscitated by standard techniques. The ABCs of trauma management, resuscitation, and physiologic stabilization must be accomplished in a timely fashion.

When a spinal cord injury has been found, a history should be obtained and an examination of the spine and a neurologic examination should be performed by a neurologic surgeon. The patient should be questioned about a lack of feeling in the extremities or inability to move them, pain, paresthesias, bladder or bowel function, and the circumstances of the accident. Whenever the trauma patient complains of pain or stiffness in the neck, the physician should suspect a cervical spine injury. Pain radiating along a particular nerve root distribution in the upper extremity may be caused by nerve root compression by a cervical spine injury. The extent and level of motor and sensory dysfunction must be clearly documented. This initial neurologic examination will serve as the baseline for future examinations of the brain and spinal cord function. Any subsequent deterioration in nervous system function is secondary to a surgically treatable neurocompressive lesion until proved otherwise. If a complete transverse myelopathy is suspected, the examiner must attempt to discover any remaining sensory responses, as in sacral dermatomes, deep pain interpreted as touch or pressure, or evidence of minimal residual motor activity.

Neurodiagnostic imaging is discussed in Chapter 12.

GENERAL MANAGEMENT PRINCIPLES

Once a cervical fracture-dislocation or spinal cord injury is identified and the patient's systemic parameters are stabilized, attention must be immediately directed to realignment and stabilization of the cervical vertebral column. The most effective way of doing this is by applying skeletal traction either with skull tongs, most commonly the Gardner-Wells tongs, or the halo ring device. These devices are effective and can be quickly applied in the emergency room, with a minimum of discomfort for the patient. Varying amounts of weights are gradually added, under frequent radiographic control, to achieve satisfactory alignment. As the traction is increased, the patient's spine may be repositioned (flexed or extended) or, as in certain cervical injuries, manipulated (for example, rotated) to realign the vertebral column adequately. When satisfactory realignment is accomplished, the weights are then reduced to maintain the alignment. Restoration of a nearly normal spinal canal not only accomplishes decompression of the spinal cord from displaced bone and soft tissues, but may also alleviate pain and sensorimotor dysfunction by reducing compression or stretch resulting from tension on the nerve root as it exits through the intervertebral foramen between the dislocated or deformed vertebrae. Even when there is complete transverse cervical myelopathy, cervical realignment with restoration of the spinal canal may benefit the patient by reducing pain and restoring important function mediated by cervical nerve roots immediately above the level of spinal cord destruction.

If satisfactory realignment of the cervical spine cannot be achieved by this closed technique, open surgical internal reduction may be considered. Surgical correction may be especially necessary in patients with locked and dislocated facet joints. Other patients, particularly those with marked spinal instability or deformity due to severe osseoligamentous injury, may require surgical stabilization and fusion to permit early mobilization and rehabilitation and prevent delayed spinal deformity with neurologic complications.

The amount of weight necessary to accomplished adequate cervical spine reduction varies considerably with the level and type of spinal column injury. In general, less weight is required for upper than lower cervical spine injuries. Initially, a 5 pound weight should be applied for an upper cervical spine injury and a 10 pound weight for a lower cervical spine injury. A follow-up lateral cervical spine radiograph should then be obtained to check for the possibility of overdistraction. In severe ligamentous disruption, as little as 5 or 10 pounds could cause overdistraction of the injury site and result in neurologic injury. As a general rule, 5 pounds will be required for each cervical vertebra above the level of cervical spinal column injury in order to achieve adequate realignment. Some have suggested that the maximal amount of weight applied should not exceed about 10 pounds for each cervical vertebra above the level of injury. However, the amount of weight must be individualized, with the addition of weight contingent on repeated lateral cervical spine radiographs and neurologic examinations. Once adequate realignment has been accomplished, the amount of weight used for maintenance will have to be individualized, being dictated by the level of the injury, stability of the fracture-dislocation, the ease or difficulty of initial reduction, and follow-up neurologic and radiographic examinations.

CERVICAL SPINE ORTHOTICS

When it is desirable to protect the neural elements from spinal instability or deformity related to cervical spine trauma, external orthoses perform functions normally achieved by the intrinsic structures of the spine and the axial muscles. The efficacy of an orthotic appliance designed for the cervical spine depends on the adeqaucy of fixation at either end of the cervical spine, that is, the skull and the thorax. Cervical orthoses have been classified into four basic types, which are listed from the least to the most restrictive: the cervical collar, the poster-type orthosis, the cervicothoracic orthosis, and the halo orthosis.[84]

Cervical collars do little to restrict motion or transfer weight. They do provide warmth and psychologic comfort and support and serve as reminders that a cervical injury may be present, but they have little role in the management of cervical spine trauma. Adding an anterior and posterior reinforcement, such as in the relatively rigid Philadelphia collar, significantly restricts cervical spine motion, particularly flexion and extension, but is generally ineffective in controlling rotation and lateral bending.

A wide variety of poster-type orthoses are available. The four-post brace has adequate chin and occiput fixation, but the anterior and posterior pieces do not grip the chest firmly. The four-poster adds more control of cervical spine motion than the Philadelphia collar, particularly in restricting flexion and extension in the middle cervical segments, but is not very effective in restricting rotation, lateral bending, and sagittal plane motion in the upper cervical spine.

The cervicothoracic orthoses are reasonably comfortable and relatively easy to fabricate. They provide at least 90% restriction of flexion, extension, and rotation. Lateral bending is reduced to 50% of the unrestricted movements of normal controls. Upper cervical spine motion is less well controlled than the middle and lower cervical spine.

The halo-vest orthosis provides the most secure control of all cervical spine motions. Even these orthoses, though, do not eliminate all cervical motion. There are clinical situations in which the cervical spine is so unstable that no external orthosis will adequately control the spinal segments involved. In these cases, internal surgical fixation and fusion may be required, with supplementary external orthotic support.

SURGICAL MANAGEMENT

In the majority of patients with cervical spinal injury, satisfactory alignment can be achieved with the closed technique, and a decompressive operation is not required. After alignment has been restored with the closed technique, attention is then directed toward permanent stabilization of the spine (prevention of acute or delayed spinal instability or deformity). Stabilization is usually accomplished with external stabilization devices, such as prolonged skeletal traction, a halo-vest appliance, or cervical braces. The latter devices may allow ambulation if the patient's neurologic status permits. In addition, cervical orthoses may be important adjuncts to surgical stabilization.

If satisfactory realignment of the cervical spine cannot be achieved by this closed technique, open surgical internal reduction may be considered. Surgical correction may be especially necessary in patients with locked and dislocated facet joints. Other patients, such as those with marked spinal instability or deformity due to severe osseoligamentous injury, are likely as well to require surgical stabilization and fusion to permit early mobilization and rehabilitation and prevent delayed spinal deformity with neurologic complications.

The two indications for surgery in cervical spine trauma, decompression and stabilization, remain controversial. The goals of surgical management of cervical spine injuries are to prevent injury to the neural elements, to decompress the neural elements to maximize neurologic recovery, to prevent delayed instability and spinal deformity with their corresponding risks of pain or delayed loss of neurologic function, and to permit early mobilization and rehabilitation of patients.

A neurodiagnostic evaluation is essential for the proper evaluation of cervical spine-injured patients if operative therapy is contemplated. Depending on the location of the mass lesion compressing the neural elements, a surgical approach can be selected that will adequately decompress the neural elements. Similarly, an appropriate stabilizing procedure must be planned to achieve correction of spinal instability if one is to minimize treatment complications. The treatment selected must counteract the forces producing the spinal instability or deformity if a stable cervical spine is to be achieved and maintained.

The timing of surgical management in patients with cervical spine injuries remains controversial but, in general, operative decompression or stabilization, or both, should be delayed until the patient's general condition will allow surgery without significant additional risk. Particularly in patients with cervical spinal cord injuries, pulmonary insufficiency is often compounded by neurogenic paralysis of the chest wall respiratory muscles. Preoperative assessment of respiratory function is useful in determining the timing of nonemergent surgery; a vital capacity greater than 700 ml is needed to avoid postoperative respiratory failure. In patients without neurologic deficit, surgical management should be performed only after all major medical problems have been resolved. This would include those patients who are neurologically intact but whose spinal dislocations cannot be corrected by closed reduction.

The timing of surgery remains controversial regarding patients with neurologic deficits, both complete and incomplete, who have evidence of continued compression of the neural elements after closed reduction. Although various investigators have recommended early operative decompression,[21,80,83,86] there remains no statistically significant data that surgery within the first few hours or days after injury results in any greater recovery of neurologic function than surgery performed days or weeks later. Benzel and Larson[8] were not able to demonstrate a correlation between the timing of surgery and the degree of neurologic return in a study of 99 patients with cervical spine injuries treated surgically. Early surgical management has also been shown to be associated with a much higher rate of serious postoperative complications than delayed surgery.[10,52] Therefore available evidence suggests that the only indication for early or emergency operation is neurologic deterioration in the presence of neurologic element compression by bone, soft tissues, or hematoma.

Although there are no definitive data proving the efficacy of surgery in other patients, some surgeons will recommend delayed surgery after cervical spinal cord injuries to try to enhance a patient's recovery. After development of a traumatic central cord syndrome when congenital or spondylotic spinal canal stenosis and cord compression are present, either anterior or posterior canal decompression might allow greater recovery after the initial injury and prevent additional injuries with subsequent falls. Also, when neural foramina are compromised by bone or disk fragments, surgery for nerve root decompression can restore or improve important root function, even if the traumatic myelopathy is unchanged by operation.[7]

Protection of the neural elements preoperatively requires considerable attention on the part of the surgeon and anesthesiologist. Awake nasotracheal intubation should be performed so that the neurologic status can be constantly monitored. Positioning and turning should also be accomplished with the patient awake, maintaining the preoperative cervical spine alignment. A lateral cervical spine radiograph should be used to verify optimal position of the cervical spinal column prior to incision. If reduction and alignment were achieved preoperatively using skeletal traction, the traction should be maintained during the preparation and surgical procedure until adequate intraoperative stabilization has been accomplished and verified radiographically.

Most patients with persistent neural compression will be found by diagnostic imaging to have a lesion ventral to the neural elements. Those patients with incomplete spinal cord injuries or with nerve root dysfunction should be operated on by an anterior approach (Fig. 14–2). The posterior longitudinal ligament should be excised and the dura decompressed. It

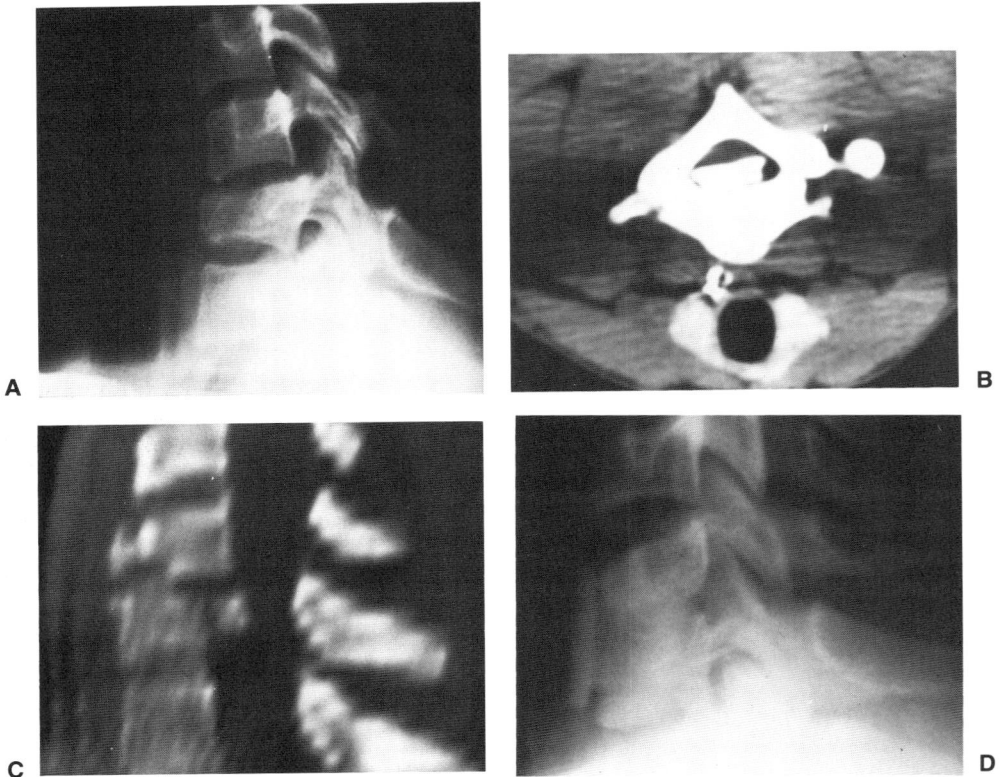

Figure 14–2.   Eighteen-year-old man who sustained a bursting fracture of C-6 and incomplete myelopathy that did not improve with adequate closed reduction using skeletal tong traction. After anterior decompressive partial corpectomy and fibula allograft reconstruction, the patient's spinal cord function fully recovered. A: Lateral radiograph; B: axial computed tomography (CT) scan; C: sagittal CT reconstruction; D: postoperative lateral radiograph.

is my opinion that the operating microscope is an important element for ensuring the success and safety of this surgical procedure. All disk, soft tissue, and bone compressing the dura must be excised. In some cases, an appropriate decompression may require corpectomy with diskectomies rostral and caudal to the involved vertebral body. On achieving an adequate neural decompression, anterior cervical fusion is generally carried out using a bone graft. Although I use an allograft fibular strut graft, many surgeons prefer the block graft technique, using iliac crest autograft or banked bone.

Anterior cervical decompression, particularly with removal of a destroyed vertebral body and posterior longitudinal ligament, will increase instability. In some such patients, the surgeon may elect to use a halo-vest orthosis postoperatively. Instability after anterior decompression and reconstruction may be of such a degree that graft dislodgement may occur despite the use of the halo-vest. In the latter circumstance, the surgeon has as alternatives performing a posterior cervical internal fixation and fusion (my preference, see Fig. 14–3), or locking the bone graft in with anterior plates and screws as described by Kaspar.[45]

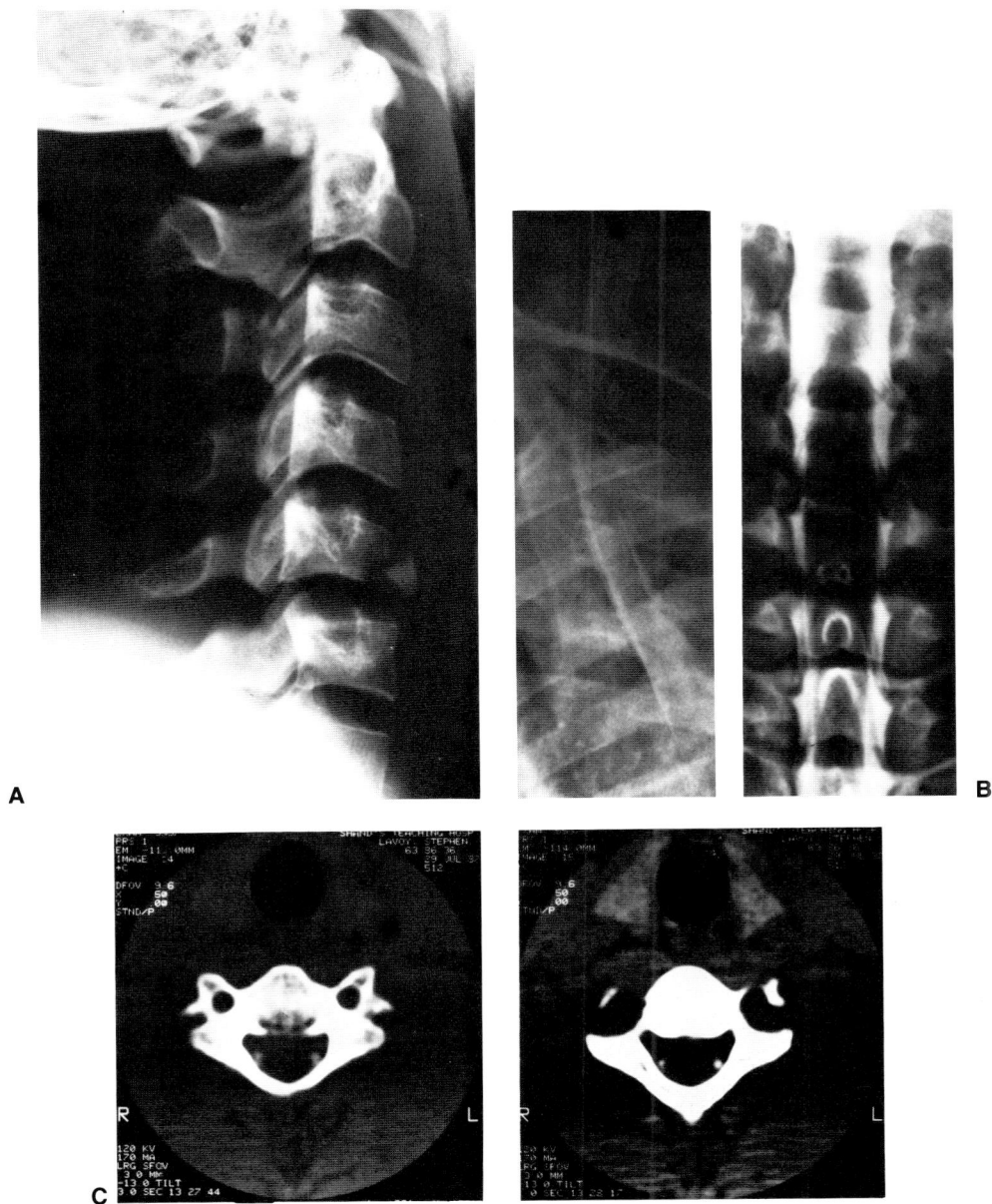

Figure 14–3. Twenty-year-old man who sustained a teardrop fracture of C-5 and an incomplete cervical myelopathy (anterior cord syndrome). Adequate skeletal reduction and immobilization failed to yield any recovery of spinal cord function. After simultaneous adequate anterior microsurgical decompressive corpectomy and fibula allograft reconstruction and posterior internal interlaminar clamp fixation and autogenous fusion, the patient's spinal cord function returned to normal. The posterior surgical fixation was performed because posterior ligamentous instability was demonstrated during closed skeletal traction (overdistraction at C5-C6). A: Lateral radiograph; B: cervical iohexol C1-C2 myelogram (note widened spinal cord); C: axial computed tomography myelogram (note large retrovertebral mass compressing the spinal cord due to epidural hematoma and swollen posterior longitudinal ligament); (Figure continued on next page)

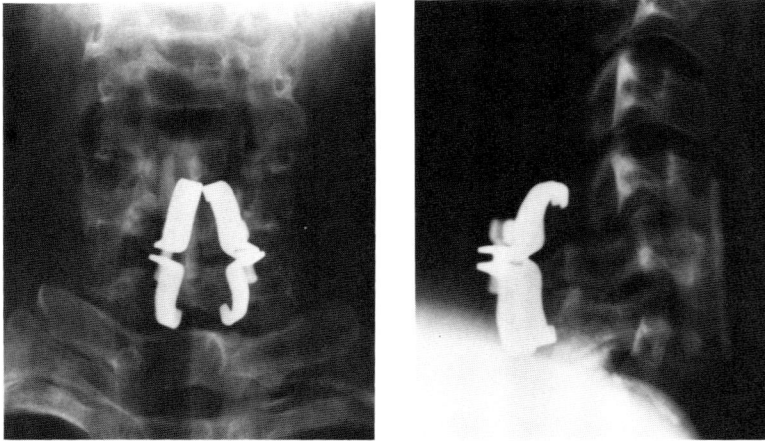

D

Figure 14–3, cont.   D: postoperative anteroposterior and lateral radiograph.

Attempted decompression of the spinal cord compressed by a ventrally located mass lesion using a posterior approach is difficult and hazardous, with the risk of inducing additional spinal cord injury. This is the most likely explanation for the neurologic deterioration reported in up to 30% of patients with cervical spinal cord injuries treated by laminectomies.[54] Posterior laminectomy is not contraindicated in all cases. On rare occasions when posterior neural compression by fractured laminar elements or hematoma is demonstrated, a decompressive laminectomy may be the preferred procedure.

In most circumstances, spinal instability requiring surgical management may be accomplished electively after the patient has been medically stable and the spinal column reduced and immobilized by external methods. Operative reduction, fixation, and fusion is indicated if the patient's cervical spine injury is such that external devices (such as, halo apparatus) are not likely to immobilize the injured segments adequately, result in a healed stable spine, or prevent fracture collapse and late deformity. Examples of such injuries include major subluxations associated with severe ligamentous disruption and major traumatic kyphotic deformities. Generally, posterior internal reduction or fixation and bony fusion is the procedure of choice for injuries with minimal or no osseous injury.[15,73,78] For patients requiring anterior surgical decompression or stabilization, or both, with bone graft, prolonged halo-vest immobilization until fusion is demonstrated, posterior fixation and fusion, or anterior plate fixation using bicortical screws should be performed to prevent graft dislocation, loss of alignment, and progressive delayed deformity.

Intraoperative radiographic verification should be obtained immediately after any bone grafting or internal spinal fixation procedure to verify satisfactory location and position of the graft and implant or implants, as well as the adequacy of spinal column reconstruction and realignment.

The following references are cited for the reader interested in the management of specific cervical spine injuries: Atlanto-occipital dislocation,[9,24,32,60,78,81] odontoid (dens) fractures,[2,3,22,25,33,36,37,50,61,63,72] combined atlantoaxial fractures,[3,22,25,36,57,61] atlas (Jefferson's) fractures,[12,38,46,47,57,70] atlantoaxial dislocations,[28,29,33,47,48,55,74] axis traumatic spondylolisthesis (hangman's fracture),[12,22,23,31,47,67,68,85] and lower cervical spine injuries: Anterior dislocation,[1,4,11,17,35,42,43] unilateral facet dislocation,[1,5,56,62] bilateral facet dislocation,[5,13,16,35,49,56,71,73,79] simple compression fractures,[4,7,9,16–18,35,53] clay-shoveler's fractures,[14] burst fractures,[59] and extension injuries.[4,26,30,51,77]

CONCLUDING REMARKS

Cervical spine injuries are a serious and complex health problem. Their optimal managment requires an extensive knowledge of the epidemiology, anatomy, phsyiology, biomechanics, pathology, and natural history of cervical spinal column and neurologic traumatic injuries as well as the benefits and limitations of the treatment methods available. Prevention of these injuries should be our most important goal. The national prevention program recently developed under the direction of the American Association of Neurological Surgeons and the Congress of Neurological Surgeons should receive strong support from all health professionals interested in spine trauma and spinal cord injury.

REFERENCES

1. Allen BL, Ferguson RL, Lehman TR, et al.: A mechanistic classification of closed, indirect fractures and dislocations of the lower cervical spine. Spine 7:1–27, 1982.
2. Althoff B, Bradholm P: Fractures of the odontoid process: A clinical and radiographic study. Acta Orthop Scand (Suppl) 177:61–95, 1979.
3. Apuzzo MLJ, Weiss MH, Ackerson T, et al.: Fractures of the odontoid process: An analysis of 45 cases. J Neurosurg 48:85–91, 1978.
4. Babcock JL: Cervical spine injuries: Diagnosis and classification. Arch Surg 111:646–651, 1976.
5. Bauze RJ, Ardan GM: Experimental production of forward dislocation in the human cervical spine. J Bone Joint Surg 60B:239–245, 1978.
6. Bedbrook GM: Some pertinent observations on the pathology of traumatic spinal paralysis. Int J Paraplegia 1: 215, 1963.
7. Benzel EC, Larson SJ: Recovery of nerve root function after complete quadriplegia from cervical spine fractures. Neurosurgery 19:809–812, 1986.
8. Benzel EC, Larson SJ: Funtional recovery after decompressive spine operation for cervical spine fractures. Neurosurgery 20:742–746, 1987.
9. Bohlman HH: Acute fracture and dislocation of the cervical spine. J Bone Joint Surg 61A:1119–1142, 1979.
10. Braakman R: Some neurological and neurosurgical aspects of injuries to the lower cervical spine. Acta Neurochir (Wien) 22:245–260, 1970.
11. Braakman R, Penning L: Mechanisms of injury to the cervical cord. Paraplegia 10:314–320, 1973.
12. Brant-Zawadski M, Miller EM, Federle MP: CT in the evaluation of spine trauma. AJR 136:369–375, 1981.
13. Burk CD, Berryman D: The place of closed manipulation in the management of flexion-rotation dislocations of the cervical spine. J Bone Joint Surg 53B:165–182, 1971.
14. Cancelmo JJ Jr: Clay shoveler's fracture: A helpful diagnostic sign. AJR 115:540–541, 1972.
15. Capen DA, Garland DE, Waters RL: Surgical stabilization of the cervical spine. A comparative analysis of anterior and posterior spine fusions. Clin Orthop 196:229–237, 1985.
16. Chan RC, Schweigel JF, Thompson GB: Halo-thoracic brace immobilization in 188 patients with acute cervical spine injuries. J Neurosurg 58:508–515, 1983.
17. Cheshire DJ: The stability of the cervical spine following the conservative treatment of fractures and fracture-dislocations. Paraplegia 7:193–203, 1969.
18. Cooper PR, Maravilla KR, Sklar FH, et al.: Halo immobilization of cervical spine fractures. Indications and results. J Neurosurg 50:603–610, 1979.
19. Denis F: Spinal instability as defined by the three-column spine concept in acute spinal trauma. Clin Orthop 189:65–76, 1984.
20. Donovan WH, Kopaniky D, Stolzmann E, Carter RE: The neurological and skeletal outcome in patients with closed cervical spinal cord injury. J Neurosurg 66:690–694, 1987.
21. Ducker TB, Russo GL, Bellegarrique R, Lucas, JT: Complete sensorimotor paralysis after cord injury: Mortality, recovery, and therapeutic implications. J Trauma 19:837–840, 1979.

22. Dunn ME, Seljeskog EL: Experience in the management of odontoid process injuries: An analysis of 128 cases. Neurosurgery 18:306–310, 1986.

23. Effendi B, Roy D, Cornish B, et al.: Fractures of the ring of the axis. A classification based on the analysis of 131 cases. J Bone Joint Surg 63B:319–327, 1981.

24. Eismont FJ, Bohlman HH: Posterior atlanto-occipital dislocation with fractures of the atlas and odontoid process. Report of a case with survival. J Bone Joint Surg 60A:397–399, 1978.

25. Ekong CEU, Schwartz ML, Tator CH, et al.: Odontoid fracture: Management with early immobilization using the halo device. Neurosurgery 9:631–637, 1981.

26. Epstein N, Epstein JA, Vallo B, Ransohoff J: Traumatic myelopathy in patients with cervical spinal stenosis without fracture or dislocation. Spine 5:489–496, 1980.

27. Fielding JW: Normal and abnormal motion of the cervical spine from C2 to C7, cineroentgenography. J Bone Joint Surg 46A:1779–1782, 1964.

28. Fielding JW, Cochran GV, Lawsing JF, et al.: Tears of the transverse ligament of the atlas. J Bone Joint Surg 56A:1683–1691, 1974.

29. Fielding JW, Hawkins RJ: Atlanto-axial rotatory fixation. J Bone Joint Surg 59A:37–44, 1977.

30. Forsyth HF: Extension injuries of the cervical spine. J Bone Joint Surg 46A:1792–1797, 1964.

31. Frances WR, Fielding JW, Hawkins RJ, et al.: Traumatic spondylolisthesis of the axis. J Bone Joint Surg 63B:400–407, 1981.

32. Fruin AH, Pirotte TP: Traumatic atlantooccipital dislocation. Case report. J Neurosurg 46:663–666, 1977.

33. Gallie WE: Fractures and dislocations of the cervical spine. Am J Surg 46:495–499, 1939.

34. Gehweiler JA, Clark WM, Schaaf RE, et al.: Cervical spine trauma: The common combined conditions. Radiology 130:77–86, 1979.

35. Glaser JA, Whitehill R, Stamp WG, et al.: Complications associated with the halo-vest. J Neurosurg 65:762–769, 1986.

36. Hadley MN, Browner CM, Sonntag VKH: Axis fractures: A comprehensive review of management and treatment in 107 cases. Neurosurgery 17:281–290, 1985.

37. Hadley MN, Sonntag V: Acute axis fractures. Contemp Neurosurg 9(2):1–6, 1987.

38. Han SY, Witten DM, Mussleman JP: Jefferson fracture of the atlas. Report of six cases. J Neurosurg 44:368–371, 1976.

39. Harris P, Karmi MZ, McClemont E, et al.: The prognosis of patients sustaining severe cervical spine injury C2-C7 inclusive). Paraplegia 18:324–330, 1980.

40. Heiden JS, Weiss MH: Cervical spine injuries with and without neurological deficit: Part I. Contemp Neurosurg 2(12):1–6, 1980.

41. Heiden JS, Weiss MH, Rosenberg AW, et al.: Management of cervical spinal cord trauma in Southern California. J Neurosurg 43:732–736, 1975.

42. Hohl M: Normal motions in the upper portion of the cervical spine. J Bone Joint Surg 46A:1777–1779, 1964.

43. Holdsworth F: Review article: Fractures, dislocations and fracture-dislocations of the spine. J Bone Joint Surg 52A:1534–1551, 1970.

44. Johnson RM, Southwick WO: Surgical approaches to the spine. In: RH Rothman, FA Simeone (eds): The Spine. Philadelphia: WB Saunders, 1982, pp 67–92.

45. Kaspar W: Anterior cervical fusion and interbody stabilization with the trapezial osteosynthetic plate technique. Aesculap Sci Information 12:1–36, 1985.

46. Keene GCR, Hone MR, Sage MR: Atlas fracture: Demonstration using computerized tomography. J Bone Joint Surg 60A:1106–1107, 1978.

47. Levine AM, Edwards CC: The management of traumatic spondylolisthesis of the axis. J Bone Joint Surg 67A:217–226, 1985.

48. Maiman DJ, Cusick JF: Traumatic atlantoaxial dislocation. Surg Neurol 18:388–392, 1982.

49. Maiman DJ, Barolat G, Larson SJ: Management of bilateral locked facets of the cervical spine. Neurosurgery 18:542–547, 1986.

50. Maiman DJ, Larson SJ: Management of odontoid fractures. Neurosurgery 11:471–476, 1982.

51. Marar BC: Hyperextension injuries of the cervical spine—the pathogenesis of damage to the spinal cord. J Bone Joint Surg 56A:1655–1662, 1974.

52. Marshall L, Knowlton S, Garfin SR, et al.: Deterioration following spinal cord injury. A multicenter study. J Neurosurg 66:400–404, 1987.

53. Mazur JM, Stauffer ES: Unrecognized spinal instability associated with seemingly "simple" cervical compression fractures. Spine 8:687–692, 1983.

54. Morgan TH, Wharton GW, Austin GN: The results of laminectomy in patients with incomplete spinal cord injuries. Paraplegia 9:14–23, 1971.

55. Mouradian WH, Fietti VG, Cochran GV, et al.: Fractures of the odontoid: A laboratory and clinical study of mechanisms. Orthop Clin North Am 9:985–1001, 1978.

56. O'Brien PJ, Schweigel JF, Thompson WJ: Dislocations of the lower cervical spine. J Trauma 22:710–714, 1982.

57. Pierce DS, Barr JS: Fractures and dislocations at the base of the skull and upper cervical spine. In The Cervical Spine Research Society (ed): The Cervical Spine. Philadelphia: JB Lippincott, 1983, pp 196–206.
58. Poldosky S, Baraff LJ, Simon RR, et al.: Efficacy of cervical spine immobilization methods. J Trauma 23: 461–464, 1983.
59. Roaf R: A study of the mechanics of spinal injuries. J Bone Joint Surg 42B:810–823, 1960.
60. Rockswold GL, Seljeskog EL: Traumatic atlantocranial dislocation with survival. Minn Med 62:151–152, 1979.
61. Ryan MD, Taylor TKF: Odontoid fractures. A personal approach to treatment. J Bone Joint Surg 64B:416–421, 1982.
62. Scher AT: Unilateral locked facet in cervical spine injuries. AJR 129:45–48, 1976.
63. Schiess RJ, Desaussure RL, Robertson IT: Choice of treatment of odontoid fractures. J Neurosurg 57:495–499, 1982.
64. Schneider RC: The syndrome of acute anterior spinal cord injury. J Neurosurg 12:95–122, 1955.
65. Schneider RC, Kahn EA: Chronic neurological sequelae of acute trauma to the spine and spinal cord. Part I. The significance of the acute flexion or "tear drop" fracture-dislocation of the cervical spine. J Bone Joint Surg 38A:958–997, 1956.
66. Schneider RC, Knighton R: Chronic neurological sequelae of acute trauma to the spine and spinal cord. Part III. The syndrome of chronic injury to the cervical spinal cord in the region of the central canal. J Bone Joint Surg 41A:905–919, 1959.
67. Schneider RC, Livingston KE, Cave AJE, et al.: "Hangman's fracture" of the cervical spine. J Neurosurg 22: 141–154, 1965.
68. Seljeskog EL, Chou SN: Spectrum of the hangman's fracture. J Neurosurg 45:3–8, 1976.
69. Shrosbree RD: Neurological sequelae of reduction of fracture dislocations of the cervical spine. Paraplegia 17:212–221, 1979.
70. Skold G: Fractures of the arches of the atlas: A study of their causation. Z Rechtsmed 90:247–258, 1983.
71. Sonntag VKH: Management of bilateral locked facets of the cervical spine. Neurosurgery 8:150–152, 1981.
72. Southwick WO: Management of fractures of the dens (odontoid process). J Bone Joint Surg 62A:482–486, 1980.
73. Stauffer ES, Kelly EG: Fracture-dislocation of the cervical spine: Instability and recurrent deformity following treatment by anterior interbody fusion. J Bone Joint Surg 59A:45–48, 1977.
74. Steel HH: Anatomical and mechanical considerations of the atlanto-axial articulations. J Bone Joint Surg 50A:1481–1482, 1968.
75. Stover SL, Fine PR (eds): Spinal Cord Injury: The Facts and Figures. Birmingham, Alabama: The National Spinal Cord Injury Statistical Center, University of Alabama at Birmingham, 1986.
76. Stover SL, Fine PR: The epidemiology and economics of spinal cord injury. Paraplegia 25:225–228, 1987.
77. Taylor AR, Blackwood W: Paraplegia in hyperextension cervical injuries with normal radiographic appearances. J Bone Joint Surg 30B:245–248, 1948.
78. Traynelis VC, Marano GD, Duncker RO, et al.: Traumatic atlanto-occipital dislocation. J Neurosurg 65:863–870, 1986.
79. Van Peteghem PK, Schweigel JF: The fractured cervical spine rendered unstable by anterior cervical fusion. J Trauma 19:110–115, 1979.
80. Wagner FC Jr, Chehrazi B: Early decompression and neurological outcome in acute cervical spinal cord injuries. J Neurosurg 56:699–705, 1982.
81. Watridge CB, Orrison WW, Arnold H, et al.: Lateral atlantooccipital dislocation: Case report. Neurosurgery 17:345–347, 1985.
82. White AA, Johnson RM, Panjabi MM, et al.: Biomechanical analysis of clinical stability in the cervical spine. Clin Orthop 109:9–17, 1975.
83. White AA, Southwick WO, Panjabi MM: Clinical instability in the lower cervical spine. A review of past and current
84. Wolf JW, Johnson RM: Cervical orthoses. In The Cervical Spine Society (eds): The Cervical Spine. Philadelphia: Lippincott, 1983, pp 54–61.
85. Wood-Jones F: The ideal lesion produced by judicial hanging. Lancet 1:53, 1913.
86. Yashon D, Tyson G, Vise VM: Rapid closed reduction of cervical fracture-dislocations. Surg Neurol 4:513–514, 1975.
87. Young JS, Dexter WR: Neurological recovery distal to the zone of injury in 172 cases of closed, traumatic spinal cord injury. Paraplegia 16:39–49, 1978.

15

Treatment of Thoracolumbar Junction Injuries

VOLKER K. H. SONNTAG
AND MARK N. HADLEY

Injuries to the thoracolumbar junction (TLJ; T11, T12, L1, and L2 vertebral bodies) are common after craniospinal trauma. TLJ fractures are the second most frequent site of vertebral column injury, after cervical spine fracture-dislocations. As with most forms of traumatic injury, motor vehicle accidents and falls represent the most common causes of TLJ fracture.

The TLJ vertebrae make up the "hinge junction" of the thoracic and lumbar spine and are particularly vulnerable to injury. Thoracic vertebral bodies rostral to T11 are provided partial protection from axial loading and rotational forces by the vertebral body apophyseal joint structure, rib articulations, and associated musculoligamentous attachments. The lower lumbar vertebrae receive relative protection from short lumbosacral-iliac bony articulations and strong intraspinous and iliolumbar ligaments.

The most frequent levels of traumatic injury are at T12 and L1. In addition, injuries at these levels are associated with the highest degree of neurologic compromise. In a review of 110 TLJ fractures at our institution, the T12 vertebral level had the highest incidence of traumatic injury and neurologic impairment (Table 15–1). The relatively low frequency of neurologic injury associated with L2 level fractures is probably due to the presence of the cauda equina. In most adults, the lower limit of the spinal cord, the conus medullaris, is located at the level of vertebral body L1. Lower, at the L2 level, the cauda equina composed of nerve roots occupies the spinal canal. This structure tolerates injury and compression better than the more rostral spinal cord.

Several injury types have been described at the TLJ based on the degree of vertebral body fracture, collapse, disruption, or dislocation. Holdsworth[9] has characterized these injuries according to the presumed mechanism of injury and described the radiographic appearance of each.

186

Table 15–1   Neurological Deficit vs Level

LEVEL	NUMBER	NUMBER INCOMPLETE/COMPLETE	% NEURO COMPROMISE
T-11	20	4/6	50%
T-12	44	17/14	73%
L-1	32	14/6	63%
L-2	14	2/1	21%
	110	37/27	58%

RADIOGRAPHIC ASSESSMENT

We recommend a diagnostic battery that includes standard anteroposterior (AP) and lateral radiographs and thin section computed tomography (CT) in the evaluation of all patients with TLJ trauma. These radiographic studies will reveal the presence of bony fracture or vertebral subluxation, will fully define the extent of bony injury, including posterior element fracture and disruption, and will identify multiple level injuries as well as bony implosion into the spinal canal.[4,14] Five to 15% of patients with one level of vertebral column fracture have a second level of vertebral column injury, so a full spine series consisting of standard AP and lateral radiographs should be obtained in suspected patients. Information learned from the standard radiographs and CT studies determines whether myelography or magnetic resonance imaging (MRI) should be done. Myelography is used to identify those patients with significant spinal cord compromise or narrowing of the thecal sac[11,12] (Fig. 15–1). Recent experience with MRI has shown that it is an excellent modality (at 1.5 tesla field

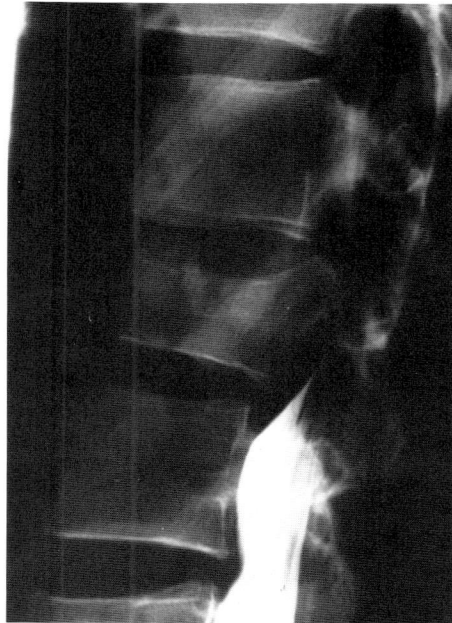

Figure 15–1.   Myelography demonstrating marked thecal sac compromise by TLJ fracture.

strength) to assess thecal sac impingement, injury to spinal cord tissue, and rupture of the posterior longitudinal ligament.

Flexion and extension radiographs are performed relatively early in the patient's hospital course if the initial studies reveal relatively minor TLJ trauma (that is, an isolated fracture of the posterior elements, a compression fracture of less than 50% vertebral body height, or a body or lateral mass fracture without fragmentation or dislocation). These dynamic studies will assess the likelihood of post-traumatic instability and will help determine subsequent therapy and follow-up.

MANAGEMENT PRINCIPLES

The treatment of patients with traumatic TLJ injuries must be individualized and must incorporate three essential features: the type of fracture, the level of injury, and the patient's neurologic condition. Several investigators have described management principles that help govern nonoperative versus operative therapy for individual lesions.[1,10,11,15,17] In general, nonoperative therapy, which may range from mild restriction of activity to complete bed rest and may include any number of external orthotic devices, is recommended for those patients with less severe TLJ traumatic injuries. This group includes those patients with TLJ fractures without spinal canal or neural element compromise, compression fractures less than a 50% reduction in the vertebral body height, and fractures without multiple column compromise or traumatic subluxation (Fig. 15–2). Patients with incomplete neurologic injuries but without neural compression by bone, disk, or blood and patients with complete neurologic injuries may also be effectively managed with nonoperative means. A caveat must be added to this last statement for the patient with a "complete" neurologic injury at the L1 or L2 vertebral level. Several reports exist describing patients with a "complete myelopathy" who recovered neurologic function after decompression of the conus medullaris or cauda equina structures. These structures may be more resistant to injury than the remainder

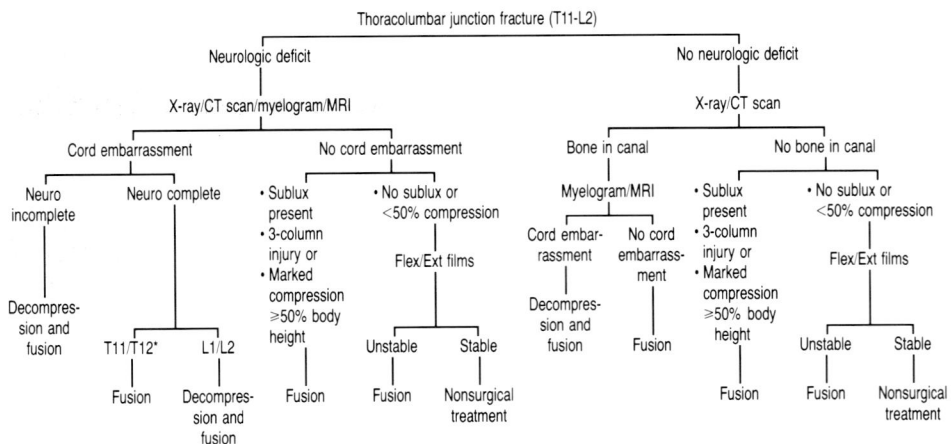

*Surgical decompression may be indicated if surgery can be performed acutely after complete neurological injury.

Figure 15–2.   Treatment algorithm for management of traumatic TLJ injuries.

of the spinal cord and may show an unexpected degree of recovery when decompressed than the more rostral central spinal cord structures.

The operative treatment of patients with traumatic TLJ injuries consists of stabilization of the vertebral column and decompression of the neural elements. There are controversies about the timing and indications for surgical intervention, but, in general, the following principles are applicable to most patients.[1–3,5,10,11,15]

Emergency surgery is rarely indicated except for the patient with neurologic dysfunction whose lesion cannot be reduced or decompressed by nonoperative traction or positioning, or for the patient with a progressive neurologic deterioration with radiographic evidence of persistent subluxation, bone, blood, or disk material compressing the spinal cord, or conus medullaris. Most investigators recommend elective surgical decompression and stabilization of TLJ fractures between 3 and 12 days postinjury. In this period, the appropriate radiographic studies may be obtained and the patient's medical status can be optimized.

The preoperative radiographic studies dictate the extent of surgical therapy in an individual patient. Patients with thecal sac compression by extruded bone fragments should undergo decompression followed by stabilization in a single-stage procedure. It is our opinion that unless there is minimal compromise of the thecal sac structures by bony fragments, distraction and stabilization with Harrington rods only is insufficient to "decompress" the spinal canal (Figs. 15–3, 15–4). Several studies have demonstrated persistent spinal canal compromise on postoperative CT scans after instrumentation without surgical decompression.[6,12,19,20]

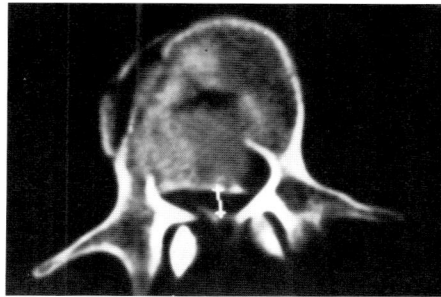

Figure 15–3. Burst fracture of T12 with marked canal and neural element compromise.

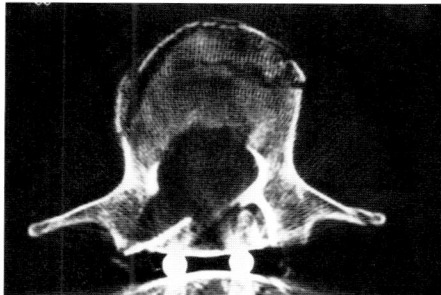

Figure 15–4. Postoperative CT reveals canal decompression achieved via modified costotransversectomy approach. Harrington rod placement does not interfere with postoperative CT assessment of the surgical decompression.

Stabilization is advocated for patients with traumatic subluxation-dislocation, those with marked compression and collapse of the TLJ vertebral segments (which produce a high incidence of progressive kyphosis with instability), those with multiple column injuries, and those with instability on dynamic flexion and extension radiographic studies. Stabilization without decompression is also advocated for those patients with no neurologic function below the T11-T12 levels (spinal cord tissue) who are greater than 24 hours after injury regardless of the disordered anatomy.

OPERATIVE APPROACHES

There are several surgical options in the treatment of traumatic TLJ injuries that require both decompression and stabilization (Table 15–2). The approach selected by the surgeon should be based on individual patient characteristics, which include the level and complexity of the traumatic fracture, the location of neural compression, the experience of the surgeon, and the availability of qualified cosurgeons (vascular, general, thoracic, or orthopedic) as required. There is no single approach applicable to all pathologic processes of the TLJ; therefore experience with more than one of the operations listed will increase the range, scope, and effectiveness of the treatment of TLJ disease.

The anterior transthoracic-transabdominal approach provides a wide exposure of the anterior portion of the spinal canal for the treatment of ventral compression at the TLJ.[6,16] Strut graft fusion procedures may be used after decompression via the anterior approach, or posterior stabilization may be performed later as a separate procedure. This operation usually requires a cosurgeon, typically a general or vascular surgeon who exposes the injured spine through the chest or abdomen, or both. The aorta and/or iliac vessels diaphragm is divided. If the pleural cavity is opened, chest tubes must be placed postoperatively. A left lateral thoracic approach may not require mobilization of the major vascular structures.[21] However, they remain in the operative field and can hinder the operative procedure with their presence.

The anterolateral approach is a lateral extracavity exposure that does not require entry into the intrapleural and intraperitoneal cavities.[13] A wide exposure of the anterolateral vertebral segments at the TLJ can be achieved, allowing decompression of the ventral spinal canal. As with the other exposures previously cited, a strut graft fusion can be performed via this approach or a second procedure done to immobilize and fuse the spine posteriorly. Typically, a thoracic or general surgeon is required to assist with the exposure.

Table 15–2   Surgical Approaches to the Thoracolumbar Junction

Anterior
  Transthoracic-transabdominal
  Left lateral thoracic
Anterolateral
  Lateral extracavity approach
Posterior
Posterolateral
  Costotransversectomy
  Modified costotransversectomy

The posterior approach should not be used for decompression of ventral spinal canal injury unless the traumatic fracture and lesion are low (L1-L2 level), compromising only cauda equina structures. At more rostral levels, the posterior approach may result in further neurologic injury by attempting to decompress a spinal canal pathologic condition that is ventral to the spinal cord and conus medullaris structures. Finally, the posterior approach for decompression may increase spinal column instability due to the wide laminectomy required. If, however, the spinal canal is narrowed by posterior element fractures, then posterior decompression is indicated. If a patient requires stabilization and fusion only (without decompression), then the posterior approach is most efficacious.

The posterolateral surgical approach combines a ventral spinal cord decompression procedure with a posterior stabilization and fusion procedure, all via the same operative exposure and at the same operative setting.[7,8,11,15,18] There is no need for a vascular, thoracic, or general cosurgeon for the posterolateral exposure. In addition, spinal cord compromise, ventral or dorsal, can be effectively treated via the costotransversectomy or modified costotransversectomy approaches. The key to these procedures is to take down the rib and transverse process at the level of injury and to resect the involved pedicle (Figs. 15–5, 15–6), gaining exposure to the ventrolateral aspect of the thecal sac. The disadvantage is that these techniques do not allow complete visualization of the full anterior aspect of the thecal sac, particularly on the side opposite the side of the exposure.

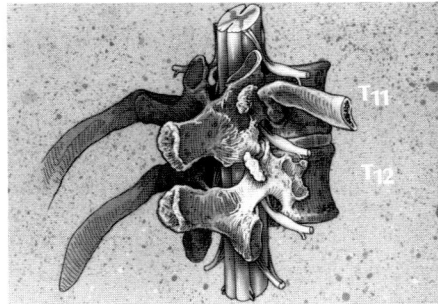

Figure 15–5. Artist's representation of approach to ventrolateral aspect of the spinal cord via posterolateral approach. The rib is removed, exposing the transverse process.

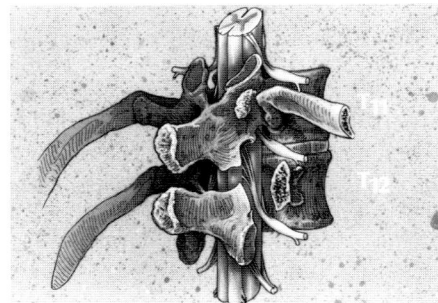

Figure 15–6. The transverse process has been resected, revealing the pedicle. The pedicle is then dissected with a high-speed drill, extending the dissection into the ventrolateral body and exposing the ventral aspect of the thecal sac.

Modified Costotransversectomy Operative Techniques

Since the modified costotransversectomy frequently accomplishes the objective of the anterior, anterolateral, and posterior approaches without the need for additional surgeons, it will be described in more detail. The patient is positioned on a tilted operating table in the prone position on a Wilson frame. Bolsters are placed under the frame on the side of the planned operative exposure (Figs. 15–7, 15–8). The side of exposure is determined by the preoperative imaging studies and is on the side of the worst ventral compression. The use of the tilted operating table and addition of the bolsters allows the patient to be rotated away from the surgeon during the posterolateral decompression to improve visualization and exposure to the ventral aspect of the spinal canal (Fig. 15–9). After the patient has been securely taped to the table, it may be tilted toward the surgeon to make the patient's back horizontal during the initial portion of the procedure.

A curvilinear paramedian skin incision is made with the center of the arc at the level of the traumatic injury (Fig. 15–10). This cutaneous flap is dissected free from the underlying musculature, carried across midline, and reflected away from the surgeon to the contralateral side. Exposure of the spinous processes and laminae similar to that of a standard posterior stabilization and fusion approach, and a single Harrington distraction rod is placed on the contralateral side, secured two levels above and two levels below the site of traumatic injury.

The ipsilateral paraspinous musculature is then incised, perpendicular to the spine directly over the ipsilateral rib and transverse process to be exposed. Dissection is carried down to the rib at the injury level or to the transverse process if at a lumbar level. The patient may now be tilted away from the surgeon and the medial 4 to 5 cm of rib is removed with

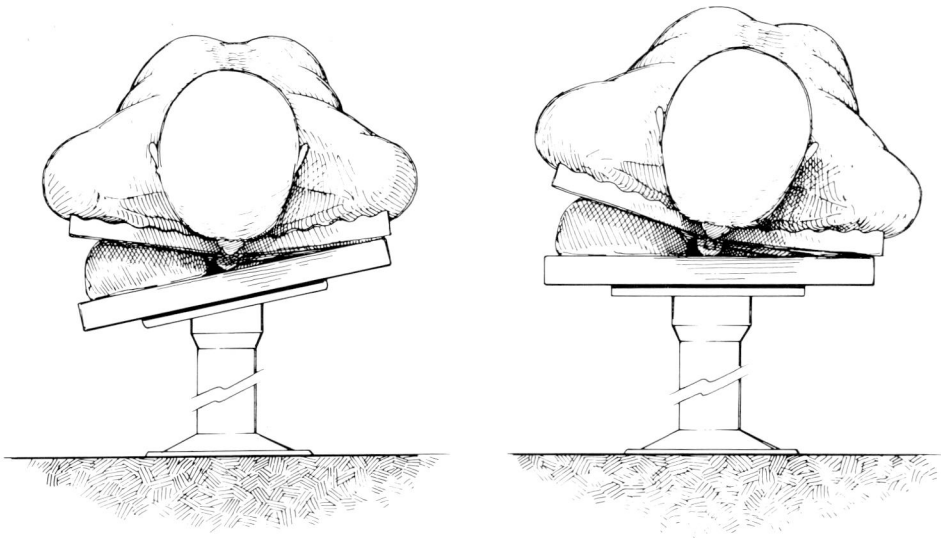

Figures 15–7, 15–8.   Patient positioned on tilted operating room table with a bolster under the frame on the side of the operative approach.

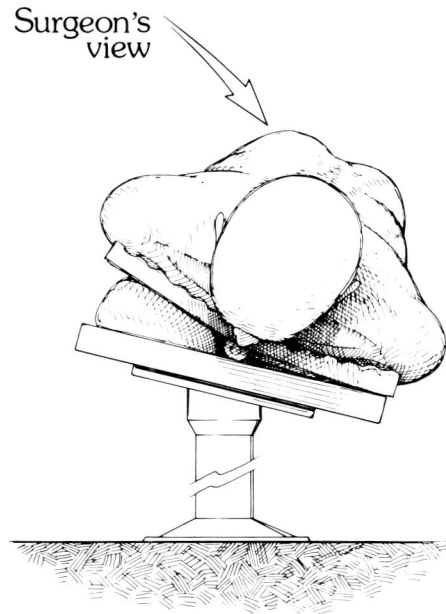

Figure 15–9. The patient may be tilted away from the surgeon, increasing the exposure to the ventrolateral aspect of the spinal canal.

caution, so as not to enter the pleural cavity or to damage the intercostal neurovascular bundle. The transverse process is the key anatomic structure for the posterolateral approach. Once exposed, the transverse process can be resected, leading the surgeon to the pedicle of the involved vertebral body. Occasionally, more than one vertebral level will require decompression. With this exposure, several involved segments may be treated at the same time.

The transverse process is resected with rongeurs, and under microscopic magnification

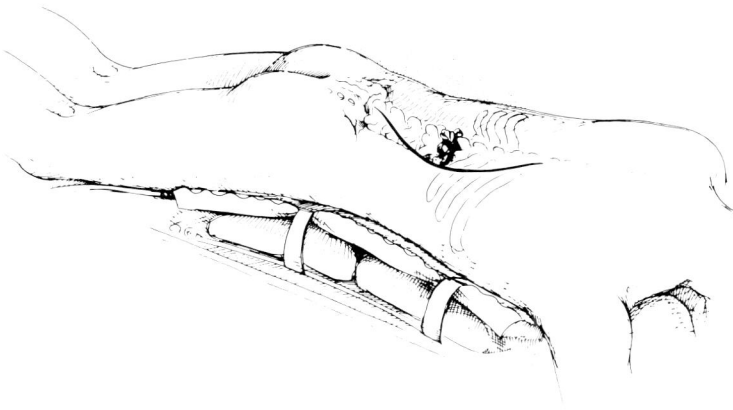

Figure 15–10. Artist's representation of curvilinear paramedian skin incision on the side of the operative approach.

(300 mm lens) and illumination, a high-speed drill is used to remove the pedicle. The ventrolateral aspect of the thecal sac can be identiifed: the intervening disk spaces (rostral and caudal) provide key landmarks. Dissection is carried into the ventral aspect of the vertebral body, and the offending compressive bone and disk fragments can be removed (Figs. 15–11, 15–12). In our experience, the rostral disk and bone fragments from the superior aspect of the fractured vertebral body typically cause the worst canal compromise. The patient may be tilted away from the surgeon, and the microscope angled to show the ventral aspect of the thecal sac. Only the contralateral ventrolateral aspect of the thecal sac cannot be seen with these techniques. The surgeon can, however, determine whether thecal sac compression is present and can eliminate it with the cautious use of reverse saddle curettes—directing the free bone fragments into the space created by the initial bony dissection of the vertebral body.

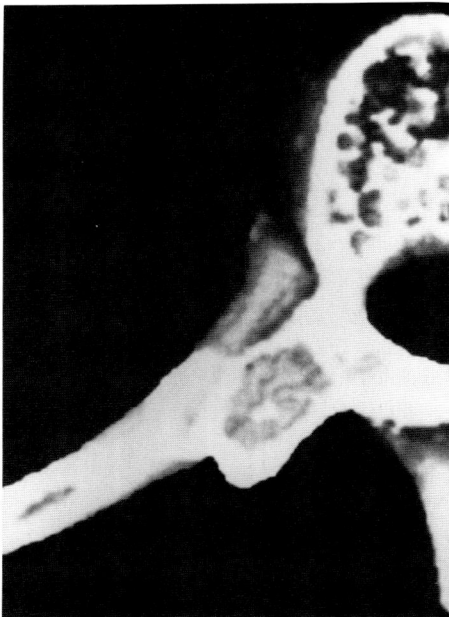

Figure 15–11.   Magnified three-dimensional CT view of T12 vertebrae focusing on the rib, transverse process, and pedicle, which must be removed to allow exposure to the ventral aspect of the thecal sac.

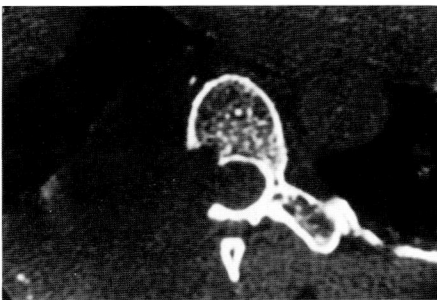

Figure 15–12.   Postoperative CT study reveals the extent of bony dissection with the modified costotransversectomy posterolateral operative approach.

Any dorsal spinal canal compression by posterior element fractures is then treated, followed by placement of the final ipsilateral Harrington rod. Autologous iliac crest bone is used for the bony fusion. We do not routinely perform intraoperative myelography, but in difficult cases when the extent of decompression is not entirely clear, intraoperative myelography may be done before placement of the second Harrington rod.

We have used this approach 30 times over the last 4 years for injury to the TLJ (Table 15-3). Twenty-three patients had traumatic TLJ fracture-dislocations with ventral fragments in the spinal canal compressing neural elements. In each case, a wide operative exposure was achieved, as just outlined. Postoperative radiographs revealed a significant decompression in every patient. No patient had an exacerbation of neurologic deficits nor did any patient develop a cerebrospinal fluid fistula. In one patient a wound dehiscence and infection developed that required reexploration and debridement, but this was the only patient in our series to require a second surgical procedure.

SUMMARY

Traumatic injuries to the TLJ vertebrae are common and may result in permanent neurologic disability and vertebral column instability. Patients with TLJ injuries must be evaluated carefully and thoroughly with serial neurologic examinations and diagnostic studies as outlined. The treatment of patients who have sustained TLJ trauma must be individualized and is determined by the type and level of fracture, the presence of dislocation or instability, and the degree of neurologic injury. Many of these patients may be managed nonoperatively; however, surgical treatment will be required in selected patients to maximize their long-term functional recovery. There are several surgical options available for the treatment of TLJ injuries, depending on specific abnormalities and the experience of the surgical team. In general, ventral compressive lesions must be approached via a ventral or ventrolateral

Table 15-3   Thoracolumbar Junction Pathologic Conditions Treated with Surgical Decompression

	NO.
Trauma	
T11	3
T12	8
L1	9
L2	3
Total	23
Herniated disk	
T10–T11	1
T11–T12	1
L1–L2	2
Total	4
Tumors	
Meningioma	1
Schwannoma	1
Metastatic	1
Total	3

exposure, allowing decompression without injury to neural structures. In our experience, the modified costotransversectomy approach is efficacious for traumatic TLJ injuries and allows both decompression and stabilization and fusion to be done at the same time.

REFERENCES

1. Bohlman HH: Current concepts review: Treatment of fractures and dislocations of the thoracic and lumbar spine. J Bone Joint Surg 67A:165–169, 1985.
2. Bohlman HH: Late, progressive paralysis and pain following fractures of the thoracolumbar spine. (Abstr.) J Bone Joint Surg 58A:728, 1976.
3. Bradford DS, Akbarnia BA, Winter RB, Seljeskog EL: Surgical stabilization of fracture and fracture dislocations of the thoracic spine. Spine 2:185–196, 1977.
4. Brant-Zawadzki M, Miller EM, Federle MP: CT in the evaluation of spine trauma. AJR 136:369–375, 1981.
5. Dickson JH, Harrington PR, Erwin WD: Results of reduction and stabilization of the severely fractured thoracic and lumbar spine. J Bone Joint Surg 60A:799–805, 1978.
6. Durward QJ, Schweigel JF, Harrison P: Management of fractures of the thoracolumbar and lumbar spine. Neurosurgery 8:555–561, 1981.
7. Erickson DL, Leider LL Jr, Brown WE: One-stage decompression-stabilization for thoracolumbar fractures. Spine 2:53–56, 1977.
8. Flesch JR, Leider LL, Erickson DL, Chou SN, Bradford DS: Harrington instrumentation and spine fusion for unstable fractures and fracture-dislocations of the thoracic and lumbar spine. J Bone Joint Surg 59A:143–145, 1977.
9. Holdsworth FW: Fractures, dislocations, and fracture-dislocations of the spine. J Bone Joint Surg 45B:6–20, 1963.
10. Jacobs RR, Asher MA, Snider RK: Thoracolumbar spinal injuries: A comparative study of recumbent and operative treatment in 100 patients. Spine 5:463–477, 1980.
11. Jelsma RK, Kirsch PT, Jelsma LF, Ramsey WC, Rice JF: Surgical treatment of thoracolumbar fractures. Surg Neurol 18:156–156, 1982.
12. Jelsma RK, Rice JF, Jelsma LF, Kirsch PT: The demonstration and significance of neural compression after spinal injury. Surg Neurol 18:79–92, 1982.
13. McAfee PC, Bohlman HH, Yuan HA: Anterior decompression of traumatic thoracolumbar fractures with incomplete neurological deficit using a retroperitoneal approach. J Bone Joint Surg 67A:89–104, 1985.
14. McAfee PC, Yuan HA, Fredrickson BE, Lubicky JP: The value of computed tomography in thoracolumbar fractures. An analysis of one hundred consecutive cases and a new classification. J Bone Joint Surg 65A:461–473, 1983.
15. McAfee PC, Yuan HA, Lasda NA: The unstable burst fracture. Spine 7:365–373, 1982.
16. Paul RL, Michael RH, Dunn JE, Williams JP: Anterior transthoracic surgical decompression of acute spinal cord injuries. J Neurosurg 43:299–307, 1975.
17. Roberts JB, Curtiss PH Jr: Stability of the thoracic and lumbar spine in traumatic paraplegia following fracture or fracture-dislocation. J Bone Joint Surg 52A:1115–1130, 1970.
18. Schmidek HH, Gomes FB, Seligson D, McSherry JW: Management of acute unstable thoracolumbar (T-11–L-1) fractures with and without neurological deficit. Neurosurgery 7:30–35, 1980.
19. Shuman WP, Rogers JV, Sickler ME, Hanson JA, Crutcher JP, King HA, Mack LA: Thoracolumbar burst fractures: CT dimensions of the spinal canal relative to postsurgical improvement. AJR 145:337–341, 1985.
20. White RR, Newberg A, Seligson D: Computerized tomographic assessment of the traumatized dorsolumbar spine before and after Harrington instrumentation. Clin Orthop 146:150–156, 1980.
21. Whitesides TE Jr, Shah SGA: On the management of unstable fractures of the thoracolumbar spine: Rationale for use of anterior decompression and fusion and posterior stabilization. Spine 1:99–107, 1976.

16

Penetrating Spinal Injuries

RICHARD K. SIMPSON, JR.,
BENJAMIN H. VENGER,
AND RAJ K. NARAYAN

Although Ambroise Paré is credited with the first description of penetrating spinal injuries (PSI) in 1567, the most famous incident occurred at the Battle of Trafalgar on October 21, 1805.[27,57] Toward the end of the struggle against the Spanish and French fleets, at approximately 1:15 PM, Admiral Horatio Nelson suddenly fell to his knees. "They have done for me at last, Hardy," Nelson exclaimed to his able flag captain. Hardy replied "I hope not." Nelson then said, "Yes, my backbone is shot through." The ship's surgeon, Dr. Beatty, rushed to his assistance and stated "My Lord, unhappily for our Country, nothing can be done for you." When victory was secured, Nelson died. Although this pessimistic attitude toward PSI has persisted over the centuries, the prognosis following such an injury is not uniformly dismal, especially if associated injuries are properly managed. However, a number of issues relating to management of PSI remain controversial, such as surgical versus nonsurgical therapy, timing of surgery, and the use of steroids.

This chapter summarizes available literature on this subject, adds to current body of knowledge from the large experience at Baylor, and concludes with our management guidelines.

HISTORICAL PERSPECTIVE

Civil War

Until recently, most PSI occurred in wartime. The earliest series of battlefield-incurred PSI can be found in records from the American Civil War. There were 642 cases of PSI documented in the *Medical and Surgical History of the War of the Rebellion*; this represented a very small proportion of the total number of casualties.[37] As shown in Table 16–1, most injuries occurred to the thoracolumbar region, although wound location often was not reported. Operative intervention was not discussed, presumably reflecting the lack of adequate surgical facilities at that time. The overall mortality was reportedly 55%.

197

Table 16–1   Civil War Statistics*

0.25% of all casualties
642 recorded cases
91 cervical injuries
137 thoracic injuries
149 lumbar injuries
5 multiple injuries
260 not specified
55% mortality
operations unknown

*Adapted from Frazier.[12]

World War I

With the introduction of aseptic surgical techniques, more battlefield PSI were treated, often by surgeons specializing in neurologic injuries (Table 16–2). Cushing suggested that mortality rates had increased whether or not an operation was performed,[7] the rates being similar to those reported for a series of 175 cases reviewed by Frazier.[12] The higher mortality, if not an artifact of data collection, was believed to be the result of more powerful and accurate missiles. Perhaps Hanson[19] represented the opinion of that era when he stated "War wounds of the spine were particularly distressing . . . one scarcely knew where to begin, if to begin at all." Indications for surgery were not well defined and treatment often consisted of debridement of the wound with little or no manipulation of the dura or cord.

World War II

There was no standard of care for PSI at the onset of World War II. The discovery of antibiotics as well as the surgical techniques developed during World War I influenced military philosophy. A policy was formulated to encourage prompt operative intervention if there was a reasonable chance that the spinal cord was not completely destroyed. Treatment consisted of laminectomy, debridement, foreign body removal, and limited exploration of intradural injuries followed by dural grafts, if necessary. According to Matson,[36] PSI, in some form, was reported in nearly 12% of battlefield injuries. Approximately half of the cases sustained severe associated chest or abdominal wounds.

Table 16–2   World War I Statistics*

32 cases
7 cervical injuries
2 thoracic injuries
8 lumbar injuries
15 not specified
8 inoperable, 100% mortality
24 laminectomies, 62.5% mortality

*Adapted from Cushing.[7]

Operative mortality decreased remarkably, compared with the preantibiotic era, and 15% of patients were reported to have improved neurologically, usually those with incomplete deficits[54] (Table 16–3). The routine placement of indwelling urethral catheters, better care of paralyzed patients, and use of blood products improved clinical outcome.

Korean War

Improvements in managing PSI during World War II and logistical advances in casualty evacuation and transportation to organized forward and base hospitals were decisive in the formulation of a new treatment policy during the Korean War.[38] Operative intervention during the acute phase of neurologic injury was thought to reduce delayed morbidity and mortality. When the patient's general condition permitted, wound debridement, laminectomy, and intradural exploration were performed in all cases of PSI. The dura was opened even if it had not been penetrated. Postponement, but not omission, of surgery was acceptable, and several cases of neurologic improvement after delayed surgery for PSI were seen.[38] The clinical outcome in 359 cases is expressed in Table 16–4. Nearly half of the patients with complete paraplegia or quadriplegia and the vast majority with incomplete deficits improved postoperatively.

Table 16–3   World War II Statistics*

1260 total cases
15.5% cervical injuries
47.7% thoracic injuries
36.8% lumbar injuries
50% associated injuries
57.1% complete deficits
42.9% incomplete deficits
35% laminectomies
15% postoperative neurologic improvement
7.1% postoperative complications
4.5% postoperative mortality

*Adapted from Spurling.[54]

Table 16–4   Korean War Statistics*

359 total cases
18% cervical injuries
53% thoracic injuries
29% lumbar injuries
100% had laminectomies
68% complete deficits, 29% improved
29% incomplete deficits, 82% improved
3% deficits not reported
3% operative mortality

*Adapted from Meirowsky.[38]

Vietnam War

Because of the reported success of spinal surgery during the Korean War, the philosophy of operating on all cases of PSI continued into the Vietnam War. There has been no compilation of all cases of PSI from this relatively recent military experience, although several smaller series have been reported.[22,23,43] A representative series by Jacobson and Bors[23] is shown in Table 16–5. Although operative mortality was slightly less than that seen during the Korean War, no neurologic improvement was observed in patients with complete neurologic injuries. Approximately 25% of patients with incomplete deficits improved postoperatively. The different results in the Korean and Vietnam wars may reflect sampling error in patient identification or differences in the definitions and documentation of deficits in the two series. Results from a recent series of battlefield injuries in Lebanon confirms the poor prognosis for postoperative neurologic recovery. In one series, neurologic improvement was seen in 50% of surgically treated cases and only 38% of those treated conservatively, a difference that was not significant and that may have represented a sampling bias.[40]

GENERAL CONSIDERATIONS

Epidemiology

The vast majority of patients sustaining PSI are young adults, mostly males aged 21 to 30 years.[52] The same age and sex distribution has been reported from very large series of gunshot wounds (GSW)[55] and stab wounds (SW).[42]

Weapon Type

Although the caliber and type of weapon is often uncertain, GSW in civilian practice are usually caused by small (.22 to .38) bullets from handguns.[39,52] Injuries from large caliber and more powerful weapons resembling those seen in military combat, such as .357, .44, .45 caliber handguns as well as bullets from rifles and shotgun pellets, are less common.[17,62] The composition of bullets can also vary, although most are made of lead. Although delayed response to injury has often been attributed to copper-jacketed fragments, which have been

---

Table 16–5   Vietnam War Statistics*

32 total cases
9% cervical injuries
44% thoracic injuries
47% lumbosacral injuries
75% complete deficits
25% incomplete deficits
100% had laminectomy
0% complete injuries improved
25% incomplete injuries improved

---

*Adapted from Jacobson.[23]

reported to cause an exaggerated granulomatous response, an inflammatory tissue reaction can also occur in response to steel and glass.[24,41,60] Lacerating injuries are usually the result of knives; however, a wide variety of weapons can be used, including scissors, bicycle spokes, and sharpened broomsticks.[31]

Wound Location

Most PSI wounds are to the thoracic spine, whereas lumbosacral and cervical injuries occur less often,[5,23,31,39,42,46] probably reflecting the relative sizes of these cord segments. Spinal injuries at more than one site are unusual in civilian PSI. Lacerating injuries (non-GSW PSI) also are most frequently seen in the thoracic region as well.[42]

Neurologic Injury

Neurologic deficits as a result of PSI may be broadly classified as: (1) complete neurologic deficit, including sensory, motor, and sphincter function, below the level of injury; (2) incomplete neurologic deficit, whereby some function remains at all cord segments; and (3) cauda equina injuries. In several series, 52 to 57% of patients had complete loss of neurologic function below the injury, 13 to 43% had incomplete injuries, and 17 to 35% had cauda equina injuries.[2,6,55,61] Lacerating PSI often results in incomplete neurologic deficits, with a Brown-Sequard lesion fairly commonly seen.[42]

Mechanism of Injury

The differences between military and civilian PSI in terms of clinical outcome, percentage of patients with complete neurologic deficits, and appearance of the cord have been attributed to the mechanism of tissue damage. Blast or concussive forces causing temporary neurologic impairment are thought to occur more frequently in PSI sustained by projectiles with high velocities.[39] Although most studies regard the kinetic energy ($\frac{1}{2}$ mv^2) released by a missile as being responsible for tissue damage, Yashon[62] has proposed that velocity is the most important factor in determining the injury potential of a projectile, expressed as a function of power (mv^3). In general, weapons used in cases of civilian PSI have muzzle velocities of 600 to 1100 ft/sec, whereas military weapons range from 2000 to 4000 ft/sec.[39,62] Shrapnel, for brief distances, also travel at high velocities and have been reported to be responsible for nearly a third of wartime PSI.[23]

Supporting the concept of concussive injury in the military setting are many reported cases of normal-appearing spinal cords at laminectomy by Frazier,[12] Haynes,[20] Meirowsky,[38] and Six et al.[52] Shock waves or indirect cord injury was thought to be responsible for neurologic impairment. The transient nature of deficits was also proposed, in part, to be the result of resolving edema. Such concussive forces are less likely to occur from weapons usually responsible for civilian PSI. Neurologic impairment in civilian PSI therefore is more likely to be the result of direct spinal cord or root damage. A patient with direct injury to nervous tissue, such as that caused by a knife, small caliber handgun, or buckshot, is less likely to show neurologic improvement. The pathologic features of spinal cords that had sustained an indirect blast injury or a direct penetrating injury have been studied in detail.[12,59]

GUIDELINES FOR MANAGEMENT

Current Controversies

For the past 20 years, the need for laminectomy, intradural exploration, and wound debridement in cases of civilian PSI has been debated. Treatment of civilian PSI has paralleled that of battlefield PSI. Since the Korean War, many surgeons have maintained that all cases of civilian PSI require exploration.[38] This philosophy is reflected by Scarff,[46] who stated that, "All compound injuries of the spine should be explored at the earliest possible moment." Recent studies have suggested that civilian PSI differ in several respects from battlefield PSI.[51] These studies conclude that the indications for neurosurgical intervention may differ from the military guidelines. Although considerable ambiguity exists, the relatively few civilian studies reported to date have concluded that neurologic deterioration or an incomplete neurologic deficit is an indication for surgery.[2,61] Wound debridement and exploration for purposes of infection prophylaxis and prevention of cerebrospinal fluid (CSF) leakage are frequently stated surgical indications,[21,55] as are decompression and fragment removal.[15,39] However, the reports concerning the actual benefits of decompressive laminectomy and intradural exploration in civilian PSI describe conflicting results.

Wound Debridement

In two series of civilian PSI, the complication rate was higher in patients subjected to surgery, with 16 to 18% of patients developing postoperative wound infections, CSF leakage, or spinal instability; none of the conservatively managed patients had such complications.[21,55]

A much higher rate of delayed infection in patients undergoing aggressive wound debridement has sometimes,[33] although not always, been seen.[4] Early operative intervention for infection prophylaxis has been advocated particularly if the abdomen has been penetrated. Infection commonly occurs (88%) when there is an associated colon injury; infections are uncommon if the gastrointestinal tract has not been entered or if penetration has been limited to the stomach or small bowel.[45] With penetrating neck wounds, the trachea or esophagus has been penetrated, patients appear to be at high risk for infection if wound exploration, thorough debridement of bone and soft tissue, and drainage are not implemented.[25]

Fragment Removal

Fragment removal has been described as an indication for operation, although there is considerable debate. Some investigators have advocated surgical intervention if bone, clot, or metallic fragments can be visualized radiographically within the spinal canal.[5,39] However, others have not seen neurologic improvement in patients subjected to surgery for fragment removal.[55,61]

No infections occurred in patients in whom fragments remained if high-dose antibiotic coverage was administered.[55] There are, however, several case reports showing delayed neurologic deterioration or radicular pain secondary to retained or migrating missile fragments.[26,60] Osteomyelitis can occur some time after PSI.[17,25,34] Radicular symptoms secondary to a herniated nucleus pulposus have occurred as a rare, yet delayed complication from GSW.[35] Several cases of delayed, acute lead intoxication from retained bullet fragments have been reported.[16,30]

Neurologic Deterioration

A worsening neurologic examination is an uncommon feature in the clinical evaluation of civilian PSI. Yashon et al.,[61] in their series of 65 patients, had two patients with progressing deficits. Both patients underwent laminectomy, neither improved, and both died of complications from their injuries. Heiden et al.[21] had a similar experience in their series of 38 patients. Only one patient had surgery for deteriorating neurologic function with no postoperative improvement. However, Wilson[58] has concluded, from his single case, that progressing neurologic injury remains an absolute indication for neurosurgical intervention. Recent reports of battle-inflicted PSI continue to support the philosophy that neurologic deterioration is a certain indication for neurosurgical intervention.[40] Guttmann[17] reviewed an extensive civilian and wartime experience and also concluded that worsening neurologic deficit was extremely uncommon and proposed that neural damage was likely the result of the immediate injury rather than delayed secondary effects.

Incomplete Deficits

There is no convincing proof that surgery improves outcome in patients with incomplete neurologic deficits after PSI. In several studies, improvement rates were similar whether or not surgery was performed.[52,55,61] In two other series, all patients who underwent surgery improved, whereas 75% of unoperated patients improved.[2,6]

Cauda Equina Lesions

Nerve root function improves in almost all patients with cauda equina injuries with or without surgery.[2] This has led some investigators to recommend only conservative management[32,61] and others to opt for surgical debridement and restoration of anatomy insofar as possible.[5,39] Surgery may be beneficial in reducing chronic pain from root herniation and in removing pressure on nerve roots from bone, bullet fragments, or herniation, although these contensions are unproved.

Lacerating Injuries

Laceration injuries of the cauda equina or spinal cord, although uncommon in the United States, occur fairly often in South Africa. Two large series have stated that the only indications for surgery were a retained knife blade, persistent CSF leakage, or abscess formation, and that only about 5% of patients developed these problems.[31,42] In these studies, no patient with complete cord or cauda equina transection improved. Of the patients with incomplete neurologic deficits, 14% recovered completely and the remainder showed some improvement. Delayed myelopathy secondary to small retained fragments of a knife blade or glass has been reported to occur up to 8 years after the initial injury. One possible exception to this generally nonoperative stance is in cases of SW to the upper cervical cord region, for which debridement, foreign body removal, and repair of dural or vascular rents are advisable.[9,47] Injuries to this region often include lacerations to the vertebral artery and veins with concomitant risk of false aneurysm formation, arteriovenous fistulas, and vascular occlusion. Delayed neurologic impairment from vascular compromise has also been reported to occur following GSW to the craniocervical junction.[14]

Shotgun Wounds

Shotgun wounds, in generally, are serious surgical injuries because considerable soft tissue loss occurs, perhaps accompanied by severe abdominal or chest injury[48,51] resulting in very long hospitalizations (up to 18 months) and multiple nonneurosurgical operations. Deficits ranged from radicular symptoms of spinal root avulsion to transection of the cord. Because these patients often have a complicated hospital course and such PSI occur infrequently, no generalizations regarding treatment have been offered. However, a recent autopsy study of a paraplegic patient who sustained a shotgun wound to the thoracic spine 14 years before his death revealed numerous intradural epidermoids and lipomas thought to be the result of traumatic implantation.[53] Delayed neurologic symptoms from buckshot can occur.[8]

Associated Injuries

Several recent reviews have concluded that associated injuries occur in only 25% of patients sustaining civilian PSI but in 67% or more of patients sustaining wartime PSI.[23] However, the current surgical management of civilian PSI has been greatly influenced by the presence of coexistent visceral, bronchial, or esophageal penetration.[5] Exploration of the spinal canal during non-neurosurgical procedures in cases of PSI, including SW and shotgun injuries, would take advantage of neck, chest, or abdominal exposures and may prevent a second operation. Debridement of devitalized tissue, immobilization of the spine when needed, wound drainage, and use of broad-spectrum antibiotics are essential to prevent complications from tracheal or esophageal penetration.[25] In GSW patients with PSI and colon injuries, abdominal exploration and debridement are indicated to prevent meningitis, discitis, and osteomyelitis, which can be delayed for months if treated conservatively.[45,58] Infections rarely occur in PSI patients when only small bowel or stomach are also injured. However, in one series delayed abscess formation and osteomyelitis were seen more frequently in patients undergoing aggressive debridement than in those treated conservatively; whether patients who had surgery also had more complicated injuries was unclear.

Injuries to other organs associated with SW are uncommon, pneumothorax or hemothorax accounting for 80% of associated injuries.[42] Complications occur more frequently if the bowel or bronchus are entered, in which cases prophylactic antibiotic administration to prevent meningitis may be indicated.[13]

THE BAYLOR EXPERIENCE

Patient Population

One hundred and sixty patients with PSI were treated at the Ben Taub General Hospital between 1980 and 1986. This series included 142 GSW, including five shotgun injuries, and 18 SW to the spinal cord or cauda equina. Twenty-seven percent of the injuries were cervical, 54% thoracic, and 19% lumbosacral cord or cauda equina injuries. The average age was 29 years, ranging from 7 to 75 years, and 94% of the patients were males.

Associated injuries of the esophagus, trachea, bronchi, or bowel occurred in 107 (67%) of patients. The most frequent associated injuries were pneumothorax followed by injury to a hollow viscus. Virtually all patients received antibiotics whether or not surgery was performed. Antibiotic type, dosage, interval, and length of treatment varied. On admission, 66% of the GSW and 22% of the SW patients had complete paraplegia or quadriplegia. Approximately 34% of GSW and 18% of SW patients had incomplete neurologic deficits. Plain radiographs were obtained for all patients. Other methods of evaluation were infrequently used (Table 16–6).

We have made some statistical comparisons between groups of patients treated in specific ways, but the patients were not randomized into treatment groups so that care must be taken in interpreting our results.

Associated Injuries

One hundred and seven patients in our series had associated injuries that required non-neurosurgical intervention. These injuries occurred to the neck in 23%, chest in 21%, abdomen in 31%, and multiple sites in 25% of cases. In our series, the presence or absence of associated injuries did not affect neurologic recovery.

Management

Neurosurgical operations were done in 22% of the GSW patients and 33% of SW patients. The stated indications for surgery were varied, and often multiple (Table 16–7). In general, the operation consisted of a laminectomy with intradural exploration and fragment removal (Table 16–8). The effects of surgery or nonoperative treatment on GSW and SW are shown in Tables 16–9 to 16–11. Dexamethasone had no effect on outcome in our patients (Table 16–12).

Table 16–6   Baylor Series: Evaluation of Patients with PSI

	NO.	%
Plain films	160	100
Myelography	20	13
CSF studies	13	8
CT scans	13	8
Tomograms	6	4
Electromyography or nerve conduction studies	4	3

Table 16–7   **Baylor Series: Stated Indications for Surgery in PSI**

	NO.	%
Exploration and debridement	19	41
Worsening neurologic status	7	19
Decompression and fragment removal	6	16
Not indicated in record	5	14

Table 16–8   **Baylor Series: Surgical Procedures Performed**

	NO.	%
Laminectomy	34	92
No laminectomy	1	3
Not clearly reported	2	5
Intradural exploration	20	57
Primary dural repair	12	60
Duraplasty (graft)	8	40
Fragment removal	20	57
Bony decompression	6	17
Wound debridement	9	26

Table16–9   **Baylor Series:**
Outcome in PSI With and Without Neurosurgic Intervention

	IMPROVED		NO CHANGE		WORSENED	
	No.	*%*	*No.*	*%*	*No.*	*%*
Complete deficits, 94 GSW						
With surgery	2	13	13	81	1	6
Without surgery	12	15	64	82	2	3
Incomplete deficits, 48 GSW						
With surgery	6	40	6	40	3	20
Without surgery	19	58	8	24	6	18
Complete deficits, 4 SW						
With surgery	1	50	1	50	0	0
Without surgery	0	0	2	100	0	0
Incomplete deficits, 14 SW						
With surgery	2	50	1	25	1	25
Without surgery	7	70	3	30	0	0

Nearly half (41%) of our operated patients underwent wound debridement and exploration. Neurosurgical intervention did not appear to influence outcome, and the complication rate was higher in surgically treated patients than those managed conservatively. Approximately 24% of the surgically treated patients in our series were operated on for removal of retained fragments, debridement, and decompression. Postoperatively, two improved and seven remained unchanged, results similar to those of the overall series. Only seven patients were operated on in our series in response to neurologic deterioration, of whom three improved, three showed no change, and one worsened.

Table 16–10   Baylor Series: Outcome from Spinal Cord Injury

	IMPROVED		NO CHANGE		WORSENED	
	No.	*%*	*No.*	*%*	*No.*	*%*
Complete (n = 91)						
With surgery	3	20	11	73	1	7
Without surgery	11	14	63	83	2	3
Incomplete (n = 39)						
With surgery	5	63	1	13	2	25
Without surgery	19	61	9	29	3	10
Total	38	29	84	65	8	6

Table 16–11   Baylor Series: Outcome from PSI to the Cauda Equina

	IMPROVED		NO CHANGE		WORSENED	
	No.	*%*	*No.*	*%*	*No.*	*%*
Complete (n = 7)						
With surgery	0	0	3	100	0	0
Without surgery	1	25	3	75	0	0
Incomplete (n = 23)						
With surgery	3	27	6	55	2	18
Without surgery	7	58	2	17	3	25
Total	11	37	14	47	5	17

Table 16–12   Baylor Series: Effect of Steroids on Outcome in PSI

	IMPROVED		NO CHANGE		WORSENED	
	No.	*%*	*No.*	*%*	*No.*	*%*
Dexamethasone (n = 66)	21	32	36	55	9	14
No steroids (n = 94)	28	30	62	66	4	4
Total	49	31	98	61	13	8

Only 7% (9 of 123) of the conservatively managed group developed neurologic complications, including meningitis, CSF leakage, pseudomeningocele, wound infection, and spinal instability (Table 16–13); 22% (8 of 37) of the surgically managed patients had these complications postoperatively. Complications occurred in 9% (10 of 107) of patients with associated injuries and in 13% (7 of 53) of patients without associated injuries, a statistically significant difference ($p < 0.05$). Associated injuries did not influence complication rates in the two groups. The mortality rate was 4% (7 of 160), with all deaths the result of severe associated injuries.

Table 16–13   Baylor Series: Neurologic Complications from PSI

	SURGICAL GROUP (n = 37)	NONSURGICAL GROUP (n = 123)
Meningitis	1	3
CSF leakage	2	2
Wound infection	3	1
Spinal instability	2	3
Pseudomeningocele	1	0
Total	8 (22%)	9 (7%)

CONCLUSIONS

The results from our large series indicate that neurosurgical operations did not clearly influence neurologic recovery from PSI. Surgical treatment did not improve outcome in any type (complete or incomplete deficits) or location of injury (spinal cord or cauda equina); the incidence of neurologic complication was higher in the surgically managed patients than in those managed conservatively. Although this analysis is limited by the retrospective, nonrandomized nature of the data, it certainly casts doubts on some traditionally held beliefs regarding management of PSI.

RECOMMENDATIONS

An accurate neurologic examination is of the utmost importance in evaluating a patient with PSI. Since many examiners will see patients after PSI, a standardized examination record would reduce interobserver variability and facilitate evaluation of treatment. Repeated observations using a single examination also will aid detection of neurologic deterioration that may indicate the need for surgery.

Although the need for urgent operative intervention as a definitive treatment of civilian PSI remains debatable, each case should be individualized, particularly when there are coexisting injuries to other parts of the body. In patients who are to undergo surgical intervention, precise localization of the bony and neural injury is paramount. Examination alone using dermatomal patterns and motor function loss, or missile entrance, exit, and trajectory have proved to be an inaccurate method of wound localization; the suspected site of cord or cauda equina injury, based on cutaneous or neurologic examination, can differ from the level of bony injury by several segments in more than 40% of patients.[28]

Plain films of the spine, both anteroposterior and lateral views, may be adequate in some patients with PSI,[12,19] but some bony injuries have been found at operation that were not seen on the radiographs.[44] Computed tomography (CT) gives better bone and soft tissue detail and may obviate myelography in some patients.[44,61] CT will not always be adequate because of the degree of artifact caused by metallic fragments and lack of precise soft tissue definition.[2] If myelography is done, water-soluble contrast agents should be used, since oil-based agents probably increase arachnoiditis when used in the presence of bloody CSF.

Standard electrophysiologic diagnostic procedures, such as an electromyogram or nerve conduction velocity, have limited utility in the evaluation of acute PSI.[29] Sophisticated techniques are currently available that may be of considerable use regarding initial assessment, intraoperative monitoring, long-term evaluation of PSI cases. Somatosensory evoked potentials and, recently, corticomotor-evoked potentials have been suggested by Simpson and colleagues[1,49,50] as offering better objective, quantitative, and reproducible neurological evaluations.

We and others recommend the immediate use of broad-spectrum antibiotics and antitetanus prophylaxis in civilians with PSI.[5,39] When indicated, surgery is performed when the patient's general medical condition permits. Life-threatening associated injuries require immediate attention and neurosurgical procedures may be performed when the patient is explored for associated chest or abdominal injuries.[4] Recommendations for the general management of acute spinal cord trauma patients have been described in detail in earlier chapters and elsewhere.[15]

Pharmacologic therapy in spinal cord injury has been recently and extensively reviewed by Yashon.[63] Many agents have been used in an attempt to reverse or limit the neurologic deficits caused by damage to the spinal cord or cauda equina. Several agents have been shown to influence neurologic recovery in experimental animals favorably. Corticosteroids have been widely used for many years in treating spinal cord injury, but we and others[3] have not demonstrated any benefit. Other pharmacologic agents, such as opiate antagonists,[11] calcium antagonists[10] and prostaglandin inhibitors,[18] are currently being evaluated for their beneficial effects on post-traumatic neurologic function but are not yet of proved benefit in humans.

Surgery

If operation is to be performed, a standard posterior approach via laminectomy is most commonly used. Although there are many variations on performing a laminectomy, several operative hazards can be encountered because of the penetrating force exerted by the missiles and consequent bone and soft tissue destruction. However, certain details that are not of concern in routine laminectomy require special attention in cases of PSI.[38]

In general, current recommendations are that a longitudinal incision be centered over the involved lamina and extended to include one intact lamina both above and below the wound. Although a subperiosteal resection of the paraspinous muscles from the lamina should be performed, sharp dissection of the muscles is recommended in the immediate area of comminution and depression. The bony damage is carefully surveyed and the interspinous ligaments are also sharply divided. Spinous processes of the involved site and the immediate cephalad and caudal processes are removed with bone-cutting instruments; great care must be taken not to disturb loose bony or metallic fragments. At this point, devitalized soft tissue can be identified and debrided, and the wound thoroughly irrigated with warmed saline. Beginning with normal tissue cephalad to the wound, small rongeurs are used to remove carefully the lamina bilaterally, and the ligamentum flavum is removed to expose intact dura. Removal of adjacent depressed and comminuted bony fragments or pieces of metal can be done easier and safer using this technique. All fragments are removed and lateral exposure is gained. Facets are spared if possible. The caudal lamina is then removed to allow visualization of the entire wounded segment.

Several surgeons advocate intradural inspection of the cord whether or not the dura has been violated to determine if an occult hematoma exists.[38] However, others recommend that if there is no evidence of CSF leakage and the dura appears intact, no intradural exploration is necessary. Intraoperative ultrasonography can help to determine if a cryptic intradural hematoma or fragment is present. If not, the wound can be closed thorough irrigation of the intraspinal compartment. If the dura was violated, it can be opened along the axis of the cord until normal tissue is visualized, and secured laterally with stay sutures. The cord is carefully inspected and hematoma or fragments are removed. Blood should be prevented from entering the subarachnoid space. The damaged dura is debrided, as are the proximal and distal ends of the damaged cord. After the intrathecal compartment is thoroughly irrigated, the dura is either closed primarily or a dural graft is used. Roots are decompressed if necessary and the wound is tightly closed to prevent CSF leakage. Spinal instability is occasionally a concern, but instrumentation for stabilization generally is not performed at the time of acute operation. Depending on the pathologic anatomy of a given case, an anterior exploration of the injured spine and spinal canal may be warranted in occasional patients.

Postoperative Care

All patients with PSI need to be followed carefully to prevent, detect, and treat complications as they arise. All patients are put on a standard care protocol used for spinal cord injury patients. Particular care is given to pulmonary, urinary, and skin care in those patients with neurologic impairment. A prospective randomized study of the use of the kinetic table (Rota-Rest bed) is currently underway at our center and should help clarify the value of such a device. Rehabilitation efforts should be initiated as soon as possible.

Concluding Remarks

In this chapter, the literature pertaining to PSI has been reviewed and supplemented with our experience at Baylor. The current diagnostic and therapeutic modalities have been described. The value of early surgical intervention in PSI remains debatable. A retrospective analysis of a large series of patients at our center did not demonstrate improved outcome in surgically treated patients with PSI, and the rate of complication seemed to be higher in that group. However, this and all other studies of PSI reported to date have been retrospective, and the groups are not strictly comparable. Likewise, the delayed benefits from surgical intervention have yet to be clearly defined. Only a large prospective randomized study with extended follow-up will be able to resolve this debate and establish optimal indications for surgery in PSI.

REFERENCES

1. Baskin DS, Simpson RK Jr: Corticomotor and somatosensory evoked potential evaluation of acute spinal cord injury in the rat. Neurosurgery 20:871–877, 1987.
2. Benzel EC, Hadden TA, Coleman JE: Civilian gunshot wounds to the spinal cord and cauda equina. Neurosurgery 20:281–285, 1987.
3. Bracken MB, Collins WF, Freeman DF, Shepard MJ, Wagner FW, Silten RM, Hellenbrand KG, Ransohoff J, Hunt WE, Perot PL, Grossman RG, Green BA, Eisenberg HM, Rifkinson N, Goodman JH, Meagher JN, Fischer B, Clifton GL, Flamm ES, Rawe SE: Efficacy of methylprednisolone in acute spinal cord injury. JAMA 251:45–52, 1984.

4. Bricker DL, Waltz TA, Telford RJ, Beall AC Jr: Major abdominal and thoracic trauma associated with spinal cord injury. J Trauma 11:63–75, 1971.

5. Carey ME: Brain and spinal wounds cause by missiles. In Long DM (ed): Current Therapy in Neurological Surgery 1985–1986. Toronto: BC Decker, 1985, pp 114–117.

6. Coleman JE, Benzel EC, Hadden T: Gunshot wounds to the spinal cord and cauda equina in civilians. Surg Forum 37:496–498, 1986.

7. Cushing H: Organization and activities of the neurological service, American Expeditionary Forces. In Hanson AM (ed): The Medical Department of the United States Army in the World War, Surgery. Washington, DC: US Government Printing Office, part 1, vol 11, 1927, pp 749–758.

8. Daniel EF, Smith GW: Foreign-body granuloma of intervertebral disc and spinal canal. J Neurosurg 17:480–482, 1960.

9. De Villiers JC, Grant AR: Stab Wounds at the craniocervical junction. Neurosurgery, 17:930–936, 1985.

10. Faden AI, Jacobs TP, Smith MT: Evaluation of the calcium channel antagonist nimodipine in experimental spinal cord ischemia. J Neurosurg 60:796–799, 1984.

11. Flamm ES, Young W, Collins WF, Piepmier J, Clifton GL, Fischer B: A phase I trial of naloxone treatment in acute spinal cord injury. J Neurosurg 63:390–397, 1985.

12. Frazier CH: Stab and gunshot wounds to the spine. In Frazier CH (ed): Surgery of the Spine and Spinal Cord. New York: D. Appleton, 1918, pp 457–497.

13. Gentleman D, Harrington M: Penetrating injury of the spinal cord. Injury 16:7–8, 1984.

14. Grant JMF, Yeo JD, Sears WR, Copeman MC: Arterial Brown-Sequard's syndrome after a penetrating injury of the spinal cord at the cervicomedullary junction. Med J Aust 142:84–85, 1985.

15. Green BA, Klose KJ: Acute spinal cord injury: Emergency room care and diagnosis, medical and surgical management. In Green BA, Marshall LF, Gallager TJ (eds): Intensive Care for Neurological Trauma and Disease. New York: Academic Press, 1982, pp 249–271.

16. Grogan DP, Buchholz RW: Acute lead intoxication from a bullet in an intervertebral disc space. J Bone Joint Surg 63:1180–1182, 1982.

17. Guttmann L: Gunshot injuries of the spinal cord. In Guttman L (ed), Spinal Cord Injuries. Comprehensive Management and Research. Oxford: Blackwell Scientific Publications, 1976, pp 177–187.

18. Hallenbeck JM, Jacobs TP, Faden AI: Combined PGI$_2$, indomethacin, and heparin improves neurological recovery after spinal trauma in cats. J Neurosurg 58:749–754, 1983.

19. Hanson AM: Management of gunshot wounds of the head and spine in forward hospitals, A.E.F. In Hanson AM (ed): The Medical Department of the United States Army in the World War, Surgery. Washington, DC: US Government Printing Office, part 1, vol 11, 1927, pp 776–794.

20. Haynes WG: Acute war wounds of the spinal cord. Am J Surg 72:424–433, 1946.

21. Heiden JS, Weiss MH, Rosenberg AW, Kurze T, Apuzzo MLJ: Penetrating gunshot wounds of the cervical spine in civilians: Review of 38 cases. J Neurosurg 42:575–579, 1975.

22. Jacobs GB, Berg RA: The treatment of acute spinal cord injuries in a war zone. J Neurosurg 34:164–167, 1971.

23. Jacobson SA, Bors E: Spinal cord injury in Vietnamese combat. Paraplegia 7:263–281, 1970.

24. Jones FD, Woolsey RE: Delayed myelopathy secondary to retained intraspinal metallic fragment. J Neurosurg 55:979–982, 1981.

25. Jones RE, Bucholz RW, Schaefer SD, Mumme M, Carder HM: Cervical osteomyelitis complicating transpharyngeal gunshot wounds to the neck. J Trauma 19:630–634, 1979.

26. Karim NO, Nabors MW, Golocovsky M, Cooney FD: Spontaneous migration of a bullet in the spinal subarachnoid space causing delayed radicular symptoms. Neurosurgery 18:97–100, 1986.

27. Keynes G: The Apologie and Treatise of Ambroise Paré. New York: Dover Publishers, 1968, pp 175, 205, 218–219.

28. Kislow VA: Clinical peculiarities of war wounds of the spinal cord. Bull War Med 4:705, 1944.

29. Lieberman JS: Neuromuscular electrodiagnosis. In Youmans JR (ed): Neurological Surgery, vol 1. Philadelphia: WB Saunders, 1982, pp 617–635.

30. Linden MA, Manton WI, Stewart RM, Thal ER, Feit H: Lead poisoning from retained bullets: Pathogenesis, diagnosis, and management. Ann Surg 195:305–313, 1982.

31. Lipschitz R: Stab wounds of the spinal cord. In Vinken PJ, Bruyn GW (eds): Handbook of Clinical Neurology, vol 25. New York: American Elsevier 1976, pp 197–207.

32. Little JW, DeLisa JA: Cauda equina injury: Late motor recovery. Arch Phys Med Rehabil 67:4547, 1986.

33. Maier RV, Carrico CJ, Heimbach DM: Pyogenic osteomyelitis of axial bones following civilian gunshot wounds. Am J Surg 137:378–380, 1979.

34. Malik GM, Sapico FL, Montgomerie JZ: Severe vertebral osteomyelitis in patients with spinal cord injury. Arch Intern Med 142:807–808, 1982.

35. Mariottini A, Delfini R, Ciappetta P, Paolella G: Lumbar disc hernia secondary to gunshot injury. Neurosurgery, 15:73–75, 1984.

36. Matson DD: The management of acute compound battle-incurred injuries of the spinal cord. In Woodall B

(ed): The Medical Department of the United States Army. Surgery in World War II. Neurosurgery. Washington, DC: US Government Printing Office, vol 2, chap 5, 1959, pp 31–65

37. Medical and Surgical History of the War of the Rebellion. In Frazier CH (ed): Surgery of the Spine and Spinal Cord. New York: D. Appleton, 1918, 464.
38. Meirowsky AM: Penetrating spinal cord injuries. In Coates JB, Meirowsky AM (eds): Neurological Surgery of Trauma. Office of the Surgeon General, Department of the Army. Washington, DC: US Government Printing Office, 1965, pp 257–344.
39. Miller CA: Penetrating wounds of the spine. In Wilkins RH, Rengachary SS (eds): Neurosurgery, vol 2. San Francisco: McGraw-Hill 1985, pp 1746–1748.
40. Ohry A, Rozin R: Acute spinal cord injuries in the Lebanon War, 1982. Israel J Med Sci 20:345–349, 1984.
41. Ott K, Tarlov E, Crowell R, Papadakis N: Retained intracranial metallic foreign bodies. Report of two cases. J Neurosurg 44:80–83, 1976.
42. Peacock WJ, Shrosbree RD, Key AG: A review of 450 stabwounds of the spinal cord. S Afr Med J 51:961–964, 1977.
43. Plaut M: War wounds of the central nervous system: Surgical results. J Trauma 12:613–619, 1972.
44. Post MJ, Green BA, Quencer RM, Stokes NA, Callahan RA, Eismont FJ: The value of computed tomography in spinal trauma. Spine 7:417–431, 1982.
45. Romanick PC, Smith TK, Kopaniky DR, Oldfield D: Infection about the spine associated with low-velocity-missile injury to the abdomen. J Bone Joint Surg 67:1195–1201, 1985.
46. Scarff JE: Injuries to the vertebral column and spinal cord. In Brock S (ed): Injuries of the Brain and Spinal Cord and their Coverings. New York: Springer Publishing, 1960, p 568.
47. Schmidek HH: Comments on De Villers JC, Grant AR: Stab wounds of the craniocervical junction. Neurosurgery 17:936, 1985.
48. Sights WP: Ballistic analysis of shotgun injuries to the central nervous system. J Neurosurg 31:25–33, 1969.
49. Simpson RK, Baskin DS: Corticomotor evoked potentials in acute and chronic blunt spinal cord injury in the rat: Correlation with neurological outcome and histological damage. Neurosurgery 20:131–137, 1987.
50. Simpson RK, Blackburn JG, Martin HF, Katz S: Peripheral nerve fiber and spinal cord pathway contributions to the somatosensory evoked potential. Exp Neurol 73:700–715, 1981.
51. Simpson RK, Venger BH, Narayan RK: Penetrating spinal cord injury in a civilian population: A retrospective analysis (1980–1985). Surg Forum, 37:494–496, 1986.
52. Six E, Alexander E, Kelly DL, Davis CH, McWhorter JM: Gunshot wounds to the spinal cord. South Med J 72:699–702, 1979.
53. Smith CML, Timperley WR: Multiple intraspinal and intracranial epidermoids and lipomata following gunshot injury. Neuropathol Appl Neurobiol 10:235–239, 1984.
54. Spurling RG: The European theater of operations. In Woodhall B (ed): The Medical Department of the United States Army. Surgery in World War II. Neurosurgery. Washington, DC: US Government Printing Office, vol 2, chap 4, 1959, pp 25–30.
55. Stauffer ES, Wood RW, Kelly EG: Gunshot wounds of the spine: Effects of laminectomy. J Bone Joint Surg 61: 389–392, 1979.
56. Vogt MW, Narayan RK: The magnetic properties of bullets and other metallic objects as they relate to MRI. Proceedings of the Annual Meeting of the Congress of Neurological Surgeons, Baltimore, October, 1987.
57. Walker D: Nelson, A biography. Trafalgar, vol 2. New York: Dial Press/James Wade, 1978, pp 499–501.
58. Wilson TH: Penetrating trauma of colon, cava, and cord. J Trauma 16:411–413, 1976.
59. Wolman L: Blast injury of the spinal cord. In Vinken PJ, Bruyn GW (ed): Injuries of the Spine and Spinal Cord. Handbook of Clinical Neurology, vol 25. New York: American Elsevier 1976, pp 221–225.
60. Wu WQ: Delayed effects from retained foreign bodies in the spine and spinal cord. Surg Neurol 25:214–218, 1986.
61. Yashon D, Jane JA, White RJ: Prognosis and management of spinal cord and cauda equina bullet injuries in sixty-five civilians. J Neurosurg 32:163–170, 1970.
62. Yashon D: Missile injuries of the spinal cord and cauda equina. In Yashon D (ed): Spinal Injury. New York: Appleton-Century-Crofts, 1986, pp 285–305.
63. Yashon D: Pharmacological treatment. In Yashon D (ed): Spinal Injury. New York: Appleton-Century-Crofts, 1986, pp 319–332.

17

Medical Management of Spinal Cord Injury

MICHAEL J. ROSNER

Medical management of the spinal cord injury patient is relatively straightforward when based on the pathophysiologic changes that occur after an injury. Although some of these changes remain vague and perhaps ill-defined, others are well-recognized and when understood will facilitate the management of patients with this type of injury.

RESPIRATORY SYSTEM

If the diaphragm is intact after a spinal cord injury, many think that respiratory function should be relatively normal. Most spinal cord injuries occur below C-4 (root level of the phrenic nerve) and, indeed, do leave the diaphragm intact.

However, the concept of "normal phrenic nerve function" coupled with the belief that intercostal muscles and accessory muscles of respiration are relatively unimportant has impeded the realization that the absence of the intercostal muscles may adversely affect the respiratory status of the quadriplegic patient. Although normal intercostal muscles provide little active ventilation during normal day to day living, they are very important in splinting and making the chest wall a relatively rigid structure against which the diaphragm can act to generate an adequate tidal volume (Vt).

The situation in the quadriplegic with paralysis of intercostal musculature is roughly analogous to a syringe with a collapsible rather than rigid barrel. When the plunger, corresponding to the diaphragm, is withdrawn, the barrel, equivalent to the chest wall in this example, puckers and collapses.

Similarly, although the diaphragm is intact in the quadriplegic, the chest wall is functionally the same as in a severe flail chest injury; the negative forces collapse the chest wall instead of generating adequate Vt.

We have measured the negative inspiratory force (NIF), the forced vital capacity (FVC), and the Vt in 25 consecutive quadriplegic and high thoracic paraplegic patients from the time of admission to the intensive care unit (ICU) until discharged from that unit. We found that admission NIF was -25 ± 5 cm H_2O, FVC about 1200 cc, and Vt approximately 350 cc. These parameters are among those used when deciding whether or not intubation is necessary (Table 17–1). The values in this group of patients are at or below the levels at which elective intubation would ordinarily be considered. In general, these profound abnormalities are almost exclusively the result of the "functional flail chest" produced by paralysis of the intercostal muscles.

The consequences of low Vt are most immediately apparent when phrased in terms of "wasted ventilation." Wasted ventilated is a very simple concept defined by the ratio of the ventilatory dead space (Vd) to the total Vt, or Vd/Vt. When this number reaches 50 to 60%, it indicates that ventilatory failure is imminent and that intubation would be appropriate. Normal respiratory Vd is approximately 2 cc/kg, or about 150 cc for the average adult male. If the Vt is only 300 cc, then wasted ventilation is already at 50%.

If the patient ventilates spontaneously with low Vt relative to Vd (high wasted ventilation) and poor (low) NIF and is unable to generate an effective cough or to take deep breaths (low FVC), the consequences are predictable. He or she soon develops diffuse microatelectasis, which can become severe even while the chest examination and radiograph remain near normal. As atelectasis worsens and becomes more generalized, the lungs will "stiffen" and "compliance" will be reduced. Compliance is defined by the ratio of the change in volume to the pressure change required to generate that volume change (dV/dP).

Practically, this means that as the lungs stiffen the pressure needed to generate a given Vt increases. However, in the quadriplegic the inspiratory force is already near the lower limits of normal and generally cannot increase significantly. Decreasing compliance with a high wasted ventilation in combination with an inability to deep breathe and cough and thereby not adequately and spontaneously reexpand the lungs potentiates atelectasis. This results in a vicious cycle of further decreasing Vt and compliance. Respiratory failure with hypoxemia quickly ensues.

This process can be followed in a patient by serially measuring weaning parameters and observing the respiratory rate. The patient, although unable to generate an adequate Vt, still can increase his or her respiratory rate. Progressive tachypnea will usually be the first sign of progressive respiratory failure. The patient will tire and eventually be unable to support his ventilation, especially since an increasingly large percentage of the ventilatory effort is wasted. The result may be acute respiratory arrest.

Blood gas determinations, which all too often are used as the primary method of assessing adequacy of pulmonary function, may be misleading. Early in the process,

Table 17–1 Indications for Continuous Mechanical Ventilation

I.	Ventilatory (mechanical) failure
	Respirations <35 to 40/min
	Inadequate alveolar ventilation with $PaCO_2$ >48 torr
	Vital capacity <10 to 15 ml/kg body weight
	Maximal inspiratory force <−25 cm H_2O
II.	Pulmonary (parenchymal) failure
	Alveolar-arterial oxygen gradient (A-aDO_2) < 300 torr (FiO_2 = 1)
	Right-to-left shunt fraction (Qs/Qt) >15 to 20%
	Wasted ventilation (Vd/Vt) >0.6
	Compliance less than 30 ml/cm H_2O

tachypnea even in the presence of high wasted ventilation, results in low arterial carbon dioxide pressure ($PaCO_2$). Tachypnea is the result of activating primary pulmonary receptors that produce dyspnea (via vagal afferents) and increase the drive to ventilation with very little if any input from the carotid chemoreceptors and does not represent a response to hypoxemia. Hypocapnia may be interpreted (incorrectly) as evidence of perfectly adequate respiratory reserve when, in fact, it represents a response to respiratory distress. $PaCO_2$ may continue to decrease with increasing tachypnea. Hypoxemia may develop, although it tends (early on) to be mild. Many of these patients are started on supplemental oxygen, which further masks the profound nature of their pulmonary impairment and does not address nor alter the basic pathophysiologic events.

As the patient tires, wasted ventilation increases further and microatelectasis continues to develop. The patient's respiratory rate can no longer be sustained, and his or her effective alveolar ventilation reaches low levels. Hypoxemia becomes profound on the basis of inadequate alveolar ventilation and atelectasis, and the patient may well have a respiratory arrest as the $PaCO_2$ finally increases.

Another key to the early detection of these events is examination of the arterial oxygen pressure (PaO_2). If a patient is receiving supplemental oxygen, so that his fraction inspired oxygen (FiO_2) is 0.35 or 0.40, then normal respiratory function would suggest that his PaO_2 should be close to 200 mmHg. If this is not the case, it represents a large alveolar-arterial (A-a) oxygen gradient. A large A-a gradient suggests pulmonary dysfunction and, in particular, a failure of oxygen-diffusing capacity. If the respiratory rate is high, the $PaCO_2$ and the PaO_2 are low, and the patient is dyspneic, then optimal treatment is not to add nasal prongs and low-flow oxygen, although this may transiently improve the PaO_2. Therapy should be directed at the underlying pathophysiologic condition, which is failure to expand the lungs adequately.

Concomitant with the inability to take deep breaths and to cough is the inability to clear airway secretions. If airway secretions accumulate, then there is progressive obstruction of small bronchioles; pulmonary segments distal to this obstruction will become atelectatic and contribute to decreasing pulmonary compliance and hypoxemia.

The use of additional oxygen to treat the mild hypoxemia associated with this early form of respiratory embarrassment may actually potentiate the development of atelectasis, especially absorption atelectasis from alveolar volume reduction with absorption of oxygen.

When a patient breathes room air, the gas composition is approximately 80% nitrogen, which is not well absorbed. If the patient is placed on an inspired oxygen concentration ($FiO_2 = 0.4$) of 0.40, then effectively the volume by which the alveolus can be expected to decline or collapse has doubled. The use of supplemental oxygen must be considered very carefully in these patients.

So far, the interaction of pulmonary contusion, aspiration, hemopneumothorax, and other pulmonary injuries, which may occur in 20 to 40% of spinal cord-injured patients, has not been discussed. Even those patients with initially clear chest radiographs may have aspirated or have a pulmonary contusion that has not yet resulted in visible change. Initially, the physical signs may be normal or nearly normal or masked by rhonchi, the noise of tubes and ventilators, and ambient sound. Helpful clues may include the presence of hypoxemia that is more profound than one would normally expect, decreased pulmonary compliance, and chest radiographic abnormalities, such as fractured ribs, clavicles, or thoracic vertebrae.

Neglect of these changes produces problems greater than simple respiratory failure that can be corrected by intubation. As the process continues, it becomes much more difficult to reexpand the lungs even in the presence of intubation and mechanical ventilation. The lungs become extremely stiff, with greatly decreased compliance; secretions accumulate, thicken, and are often colonized, and infection promptly develops.

The interaction of bronchopulmonary infection, profoundly atelectatic lungs, pulmonary contusion, or factors such as aspiration and chest injury in the patient whose immune response may already be depressed can result rapidly in the development of the adult respiratory distress syndrome (ARDS). Mortality from this entity continues to be 40% or greater. Also associated with this condition is prolonged morbidity during which assisted ventilation is required to reverse the pulmonary capillary changes that may take as long as 4 weeks, even in the neurologically normal patient. The consequences of ARDS in the quadriplegic patient can be devastating or fatal, and extraordinarily expensive. In spinal cord-injured patients this disease may cause a patient who would otherwise have become independent to become permanently ventilator dependent.

Prevention of ARDS includes maintenance of the functional residual capacity (FRC) of the lung, that is, keeping the lungs adequately expanded. This may be accomplished by frequent coughing by the patient. In the quadriplegic patient, though, turning, coughing, and deep breathing should not be relied on to keep the lungs expanded. After spinal injury, inspiration and cough are hampered by a relatively flaccid chest wall and the high positive pressures that could be generated in the normal person by coughing are not achieved. Nonetheless, these measures, particularly in the partially injured patient, should be encouraged to help clear secretions. Nasotracheal or orotracheal suctioning and other standard measures to clear secretions should always be used aggressively, especially in the early phases before obvious pulmonary dysfunction develops.

The use of alternative methods of maintaining FRC, such as continuous positive airway pressure (CPAP) by mask, is encouraged. In a recent comparison of coughing, deep breathing, turning, incentive spirometry, and CPAP by mask, the pulmonary complications in the CPAP by mask group were markedly reduced. Similarly, just as the cough and deep breathing technique have intrinsic limitations because of the pulmonary changes brought about by the cord injury, so does the use of incentive spirometry. Expecting a patient to generate 1.5 or 2.5 liters of vital capacity using one of the bedside instruments when the best he can do is only 700 cc will not maintain pulmonary expansion, alveolar expansion, and the FRC.

Mobilizing secretions is extraordinarily important. The use of mechanical techniques such as suctioning either via endotracheal or nasotracheal routes is mandatory in many patients with severe cord injuries. Equally important is maintenance of those secretions in a fluid and liquid state so they can be easily removed. Airway humidity is critically important; adequate humidity can be delivered by nebulizers as either cold or warm mist. The former is usually adequate. However, there are times when a warm mist will produce a much better result because the partial pressure of water is related to temperature. It is the water vapor that can reach the small microscopic airways and help liquefy secretions in those difficult to penetrate areas.

Bronchodilatory therapy will not only help mobilize secretions by keeping airways open, but also may improve the activity of the pulmonary cilia. The cautious use of acetylcysteine (Mucomyst) can be helpful, but it can also induce bronchospasm and irritate the tracheal or bronchial epithelium in many patients. Intratracheal instillation of saline or half-strength sodium bicarbonate may be useful. Oscillating beds may be very useful to help clear secretions. The patient is rocked from side to side and presumably this helps to drain secretions and to decrease ventilation and perfusion abnormalities.

Chest auscultation may be "clear" in a patient who has thick or dried secretions. If secretions are too thick to move about with breathing, no rhonchi are heard. Atelectasis may be so diffuse that areas of reduced breath sounds are either not heard or are masked by ambient noise. Therefore in a patient who is on a ventilator and hypoxic in the presence of increased inspired oxygen but in whom auscultation reveals clear lung fields, airway humidification and mobilization of secretions may be inadequate.

Similarly, wheezes may not be heard when CPAP or positive end-expiratory pressure (PEEP) are used. The positive airway pressure maintains FRC by preventing collapse of the terminal bronchioles and alveoli. At the same time, terminal flow velocity may be decreased and wheezing from early, delayed bronchospasm may be missed or misinterpreted. If this process continues unchecked and unrecognized, the patient can develop severe problems with acute asthma. If appropriate bronchodilator therapy is not instituted, the patient can continue to deteriorate with increasing $PaCO_2$ and peak inspiratory pressure and hyperinflation of portions of the lung. This can cause a pneumothorax and at an end-stage can produce severe bullous emphysema. These changes are not necessarily reversible.

It is easy to ascribe a deteriorating pulmonary condition to either developing ARDS or to some concomitant pulmonary injury, such as aspiration pneumonia or pulmonary contusion. These, in general, are best treated with increasing PEEP and mechanical ventilation. However, the patient with acute bronchospasm may be worsened by these treatments, which are only directed at increasing ventilatory pressures.

In summary, severe pulmonary failure in patients with spinal cord injuries is best prevented by a careful plan, which includes maintenance of FRC, as already discussed, clearing secretions, which will begin to accumulate from the time of injury onward, and repeated evaluation of the need for intubation. It is also important to remember that in the unintubated patient, objective indications for elective intubation are not blood gas results, but progressive tachypnea, inadequate or declining FVC, low Vt associated with high wasted ventilation, and low and declining NIF. If the patient has a Swan-Ganz catheter, then pulmonary dysfunction may be signaled at an early stage by an increasing pulmonary shunt fraction (Qs/Qt). Fluid management and its interaction with some of these parameters will be discussed in the section on cardiohemodynamics.

Pulmonary Infections

It is imperative to treat infection at an early stage in patients with spinal cord injuries. However, the use of prophylactic antibiotics is controversial. By their very nature, quadriplegic patients are long-term patients. Within several days of hospitalization, almost all patients, even those in good health, will begin to change their normal flora. Especially if the patient is intubated, normal oral flora will begin to contain increasing numbers of nosocomial organisms.

This cannot be prevented and may be potentiated by the use of prophylactic antibiotics, with development of resistant organisms selected for their ability to colonize the particular patient. Antibiotics cannot sterilize the tracheobronchial tree, but rather should be used to treat known pulmonary infection. Fever, assessment of secretions, evaluation of predominant flora on Gram's stain, and presence of infiltrates on chest radiograph should all be taken into account in judging whether or not a given bacteriologic report from the laboratory forms the basis for instituting antibiotics.

In the presence of obvious pneumonia, sepsis, developing ARDS, or other infection, antibiotics should be instituted immediately. They should be directed at the most likely organisms, which will always be nosocomial and often require a broad-spectrum approach, and should never be withheld until culture results are returned from the laboratory while a patient deteriorates with progressive infection.

Antibiotics should be stopped after 5 to 7 days if the pneumonia has cleared by chest radiograph, by physical examination, by sputum criteria, by fever reduction, or by decreasing white count and normalization of the differential. If the patient develops a new fever while on seemingly appropriate antibiotics, it may be best to stop treatment until new cultures can be taken and a clear source of the fever identified. This may be an infected intravenous site, a central catheter site, a urinary tract infection, epididymitis or perirectal abscess, sinusitis, or another source. Heterotopic ossification must also be considered as a source of fever once the patient has been immobile 2 to 3 weeks.

Discontinuing Mechanical Ventilation

When a patient is ready for weaning from a ventilator, several principles can be used. Serial measures of FVC, NIF, Vt, augmented by blood gas determinations, physical examination, and respiratory rate evaluation, provide the objective basis for allowing weaning to continue at a faster or slower rate. We prefer to wean patients by gradually decreasing the intermittent mandatory ventilation (IMV) rate to about four breaths per minute. For the majority of the day and night, the patient provides most of his own ventilation. However, because his work of breathing has been reduced by positive airway pressure (CPAP or PEEP) and the reduced dead space of an endotracheal tube or tracheostomy, the cord-injured patient may not tolerate further IMV reduction or extubation without further "weaning." The IMV rate may be reduced further to zero while CPAP equal to 5 to 10 cm H_2O is maintained. The patient thereby breathes on his or her own without ventilator support for a variable period of time. Some patients will maintain their own ventilation without further problems; other patients will tolerate only a few minutes of this and will require mechanical support again very quickly. Essentially, these periods of low or no IMV should be lengthened, depending on the patient's ability to tolerate them. As this process continues, patient fatigue may require us to place patients back on an IMV rate of 10 to 14 for 6 to 8 hours (usually at night) in order to provide adequate rest.

When the patient can breathe adequately for a day or longer, we gradually reduce CPAP to zero, effectively a T-tube trial. The presence of CPAP as previously discussed helps to maintain as well as reestablish the FRC of the lung. The patient without CPAP must work much harder than with CPAP. Clearly, then, a T-tube trial with no CPAP is a better test of a patient's ability to tolerate extubation than is the fact that he may have tolerated 12 or 24 hours of CPAP alone.

In addition to weaning parameters that can be easily and inexpensively obtained in any ICU, the use of continuous measurement of end-tidal carbon dioxide (ET-CO_2) and pulse oximetry can make the weaning process safer and more objective. Many quadriplegic patients become anxious when IMV rates are slowed to low levels, even though they may tolerate this physiologically, and demand to be placed back on the ventilator. ET-CO_2 monitoring can be very effective in helping to determine when to place a patient on a ventilator.

In addition, most ET-CO_2 monitors have high and low respiratory rates as well as high and low ET-CO$_2$ alarms. As already discussed, the initial response to inadequate pulmonary reserve is tachypnea, and after one knows a given patient's "baseline" parameters, weaning can be more objectively based on respiratory rate. Respiratory rates that increase from 15 to 20 to 35 to 40 breaths per minute may well not be tolerated for very long. Similarly, if they are associated either with significant hypocapnia or carbon dioxide retention, then the signal is clear that the patient is beginning to decompensate and he should be allowed to rest before trying again. Some patients move through this stage very rapidly, others very slowly. This is a function of their age, the severity of their neurologic as well as pulmonary disease, preexisting factors, and concomitant injuries.

Psychologic dependence on the ventilator should not be underestimated, but attributing all weaning difficulties to psychologic factors is dangerous. Behavioral explanations should be accepted only after physiologic abnormalities have been eliminated as explanations for the difficulty.

Tracheostomy

If the patient has been treated with continuous endotracheal or nasotracheal intubation and fails weaning trials, a tracheostomy should be considered. Tracheostomy reduces physiologic dead space and therefore wasted ventilation will decrease. If the patient's Vt is 200 cc and dead space with intubation is 100 cc, then wasted ventilation is 50%. If a tracheostomy can reduce dead space to 50 to 75 cc, then wasted ventilation will only be 25 to 30%, even though the Vt has not changed. This represents a substantial improvement in effective use of the weakened pulmonary and chest wall structures and may allow the previously ventilator-dependent patient to become independent.

The consequences of premature extubation even when the patient appears to be doing well can be reintubation, perhaps preceded by respiratory arrest. Extubation will increase dead space and usually will decrease FRC because of the inability to expand the lungs fully. Secretions are less well removed by suctioning, and CPAP has been withdrawn: atelectasis may recur. So, even after extubation, the patient may be helped to maintain FRC by periodic CPAP delivered by mask. Respiratory treatments, nasotracheal suctioning, bronchodilators, and airway humidification also can still be used. These treatments may differentiate successful extubation in the marginal patient from extubation that is quickly followed by reintubation and repetition of the entire cycle.

HEMODYNAMIC MANAGEMENT

The most important hemodynamic responses of the spinal cord-injured patient are due to sympathectomy combined with intact vagal efferents and afferents (Table 17–2).

The typical quadriplegic patient presents to the emergency room with mild hypotension with a mean arterial pressure (MAP) of about 70 to 75 torr, and a pulse rate of about 70. These blood pressures often persist despite 4000 to 6000 cc of fluid administered during resuscitation and transport of these patients; admission central venous pressures often are in the normal to high normal range. Hypovolemia does not (usually) explain this hypotension.

Although one might suspect that cardiac output is depressed in these patients, direct observations using flow-directed pulmonary artery catheters show that the cardiac index is

**Table 17–2   Admission Cardiopulmonary Values
in 24 Acutely Quadriplegic Patients**

	MEAN ± SD	RANGE
Vt	360 ± 190	150–635 cc
FVC	1186 ± 650	400–2640 cc
NPIF	−29 ± 17	−10 to − 60 mmHg
Qs/Qt	28 ± 15	11–52%
PCWP	13.5 ± 3.7	7–20 mmHg
Pulmonary artery pressure	22 ± 5	13–21 mmHg
Central venous pressure	11 ± 4	4–23 mmHg
Cardiac output	7.7 ± 1.9	5.2–12.5 liter/min
Systemic vascular resistance	800 ± 220	350–1200 dyne-sec-cm^{-5}
MAP	83 ± 11	53–107 mmHG
Heart rate	72 ± 13	50–100 beats/min

actually 50 to 100% above normal, associated with low systemic vascular resistance values (400 to 800 dyne-sec/cm^5), consistent with a nearly complete sympathectomy. The injured sympathetic nervous system is unable to shift vascular volume from the musculoskeletal system to the splanchnic or renal beds as may be required. This can decrease renal perfusion despite nearly normal arterial, central venous, and pulmonary capillary wedge pressures (PCWPs) and adequate fluid administration.

Since intravascular volume usually is adequate in the resuscitated quadriplegic patient, low urine output and mild hypotension may not improve after further fluid loading. While these patients may require additional fluids early in their course, once the PCWP increases to about 15 mmHg then administration of additional fluids can cause pulmonary edema. Even if fully developed pulmonary edema and congestive failure do not occur, increases in lung water can decrease pulmonary compliance and may precipitate respiratory failure in these marginally compensated patients.

The ideal blood pressure for a patient with a spinal cord injury is that which supports adequate mentation and urinary outputs above 0.5 cc/kg/hr. The exact method of support will vary according to both local practice and the specific circumstances of an individual patient.

We typically treat oliguria with relatively low doses of dopamine (2 to 3 μg/kg/min, a so-called renal dose). This dose usually has no blood pressure effect, but urine output will usually increase by stimulation of dopamine receptors with dilation of afferent renal arterioles. This agent is also mildly chronotropic and may help to control bradyarrhythmias.

Alpha agents, such as phenylephrine or norepinephrine, can reverse the relative hypotension caused by peripheral vasodilation seen after cervical spinal cord injuries. However, these drugs may cause vasoconstriction in the renal arterial bed and produce ischemic nephrotoxicity, so urine output must be monitored closely during their use. Also, high doses of phenylephrine may increase systemic blood pressure sufficiently to stimulate aortic and carotid baroreceptors and lead to reflex bradycardia. Vagal efferents are intact in most spinal cord-injured patients, and alpha agents can potentiate bradyarrhythmias in some patients. Renal doses of dopamine may be combined with alpha agents to help avoid the nephrotoxic effects of prolonged phenylephrine administration, although the need for this in the quadriplegic is not frequent.

Furosemide, mannitol, other diuretic agents, and cardiotonic drugs may be used as necessary. The latter can have a detrimental effect on heart rate. Although bradyarrhythmias are unusual in the young quadriplegic patient, they are frequent and life-threatening in older patients, particularly those with preexisting coronary artery disease and can result in hypotension and asystole.

Anticholinergic drugs such as atropine are used commonly to block vagal efferents. Although this may be life-saving, atropine can cause drying and thickening of pulmonary secretions and potentiate concurrent respiratory problems and can cause or prolong paralytic ileus. Chronotropic agents, such as dopamine and other catecholamines, have fewer of these side effects and their effects are more easily controlled and titrated. Occasionally, bradycardia may be sufficiently severe that a pacemaker is required.

Heart failure occurs rarely in patients with spinal cord injuries. However, when it does, this failure is atypical in that these patients often have cardiac outputs that are high or near normal, although they do have a low urine output, prerenal azotemia, and hyponatremia with low urinary sodium. Abnormal lung findings may be absent in ventilated patients, since high inspiratory pressure and even relatively low levels of CPAP or PEEP may prevent the development of rales and other pulmonary findings consistent with congestive failure. If suspected, pulmonary artery catheters are useful in the diagnosis and management of congestive heart failure.

Congestive heart failure in younger patients often can be reversed with diuretics, but in older patients management can be extremely difficult. Digitalization may be required but can potentiate bradyarrhythmias. Beta-adrenergic agents may improve cardiac contractility and improve heart function. A combination of these various agents along with diuretic therapy may be necessary. In older patients, a pacemaker can help to increase heart rate and cardiac output. Older spinal cord-injured patients with cardiac failure have a particularly poor prognosis.

GASTROINTESTINAL MANAGEMENT

Early abdominal examinations in patients with spinal cord injuries may reveal intact or even hyperactive bowel sounds. However, persistalsis is not effective without sympathetic modulation and ileus develops, sometimes as late as 2 or 3 days after injury. Experimental evidence suggests that peristalsis is ineffective in both the large and the small bowel so that either or both may be involved.

Patients with spinal cord injuries, with or without endotracheal tubes, will often swallow large amounts of air, which can cause gastric and bowel dilation and possibly lead to reflex bradycardia and asystole. As the abdomen distends, the diaphragm is pushed into the chest cavity, reducing total lung volume and FRC. As ileus develops, third space and nasogastric fluid losses via suction can adversely alter fluid and electrolyte balance.

It is generally wise to delay enteral feeding until flatus and bowel movements have returned. Enemas, bowel, and gastric stimulants rarely hasten recovery of stomach and bowel function and should be used cautiously. Since the large bowel is also dyssynergic, paralytic ileus may appear as a bowel obstruction on radiographs. Such obstruction would be rare after spinal cord injury, and an unnecessary laparotomy could be catastrophic in this fragile group of patients.

GENITOURINARY SYSTEM

During "spinal shock" the urinary bladder is atonic and flaccid. Although the bladder, typically becomes hyperactive ("upper motor neuron" bladder) with automatic function in spinal cord injuries above the conus medullaris, inappropriate early management of urinary abnormalities may delay return of bladder function or prevent it entirely.

To prevent bladder distention and to monitor fluid output in the early postinjury phase, we place an indwelling catheter. After the patient has become stable medically and fluid management is not a problem, we begin intermittent bladder catheterization three to six times daily to keep maximum bladder volume below 350 to 500 cc. Intermittent catheterization reduces the incidence of bladder and kidney infections and is preferred over indwelling catheters for chronic use. We generally do not use suppressant antibiotics, but rather treat specific urinary infections. If fever develops, urine cultures must be obtained and selective antibiotics used for a relatively short period. However, most bacteriuria is not an adequate explanation for "fever" and inappropriate antibiotic use may cause more complex problems.

With injuries to the conus medullaris or cauda equina, urodynamic testing will help define the degree of urinary dysfunction and possible methods of reestablishing urinary continence. Prolonged follow-up of urinary problems is mandatory to prevent chronic infection and eventual injury to the kidneys and the renal failure that was a primary cause of death of patients with spinal cord injuries in the past.

INTEGUMENT

The spinal cord-injured patient is extremely susceptible to the development of decubitus ulcers, probably related to a combination of low blood pressure and reduced skin perfusion and to reduced body movement, which ordinarily would relieve pressure on the skin. Positioning and turning ("log rolling") are valuable in preventing skin breakdown, although careful turning may cause some movement of the unstable spine. Oscillating and air flotation beds are also useful in the care of patients with spinal cord injury.

Sheepskin or other padded booties can reduce pressure on a patient's heels but may not prevent decubitus ulcers. A pillow placed beneath the calves of the patient distributes the weight of the leg over the entire area of the calf-pillow interface and eliminates heel pressure entirely. None of these measures eliminates the need for frequent inspection, cleanliness, and good nursing care to prevent decubitus ulcers.

VENOUS SYSTEM AND PULMONARY EMBOLI

Quadriplegic and paraplegic patients are at a very high risk for venous thrombosis, as has been demonstrated using radioactive fibrinogen. In contrast, neurologically intact patients with spinal fractures treated with bed rest have a low incidence of venous thrombosis.

The best method of prophylaxis against pulmonary emboli is not certain. Minidose heparin (such as 5000 U subcutaneously twice daily) is commonly used but unproven. Volume expansion with some anticoagulation can be achieved by the use of dextran 40 in normal saline or glucose. Depending on the fluid and electrolyte status of the patient, this may well be useful. Aspirin administration has some theoretical utility, but there is no proof of efficacy in the quadriplegic patient. Thigh-length, fitted hose significantly reduces venous thrombosis in the lower extremities of certain susceptible persons but have not been well evaluated in quadriplegic patients. Pneumatic antiembolism stockings might have greater benefit, but proof of this is lacking. None of these mechanical treatments can prevent thrombosis in the pelvic venous systems so that anticoagulation or antiplatelet therapy probably should be considered in addition to mechanical therapies.

We currently recommend the use of minidose heparin and adequate hydration of the patient as the best and simplest approach. In selected patients, we may also use compressive stockings or oscillating beds, or both, and occasionally administer antiplatelet agents as well. We consider this practice reasonable but unproven.

If pulmonary emboli occur and the patient is not a candidate for heparinization because of systemic disorders, sepsis, or gastric bleeding, placement of a vena cava filter device should be considered. In experienced hands, this procedure can be performed quickly and with low morbidity using fluoroscopy.

EMOTIONAL REACTION

A patient's emotional response after a spinal cord injury is a major concern. Usually, both patients and his or her family experience a period of grief; the rate at which each person successfully resolves this grief varies. The stages of this reaction are stereotyped and begin with denial of the injury followed by anger and hostility. Situational depression then is prominent, moving finally toward resolution and acceptance. As the injury is accepted, the patient begins to plan realistically and participate actively in his or her rehabilitation. Family members usually go through the same process. To complete the process successfully, the patient must experience and resolve each phase before "grieving" ceases.

Denial is especially profound in the quadriplegic patient, since these are often very young persons who have not yet accepted their own mortality. Family members demonstrate this same phase as they cheerfully express to the medical staff that the patient is a "fighter." Treatment of acute problems soon after injury makes it easy for both the family and the patient to concentrate on items and events other than how they are going to deal with this terrible loss. The preoccupation of the doctors and nurses with medical and surgical management increases this distraction. Often, the patient and family during this phase of his or her illness are compliant and grateful for all the activity and attention. The basic question: "Is the neurologic deficit permanent?" may not be asked. The physician, trying not to eliminate hope, may avoid discussion of the injury's permanence and thus enhance the denial reaction.

As denial begins to resolve and the facts of the situation are more obvious, the family and patient can become angry and hostile. Often, this may be expressed as frustration with the "unfairness" of the whole situation. Anger may be directed at someone who may have been responsible for the injury. Alternatively, anger may be diffuse and undirected. The patient or his family can become extremely demanding of the nursing and physician staff— becoming angry and intolerant of minor delays in the delivery of physical therapy, occupational therapy, and other vagaries of hospitalization. They may focus this hostility on a particular person, on the housestaff or nursing staff and refused to be cared for by "that doctor." However, they rarely direct this hostility at the attending or primary physician. Failure to resolve anger and hostility in a systematic fashion will not only prevent the patient and his family from moving on to a useful and productive approach to the illness, but also can lead to litigation.

If and when anger and hostility resolve, depression and sadness follow. The patient becomes more withdrawn and passive. He may require "narcotics for severe pain" that is ill-defined and not obviously related to his or her injuries. The medical and nursing staff must be especially aware of this tendency because "it is easy to quiet the patient down" with narcotics. The family becomes less demanding as the patient becomes more comfortable, and everyone finds it easier to care for the quadriplegic patient. Although it is important to treat the patient's pain appropriately, it is equally important not to allow a psychologic dependence on narcotics to become a physical addiction.

Resolution and acceptance of the injury with effective planning may not be seen until the patient has been transferred to a rehabilitation unit or is in the more chronic phases of the illness. Because successful adaptation to the injury depends on completion of the grief process, the medical and nursing staff have a responsibility to be aware of this process and to foster and guide it rather than delaying or diverting it. Requests by family members to "not tell the patient" that he may be permanently injured are generally not helpful and usually represent the family's inability to accept the injury.

Although there is no ideal time to educate the patient, little is to be gained by allowing denial, ignorance, and misinformation to prolong denial. In speaking to families and patients with acute quadriplegia and paraplegia, it is important to stress that the outcome of such an illness is variable, particularly with incomplete injuries. With complete loss of spinal cord function, it is unwise to hold out undue hope for recovery, and an honest appraisal, including reasonable statements of uncertainty, is best. A compassionate approach should be adopted early to educate the patient and family, explaining what the deficit is and how it was incurred, and providing an overall plan for management. Initially, the patient and family reliably will not understand and reliably will not remember what is said. Eventually, they must and will begin to hear a clear and accurate message as the process that has been described to them unfolds. As this occurs, confidence in the medical staff will improve.

REFERENCES

1. Blaisdell FW, Lewis FR Jr: Respiratory Distress Syndrome of Shock and Trauma: Post Traumatic Respiratory Failure. Philadelphia: WB Saunders, 1977.
2. Bloch RF, Basbaum M (eds): Management of Spinal Cord Injury. Baltimore: Williams & Wilkins, 1986.
3. Bourden SE: Psychological impact on neurotrauma in the acute care setting. Nurs Clin North Am 21:629–640, 1986.
4. Caplan B, Gibson CJ, Weiss R: Stressful sequela of disabling illness. Int Rehabil Med 6:58–62, 1984.
5. Dantzker DR (ed): Cardiopulmonary Critical Care. Orlando, FL: Grune & Stratton, 1986.
6. El Masri WS, Silver JR: Prophylactic anticoagulant therapy in patients with spinal cord injury. Paraplegia 19: 334–342, 1981.
7. Erickson RP: Autonomic hyperreflexia: Pathophysiology and medical management. Arch Phys Med Rehabil 61:431–440, 1989.
8. Fealey RD, Szurszewski JH, Merritt JL, DiMagno EP: Effect of traumatic spinal cord transection on human upper gastrointestinal motility and gastric emptying. Gastroenterology 87:69–75, 1984.
9. Frank RG, Elliott TR: Life stress and psychologic adjustment following spinal cord injury. Arch Phys Med Rehabil 68:344–347, 1987.
10. Frisbie JH, Sarkarati M, Sharma GV, Rossier AB: Venous thrombosis and pulmonary embolism occurring at close intervals in spinal cord injury patients. Paraplegia 21:270–271, 1983.

11. Jarrell BE, Posuniak E, Roberts J, Osterholm J, Cotler J, Ditunno J: A new method of management using the Kim-Ray Greenfield filter for deep venous thrombosis and pulmonary embolism in spinal cord injury. Surg Gynecol Obstet 157:316–320, 1983.

12. Lloyd LK, Kuhlemeier KV, Fine PR, Stover SL: Initial bladder management in spinal cord injury: Does it make a difference. J Urol 135:523–527, 1986.

13. Mackenzie CF, Shin B, Krishnaprasad D, McCormack F, Illingworth W: Assessment of cardiac and respiratory function during surgery on patients with acute quadriplegia. J Neurosurg 62:843–849, 1985.

14. Maynard FM, Glass J: Management of the neuropathic bladder by clean intermittent catheterization: 5 year outcome. Paraplegia 25:106–110, 1987.

15. Meshkinpour H, Harmon D, Thompson R, Yu J: Effects of thoracic spinal cord transection on colonic motor activity in rats. Paraplegia 23:272–276, 1985.

16. Montgomerie JZ, Madorsky JG, Gilmore DS, Graham IE: Colonization of patients with spinal cord injury with Pseudomonas aeruginosa and Klebsiella pneumoniae at different institutions. J Hosp Infect 10:198–203, 1987.

17. Myllynen P, Kammonen M, Rokkanen P, Bostman O, Lalla M, Laasonen E: Deep venous thrombosis and pulmonary embolism in patients with acute spinal cord injury: A comparison with nonparalyzed patients immobilized due to spinal fractures. J Trauma 25:541–543, 1985.

18. Pederson E: Regulation of bladder and colon-rectum in patients with spinal lesions. J Auton Nerv Syst 7:329–338, 1983.

19. Rosner MJ, Coley I, Elias Z: Pulmonary shunt fraction (Qs/Qt) in acute quadriplegia. In: Green BA, Summer WR (eds): Continuous Oscillation Therapy: Research and Practical Applications. Coral Gables, FL: University of Miami Press, 1986, pp 31–38.

20. Rosner MJ, Elias Z, Coley I: New principles of resuscitation for brain and spinal injury. NC Med J 45:701–708, 1984.

21. Saltzstein R, Melvin J: Ventilatory compromise in spinal cord injury—a review. J Am Paraplegia Soc 9:6–9, 1986.

22. Shoemaker WC, Ayres S, Grenvik A, Holbrook PR, Thompson WL: Textbook of Critical Care, ed 2. Philadelphia: W.B. Saunders, 1989

23. Stanton GM: Spinal cord injury: Psychological adaptation. J Neurosurg Nurs 15:306–309, 1983.

24. Varma JS, Binnie N, Smith AN, Creasey GH, Edmond P: Differential effects of sacral anterior root stimulation on anal sphincter and colorectal motility in spinally injured man. Br J Surg 73:478–482, 1986.

18

Delayed Sequelae of Spinal Cord Injury

MICHAEL C. ROWBOTHAM
AND NICHOLAS M. BARBARO

Although the majority of patients with traumatic spinal cord injury (SCI) have a stable neurologic deficit that does not change appreciably with time, some patients develop a progressive loss of function some time after the acute phase of their injury. The two most common causes of delayed deterioration are progressive spinal deformity at the site of trauma and post-traumatic syringomyelia (Fig. 18–1). Still other patients, who do not develop an objective loss of function, become disabled from either pain, spasticity, or both. These are among the most debilitating and challenging aspects of the long-term care of patients with SCI.

SPASTICITY

Spasticity is a hyperactivity of tendon stretch reflexes as a result of decreased tonic inhibition (upper motor neuron syndrome). However, this does not adequately describe the severe spasticity that can reduce function or even result in further injury. In this form, the spasm may be accompanied by pain, thereby adding to the patient's disability. In addition, many patients describe such "spasms" as painful, so that pain and spasticity can produce additional disability.

A number of pharmacologic and surgical manipulations are available for treating spasticity. Before these therapies are discussed, a brief review of the relevant pharmacology is warranted.

Pharmacologic therapy for spasticity focuses on three types of drugs, two of which probably work similarly. Baclofen is a derivative of gamma aminobutyric acid (GABA), which inhibits motoneurons. Both mono- and polysynaptic reflexes are thought to be inhibited by baclofen. Benzodiazepines, such as diazepam, enhance the efficiency of GABAergic transmission and, thus, probably work through a mechanism similar to that for baclofen. The third drug is dantrolene, which directly reduces muscle contraction by decreasing the amount of calcium released from the sarcoplasmic reticulum and may reduce reflex-associated contractions more than voluntary ones.[16]

226

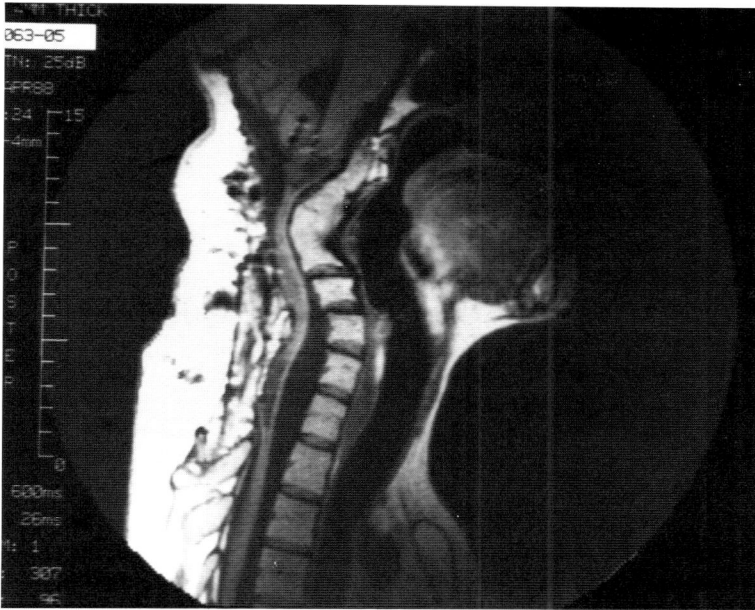

Figure 18–1.   Midsagittal MRI showing severe spinal deformity at C-2 and cystic lesions in brainstem and spinal cord (arrows).

In general, one drug is used in gradually increasing doses until either the desired effect is achieved or side effects make it impossible to increase the dosage further. One such side effect is weakness. Patients with SCI often take advantage of their spasticity to stand, walk, or transfer. Elimination of spasticity can therefore adversely affect important functions. Another frequent limiting effect is sedation. Because GABAergic inhibitory effects can occur throughout the nervous system, it is difficult to limit the action of these agents to the spinal cord.

To limit this problem, baclofen has been injected directly into the spinal subarachnoid space[16,38] with reportedly fewer side effects than seen when it is administered systemically. Although promising, this treatment must still be considered experimental.

A number of surgical approaches have been developed in an effort to treat spasticity after SCI. Most of these have centered around interrupting the spinal reflex arc. The simplest but least selective approach has been the use of intrathecal phenol to damage the spinal roots. The potential benefit of this procedure must be weighed against the possibility of functional loss. For example, loss of the bladder-emptying reflex must always be considered a possible complication with such therapy.

The reflex arc can be interrupted more selectively by destroying one or more nerve roots at the intervertebral foramen using a radiofrequency probe.[22] This enables the surgeon to select individual roots involved in a particular spastic reflex. It is usually not possible to spare the motor function of the particular root involved. If motor function is necessary, a more selective dorsal rhizotomy is required.

Selective dorsal rhizotomy enables one to interrupt particular reflex arc selectively without eliminating the voluntary movement. If the entire dorsal root is sectioned, there is loss of proprioceptive function, which may be as disabling as a motor lesion. It may be possible to avoid this problem by intraoperative stimulation of individual dorsal rootlets with visual and/or electromyographic observation of muscle contraction.[13] Only those rootlets that appear to be involved in the spastic reflex are sectioned. A second approach has taken advantage of the anatomic division in the dorsal root. Selective section of the lateral root as it enters the spinal cord interrupts important pain fibers and has been reported to be effective in elimination of painful spasticity after SCI.[32]

The best treatment for spasticity is the recognition and elimination of a simple urinary tract infection or of an enlarging syrinx in the spinal cord. When this is not possible, efforts must be made to reduce spastic reflexes to the minimal level, which will still maximize the patient's function. Generally, this can be done through pharmacologic means, although elimination of spasticity should not be done at the expense of excessive sedation or weakness. Ablative approaches should be reserved for those patients in whom medical management is not effective, and only after careful consideration is given to the potential loss of function with each technique.

PAIN

Survival after SCI has improved dramatically in this century. In World War I, only 10% of patients with SCI survived 1 year. The figures improved during World War II, and in a series of 300 consecutive patients treated during the Korean War, the overall mortality was only 1%.[34] With the survival of increasing numbers of patients with SCI associated with the advent of antibiotics, rapid transportation, and better rehabilitation methods, the problem of persistent pain after SCI has become obvious. Using various definitions of chronic pain, the incidence of pain after cord injury has been reported to be between 6 and 90%[7,11] and in large series from World War II and the Korean War, the incidence averaged 45%. In the civilian population, chronic pain severe enough to limit activities is present in more than 50% of patients with SCI, and chronic severe pain in 5 to 10% of patients.

Types of Pain After Spinal Cord Injury

There is no uniform nomenclature for the different forms of pain after SCI. Pain may be transient or permanent, immediate or delayed, well-localized or diffuse. It may occur in multiple forms in the same patient and even evolve from one form into another over time, all without objective evidence of further neurologic deterioration. Eight distinct forms of chronic pain are presented in Table 18–1.

Nerve root pain is asymmetric, well-localized to segments near the level of injury and felt as sharp, knifelike, or cramping and radiates in a reproducible pattern. With the original SCI, nerve roots or dorsal root ganglia may be damaged and arachnoidal scarring can further aggravate the problem by binding the roots. Nerve root pain is most common after cauda equina injuries and infrequent after cervical cord injuries. Physical examination may show allodynia (pain from non-noxious stimulation or summation, pain from repetitive stimulation) in areas with sensory deficits that may range from mild to profound. The pain evoked may be burning, sharp, or electrical in quality and may radiate widely within the territory of

Table 18–1   Classification of Pain After SCI

Nerve root pain
Dysesthetic pain syndrome
Painful phantoms
Hyperalgesic border pain
Reflex sympathetic dystrophy
Musculoskeletal pain
Visceral pain
Autonomic dysreflexia
Lhermitte's sign

that nerve root. Traction on nerves and nerve roots, such as straight leg raising, will produce pain. Progressive spinal deformity or degenerative spine changes, such as facet hypertrophy or herniated nucleus pulposus, may produce nerve root compression and pain as late sequellae of cord injury.

Dysesthetic pain syndrome (DPS) is a diffuse pain below the level of injury, variously called diffuse causalgia, diffuse burning pain, or spinal cord dysesthesia.[10,12,15,27,29] DPS is the most common pain syndrome following complete or incomplete cord injuries. It usually occurs within 1 year of injury and occurs in most SCI patients in at least a mild form. DPS is diffuse and nonradicular, and affected areas have some degree of abnormal sensation. Common features include unpleasant sensations of burning, stinging, or stabbing that are usually continuous. Cutaneous stimulation or movement of deeper structures may aggravate the pain, but focal trigger points, if present, will not reproduce the entire pain syndrome. Cutaneous sensitivity may cause the patient to wear gloves or other protective clothing to prevent inadvertent skin stimulation. There is no obvious relationship between the etiology, completeness, or level of cord injury and the development and severity of DPS. Patients with DPS frequently report that their pain increases in intensity with anger or depression, and other variables such as weather. Because the pain is diffuse and difficult to describe, patients may be misdiagnosed as having psychogenic pain, especially in cases where motor recovery is nearly complete, as in some cases of cervical central cord injury.[20]

Painful phantoms are a diffuse pain felt below the level of injury, usually a complete cord injury. The distinction between a painful phantom and DPS may relate as much to the patients' perception of their sensory loss and to the inquisitiveness of the examiner than to a physiologic difference between the two syndromes. Phantom sensations are usually noticed soon after the original injury similar to postamputation phantoms, but may fade into the diffuse burning sensations characteristic of DPS.

Hyperalgesic border pain is easily confused with nerve root pain. Complaints of tingling, burning, or a tight band-like sensation are localized to the rostral border of the sensory level. Physical examination shows a 1 or 2 segment wide band of hyperpathia separating normal from deafferented, paralyzed segments.[11] A variant of this, called "endzone" pain, appears early after injury and is thought to presage a good recovery. As the recovery progresses, the band of hyperpathia moves caudally, eventually disappearing at the toes. When recovery is incomplete, the band persists at a definitive sensory level. This phenomenon occurs most often in conus medullaris and cauda equina lesions. When injury level pain such as already described occurs late after cord injury, especially if it is asymmetrical and ascends, syringomyelia must be considered.

Reflex sympathetic dystrophy (RSD) is not well established as a distinct type of pain following spinal cord injury.[2,35] There is overlap in symptoms and examination findings with the other pain categories already described. The pain unilaterally affects a limb that is otherwise not severely impaired, and characteristic features, such as cool skin, mottled coloring, increased sweating, and trophic changes in nails, hair, and joints are present. In cases of RSD without peripheral nerve or SCI, sympathetic blockade relieves pain at least temporarily in up to 90% of cases.

Musculoskeletal pain occurring at or near the level of injury is very common early after traumatic cord injury. When pains of this type occur as late sequelae, diagnostic evaluation is indicated. These pains are similar to nerve root pain in that they are frequently asymmetrical, improved by rest, and exacerbated by specific postures and movements. Headache and neckache are common, even though the level of injury may be many segments below. The origin of the pain is in bones, intervertebral disks, joints, ligaments, and muscles in persistent spasm. In incomplete cord lesions, pain of musculoskeletal origin may occur in any body area. Muscles in persistent spasm can be tender and produce pain that radiates in characteristic patterns. Spasticity can contribute to spinal deformity, especially in children and patients with high, complete lesions. Spasticity reduces the mobility of functionally important joints, such as the shoulder, and is an important and treatable source of pain. Paraplegic patients, who must depend on their arms for transfers and for use of a wheel chair, are particularly prone to develop bursitis, tendonitis, rotator cuff injuries, and myofascial pain syndromes of the head, neck, and shoulder.

Visceral pain must be separated into two categories: those akin to painful phantom sensations and those due to tissue damaging processes in which nociceptive input from the viscera and abdominal wall is misperceived because of the cord injury. Body phantoms may include unpaired structures, such as the penis and rectum, and all visceral organs.[6] Unpleasant spontaneous sensations such as fecal urgency, bladder fullness, and a burning feeling in the bladder are common and occur in the absence of a full bladder or rectum or a urinary tract infection. These sensations are longlasting and usually continuous, but are easily confused with sensations caused by visceral disease.

Many authors have documented that spinal cord-injured patients do not detect intra-abdominal disease until much later than normal persons. Pollock et al.[28] described patients unable to experience pain from cystitis, epididymitis, kidney, and bladder stones, among other conditions.[29] The situation is complicated by a 5% incidence of acute intra-abdominal disease in the first month after SCI. Berlly and Wilmot[4] found peptic ulcers (including perforation), pancreatitis, cholelithiasis, and fecal impaction to be particularly common, and all presented similar diagnostic problems.[5]

When confronted with a patient with possible visceral disease, the examiner must consider the level and completeness of the cord lesion. Sweating, fever, and changes in pulse and blood pressure are particularly important. Careful abdominal and rectal examination is mandatory. The absence of abdominal tenderness does not rule out disease, nor do other negative findings so reassuring in noncord-injured patients. Blood, urine, and imaging studies may be indicated. Referred pain, especially in the neck and shoulder due to diaphragmatic irritation is an important sign. With a rigorous diagnostic approach and frequent reexamination as symptoms change, the physician can diagnose and treat serious illnesses before complications occur.

If no explanation can be found after a careful search, one must assume that the pain is a "visceral vision" of one of the syndromes described.

Autonomic dysreflexia (AD) is a syndrome of sympathetic overactivity that can be life threatening, most commonly occurring after high thoracic and cervical SCI. AD is a paroxysmal syndrome of severe hypertension, bradycardia, sweating, facial flushing, and headache. Seizures, aphasia, and subarachnoid hemorrhage have all been reported as sequelae of AD.[24] Piloerection, nasal obstruction, and paresthesias may also occur. AD is common; in one series 48% of 213 consecutive patients with lesions above T6 had AD at some time, usually more than 2 months after injury.[25] Trigger stimuli include bladder distention and infection, defecation and rectal distention, cutaneous stimulation, muscle spasm, and exercise. Paroxysmal headache is an important feature of AD, and the risk of malignant hypertension is significant. Treatment is directed toward finding and eliminating the trigger stimulus and reducing hypertension. A severe episode may require treatment in an intensive care unit.

Lhermitte's sign consists of electric shocklike paresthesias radiating into the trunk or limbs during flexion of the neck[17] and virtually always indicates cervical spinal cord disease. Lhermitte's sign is important to recognize because it has localizing significance and, when persistent, may be an important clue to the presence of a treatable underlying cause.

TREATMENT OF PAIN AFTER SPINAL CORD INJURY

Optimum pain management begins with a thorough diagnostic evaluation. A multidisciplinary approach, which includes contributions from the fields of medicine, neurology, neurosurgery, psychiatry, anesthesiology, orthopedics, rehabilitation medicine, and physical therapy is preferred. Diagnostic studies may be indicated, especially in evaluation of nerve root pains, visceral pain, pain of musculoskeletal origin, and persistent Lhermitte's sign. Neurologic deterioration and new pain above the level of injury are particularly important; the possibility of synrigomyelia should always be considered.

Medical problems, such as infections, should be treated and psychologic factors that impair a patient's ability to aid in his own rehabilitation (such as depression, family conflicts, and unresolved litigation) must be addressed. Transcutaneous nerve stimulators (TENS) have been valuable for pain at the site of spinal injury and nerve root pain, and occasionally for painful phantoms and dysesthetic pain syndromes.[11,14] Physical therapy, bracing, prosthetic use, and treatment of myofascial trigger points may improve pain dramatically in some patients.

Medications useful in pain management include nonsteroidal anti-inflammatory drugs (NSAIDs), acetaminophen, opioid analgesics, antidepressants, anticonvulsants, neuroleptics, benzodiazepines and other antispasticity agents (Table 18–2). NSAIDs and acetaminophen can be used at any time. Because of the long-term nature of many pain problems after SCI and the potential for development of dependence, opioids present special problems that should be addressed before they are prescribed.[18] Antidepressants are useful for a wide variety of pain syndromes and supervised trials of these medications are indicated in most patients with pain after SCI. Anticonvulsants are useful for neuropathic pain that has prominent lancinating qualities. Neuroleptics should be held in reserve with few exceptions. The pharmacologic management of chronic pain in patients with SCI requires frequent patient follow-up, knowledge of each drug's actions, skill, and patience. Whenever possible, a single drug should be used at the lowest effective dose. This can be determined by asking

Table 18–2   Drug Classes Useful in Management of Chronic SCI Pain

NSAIDs
    Acetaminophen, aspirin, diflunisal, ibuprofen, naproxen
Opioid analgesics
    Morphine, methadone, hydromorphone, levorphanol, codeine, oxycodone
Antidepressants
    Amitriptyline, nortriptyline, imipramine, desipramine, doxepin, trazodone
Anticonvulsants
    Carbamazepine, phenytoin, clonazepam, valproic acid
Antispasticity Agents
    Diazepam, lorazepam, baclofen, dantrolene, cyclobenzaprine
Neuroleptics
    Methotrimeprazine, chlorprothixene

the patient how much pain relief was obtained and how long it lasted. The physician should allow an adequate trial of any medication before giving up on that drug or class of drugs.

Unfortunately, clear guidelines do not exist for determining minimum dose and duration of treatment for an adequate trial of any of the medications listed here (Table 18–3). For acetaminophen, aspirin, and other NSAIDs, some benefit should be apparent within the first few doses if an adequate amount is administered. For opiates, if the dose and route are correctly chosen, some benefit should be quickly apparent. Other agents such as antidepressants, anticonvulsants, neuroleptics, benzodiazepines, and other antispasticity agents require a small initial dose and a slow build up to the desired daily dose because of the frequent occurrence of dose-related side effects. In addition, therapeutic effects of a given dose may not be apparent for days or even weeks, particularly for tricyclic antidepressants. An adequate trial requires that the patient takes the drug (drug levels are readily available for several antidepressants, all anticonvulsants, and some benzodiazepines) and slowly increasing the dose until pain relief is achieved or dose-limiting adverse effects occur. For antidepressants, anticonvulsants, and antispasticity agents, more than one drug of that class should be tried if the first agent is not efficacious.

Table 18–3   Pharmacologic Management of Chronic SCI Pain

PAIN TYPE	DRUG CLASS					
	NSAIDs	Opioids	Anti-Depressants	Anti-Convulsants	Anti-Spasticity Agents	Neuro-leptics
Nerve root pain	+ +	+	+ +	+ +		+
Dysesthetic pain syndrome		+	+ +	+ +		+
Painful phantoms		+	+ +	+ +		+
Hyperalgesic border pain		+	+ +	+ +		+
Reflex sympathetic dystrophy		+	+			+
Musculoskeletal pain	+ +	+ +	+		+ +	
Visceral pain		+	+			
Lhermitte's sign			+	+ +		

+ = possibly useful and may occasionally be very useful, but not a first choice; + + = first choice or a major alternative.

More than one medication is often necessary for optimum pain control. Combining opiates and NSAIDs with the other drug classes presents no major problems except for added sedation. Combinations of antidepressants, anticonvulsants, and neuroleptics are frequently encountered in clinical practice. Because of additive sedation, cardiac conduction effects, anticholinergic activity, and anti-α-adrenergic effects, caution is necessary when combining antidepressants and neuroleptics. Anticonvulsants and benzodiazepines may each produce excessive sedation. Physical and psychologic dependence and mood disorders can follow long-term benzodiazepine use.

ANESTHESIOLOGIC APPROACHES

Anesthesiologic approaches to management of chronic pain after SCI are in widespread use but their role and indications are not completely clear. This is a controversial area and controlled studies are not available to provide guidance.

Local anesthetic injection into specific nerves or musculoskeletal structures may produce dramatic but temporary pain relief. In normally innervated areas, this may sometimes provide long-lasting or even permanent relief, especially of myofascial trigger points. In partially or completely deafferented areas, local anesthetic injection rarely provides more than temporary relief but can aid in determining the source of pain. Long-lasting nerve blocks using alcohol, phenol, or ammonium sulfate can be used to provide pain relief that may last for months when temporary local anesthetic blockade of a structure is effective. These blocks usually do not provide long-lasting relief when the target structures are deafferented or when the nerve arises from below the level of the spinal cord lesion. Epidural local anesthetic blockade may produce excellent temporary relief of nearly all pain types, including hyperalgesic border zones and DPS. Unfortunately, the initial traumatic injury may have permanently disrupted the epidural space in the target areas. Also, although this technique may produce complete pain relief, the relief is often temporary and little useful information is gained. Steroids are often added to local anesthetic agents in all the previously mentioned techniques, but proof of additional benefit is lacking. The use of intrathecal phenol or alcohol for pain and spasticity is something of a "sledgehammer" method, but it may be permanently effective.[36] Increased neurologic impairment, especially of bowel and bladder function, is a major risk. Surgical techniques have largely replaced this type of nonselective destructive therapy.

OPERATIVE APPROACHES

A number of operations have been attempted to relieve pain that follows SCI with only limited success. One reason is that most series combine the various pain syndromes and cannot show a beneficial effect of any one procedure on the entire patient population. One ablative technique that is useful for some post-traumatic pain syndromes is the lesioning of the spinal dorsal root entry zone (DREZ) with reduced pain in 50% of patients in one series.[37] When only cases of hyperalgesic border pain were considered, the effectiveness was reported as 74%, but only 20% of patients with "diffuse" pain (dysesthetic pain syndrome on painful phantoms) were helped by DREZ lesions. Other ablative techniques are not frequently used in the treatment of pain after SCI. Cordotomy and even cordectomy have not met with long-term success in these syndromes.[3] Although the exact reason for this is not known, the generation of central pain mechanisms at higher levels has been postulated. Electrical stimulation of the spinal cord and brain have also been tried for SCI pain syndromes with mixed results.[36] Although stimulation of deep brain structures might be expected to be most beneficial for "central" pain syndromes, this technique has not proved to be effective in this group of patients.[40,41]

POST-TRAUMATIC SYRINGOMYELIA

Post-traumatic syringomyelia, or cystic myelopathy, is discussed separately because of its unique constellation of features and morbidity if untreated. The widespread use of magnetic resonance imaging (MRI) has dramatically improved our ability to diagnose these cystic lesions after SCI and will help us define the real incidence of post-traumatic syringomyelia. Patients with complete cervical lesions have the highest chance of developing a syrinx as a late complication, about 8% in one series.[42] Paraplegics with incomplete lesions have a 2% incidence of syrinx formation. Syringomyelia may not be recognized for months to years after SCI, with a mean of 9 years. Pain is the most common initial symptom and is present in 70% of patients by the time a syrinx is diagnosed. The pain often is aggravated by coughing, sneezing, straining, or change in posture, most often at or above the level of the lesion. It is dull, aching, or burning in character. Other common symptoms are increased motor or sensory deficits, increased spasticity, increased sweating, and AD.

In patients with an ascending sensory level, the sensory loss is dissociated between proprioception and pain/temperature. If the original lesion is incomplete, a descending sensory level can sometimes be demonstrated. Increased weakness is common. Trigeminal involvement sparing the central portions of the face indicates syrinx extension into the brainstem.

Surgery for post-traumatic syringomyelia is recommended when patients demonstrate pregressive loss of neurologic function or worsening pain, spasticity, or AD. One must be cautious not to "overinterpret" small cystic spinal cord lesions, which probably represent myelomalacia and which are not responsible for the patient's syndrome. Spinal cord widening on MRI is sought as an important feature in determining whether or not to recommend surgery. The most common current operation is a myelotomy and placement of a shunt into the syrinx[42–44] with cyst drainage either into the adjacent subarachnoid space or into the pleural or peritoneal cavities (Table 18–2). Advocates of extraspinal shunting argue that the subarachnoid space in these cases is not normal and that the syrinx is created by the pressure differential above and below the level of SCI. Further evidence for this is that some patients with post-traumatic synringomyelia develop arachnoid loculations that compress the spinal cord and that can be in a dynamic equilibrium with their syrinx.[45] Syrinx shunts have all of the problems of other shunt systems and require evaluation for patency when clinically indicated.

SUMMARY

SCI is associated with a number of complex delayed effects. These include mechanical effects, such as progressive spinal deformity, and pathophysiologic effects, such as pain and

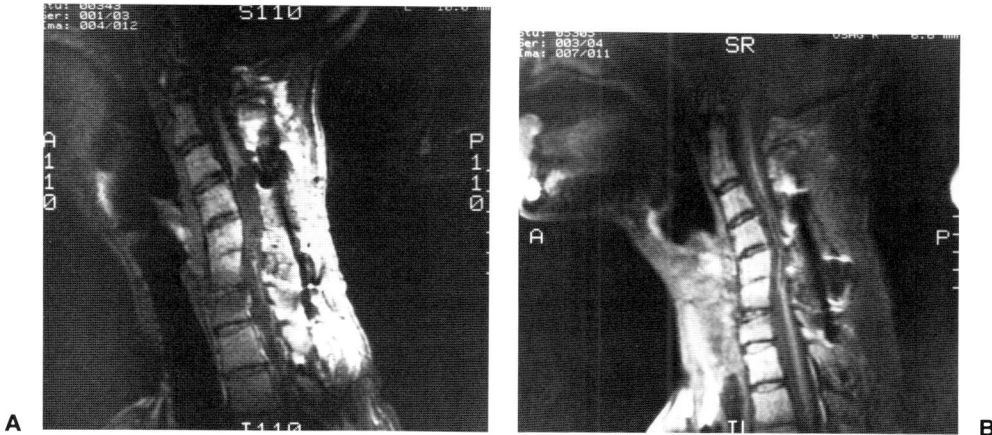

Figure 18–2. A: Sagittal MRI showing focal syrinx expanding the upper cervical spinal cord (arrows). B: Sagittal MRI of same patient following placement of two syringoperitoneal shunts. Spinal cord is now flattened and two residual cavities are seen (arrows). Shunting resulted in improved deltoid muscle strength and reduced shoulder pain.

spasticity. Commonly, these problems are interrelated, as when post-traumatic syringomyelia results in increased spasticity and pain. The development of a new syndrome in a patient with an SCI warrants a prompt and complete evaluation.

Appropriate medical therapy requires an understanding of spinal cord physiology and pharmacology. In addition, application of medical therapy, especially for pain syndromes, requires painstaking empirical trials with attention to side effects and drug interactions. Only after medical management has failed should operative approaches be tried. A possible exception is with syringomyelia, for which operative approaches appear to offer the best chance for reversal or stabilization of cord deficits. All of these complex issues are best addressed by a multidisciplinary team of physicians committed to the care of the patient with SCI.

Acknowledgments

The authors thank Howard L. Fields, M.D., Ph.D. for manuscript review and Lael Carlson for word processing. This work is supported in part by the Pain Research Training Program, National Institute of Neurological and Communicative Disorders and Stroke grant NS-07265.

REFERENCES

1. Andrews BT, Weinstein PR, Rosenblum ML, Barbaro NM: Intradural arachnoid cysts of the spinal canal associated with intramedullary cysts. J Neurosurg 68:544–549, 1988.
2. Andrews L, Armitage K: Sudeck's atrophy in traumatic quadriplegia. Paraplegia 9:159–165, 1971.
3. Barbaro NM, Wilson CB, Gutin PH, Edwards MSB: Surgical treatment of synringomyelia. Favorable results with syringoperitoneal shunting. J Neurosurg 61:531–538, 1984.
4. Berlly M, Wilmot C: Acute abdominal emergencies during the first four weeks after spinal cord injury. Arch Phys Med Rehabil 65:687–690, 1984.

5. Bloch R: Autonomic dysfunction. In Bloch R, Basbaum M (eds): Management of Spinal Cord Injuries. Baltimore: Williams & Wilkins, 1986, pp. 149–163.
6. Bors E: Phantom limbs of patients with spinal cord injury. Arch Neurol Psychiatry 66:610–631, 1951.
7. Boshes B: Trauma to the spinal cord. In Baker A, Baker L (eds): Clinical Neurology, vol 3. Philadelphia: Harper & Row, 1982, Chapter 35.
8. Burke D, Woodward J: Pain and phantom sensation in spinal paralysis. In Vinken P, Bruyn G (eds): Handbook of Clinical Neurology, vol. 26. Amsterdam: North-Holland, 1976, pp 489–499.
9. Cain H: Subarachnoid phenol block in the treatment of pain and spasticity. Paraplegia 3:152–160, 1965.
10. Davidoff G, Roth E, Guarracini M, Sliwa J, Yarkony G: Function-limiting dysesthetic pain syndrome among traumatic spinal cord injury patients: A cross sectional study. Pain 29:39–48, 1987.
11. Davis L, Martin J: Studies upon spinal cord injuries. J Neurosurg 4:483–491, 1947.
12. Druckman R, Lende R: Central pain of spinal cord origin. Neurology (Minneap) 15:518–522, 1965.
13. Fasano VA, Barolat-Romana G, Zeme S, Sguazzi A: Electrophysiological assessment of spinal circuits in spasticity by direct dorsal root stimulation. Neurosurgery 4:146–151, 1979.
14. Fields H: Pain. New York: McGraw Hill, 1987.
15. Friedman AH, Nashold BS: DREZ lesions for relief of pain related to spinal cord injury. J Neurosurg 65:465–469, 1986.
16. Goodman AC, Gilman LS, Rall TW, Murad F: The Pharmacological Basis of Therapeutics, 7th ed. New York: Macmillan, 1985, pp 486–489.
17. Hachen H: Psychological, neurophysiological and therapeutic aspects of chronic pain: Preliminary results with transcutaneous electrical stimulation. Paraplegia 15:353–367, 1977.
18. Heilporn A: Two therapeutic experiments on stubborn pain in spinal cord lesions: Melitracen-flupenthixol and the transcutaneous nerve stimulation. Paraplegia 15:368–372, 1977.
19. Holmes G: Pain of Central Origin. In: Contributions to Medical and Biological Research, vol 1. New York: Hoeber, 1919, pp 235–246.
20. Hopkins A, Rudge P: Hyperpathia in the central cervical cord syndrome. J Neurol Psychiatry 36:637–642, 1973.
21. Hosobuchi Y: Subcortical electrical stimulation for control of intractable pain in humans. J Neurosurg 64:543–553, 1986.
22. Kasdon DL, Lathi ES: A prospective study of radiofrequency rhizotomy in the treatment of post-traumatic spasticity. Neurosurgery 15:526–529, 1984.
23. Levy RM, Lamb S, Adams JE: Treatment of chronic pain by deep brain stimulation: Long term follow-up and review of the literature. Neurosurgery 21:885–893, 1987.
24. Lindan R, Joiner E, Freehafer A, Hazel C: Incidence and clinical features of autonomic dysreflexia in patients with spinal cord injury. Paraplegia 18:292, 1980.
25. Little S: Electrical paresthesias in extremities following injury to central nervous system. Arch Neurol Psychiatry 56:417–427, 1946.
26. Melzack R, Loeser J: Phantom body pain in paraplegics: Evidence for a central "pattern generating mechanism" for pain. Pain 4:195–210, 1978.
27. Pagni C: Central pain due to spinal cord and brain stem damage. In Wall P, Melzack R (eds): Textbook of Pain. London: Churchill Livingstone, 1984, pp 481–495.
28. Pollack L, Brown M, Boshes B, et al.: Pain below the level of injury of the spinal cord. Arch Neurol 65:319–322, 1951.
29. Richardson RR, Meyer PR, Cerullo LJ: Neurostimulation in the modulation of intractable paraplegic and traumatic neuroma pains. Pain 8:75–84, 1980.
30. Rossier AB, Foo D, Shillito J: Post-traumatic cervical syringomyelia. Brain 108:439–461, 1985.
31. Sindou M, Millet MF, Mortanais F, Eyssette M: Results of selective posterior rhizotomy in the treatment of painful and spastic paraplegia secondary to multiple sclerosis. Appl Neurophysiol 45:335–340, 1982.
32. Tunks E: Pain in spinal cord injured patients. In Bloch R, Basbaum M (eds): Management of Spinal Cord Injuries. Baltimore: Williams & Wilkins, pp 180–211.
33. Wannamaker G: Spinal cord injuries: A review of the early treatment in 300 consecutive cases during the Korean conflict. J Neurosurg 11:517–524, 1954.
34. Weinapel S, Freed M: Reflex sympathetic dystrophy in quadriplegia: case report. Arch Phys Med Rehabil 65:35–36, 1984.
35. Williams B, Page N: Surgical treatment of syringomyelia with syringopleural shunting. Br J Neurosurg 1:63–80, 1987.
36. Penn RD, Kroin JS: Long term intrathecal baclofen infusion for treatment of spasticity. J Neurosurg 66:181–185, 1987.
37. Young RR, Delwaide PJ: Drug therapy: Spasticity, part 1. N Engl J Med 304:28–33, 1981.
38. Young RR, Delwaide PJ: Drug therapy: Spasticity, part 2. N Engl J Med 304:96–99, 1981.

19

Neurorehabilitation

SHELDON BERROL

Rehabilitation after brain injury is a therapeutic process designed to facilitate maximal restoration of function. Careful attention must be focused on the prevention and management of those factors that impede this process. Regardless of outcome possibilities based on statistics, each patient must be individually assessed in terms of diagnosis, associated injuries, responses, and achievable goals.

Early institution of rehabilitation principles can substantially reduce the impact of such complicating factors as bed rest, spasticity, contractures, and heterotopic ossification. The process of rehabilitation can be most effective if initiated in the phase of trauma management, so that additional levels of disability due to complications do not accumulate. Unfortunately, where medical and survival problems are most acute, rehabilitation must proceed slowly.

Rehabilitation after brain injury is frequently a lengthy process that invokes many levels of intervention. Appropriate timing of these interventions, and availability of a knowledgeable rehabilitation team in a coordinated fashion, are required to identify and pursue reasonable goals whose achievement can be objectively assessed.[1]

The rehabilitation team in the acute setting should involve at least the neurosurgeon, physiatrist, nurse, physical therapist, occupational therapist, speech pathologist, and social worker. This team must be involved with early discharge planning and aid in timely and appropriate placement when the patient is medically stable.

EARLY REHABILITATION

The initial phase of management should be directed toward preventing complications such as skin breakdown, contractures, and the reduction of muscle tone. The family should be incorporated into the process, and provided with clear competent information so that they begin to understand the range of possible disabilities.

The hallmark of skin care is the prevention of excessive pressure, particularly over such bony prominences as the malleoli, knees, sacrum, occiput, and scapulae. Initially, patients will require turning at least every 2 hours, day and night. Adequate padding should be provided at all points of skin contact over bone or with bed rails, foot boards, or orthotic devices. As the patient emerges from coma and becomes restless, friction damage to epithelial tissue must be prevented.[11]

SPASTICITY

Central nervous system injury results in increased muscle tone, characterized by hyperactive deep tendon reflexes, increased resistance to passive stretch, cocontraction, and clonus. This results in contracture formation, intertrigo, skin breakdown, positioning problems, and difficulty in maintaining hygiene.

Noxious stimuli that could increase tone should be avoided. The side-lying position frequently results in temporary diminished tone because primitive motor patterns are minimally stimulated in this position. A vigorous physical therapy range of motion exercise program should be used, as well as incorporating adequate range of motion for joints to maintain maximal length of muscle fibers with all routine nursing procedures. The patient should be evaluated for seating as early as possible in an appropriately stabilized position that minimizes tone.

Patients with widespread spasticity may benefit from drug therapy to modify muscle tone. Pharmacotherapy is based on desired result balanced against side effects. Brain-injured patients are sometimes more sensitive than normal patients to sedation: diazepam and other benzodiazepines may contribute to increased confusion. Baclofen appears to be less effective in spasticity after cerebral injury than that of spinal origin and may increase the risk of seizure. Dantrolene sodium is more effective for treating spasticity of cerebral origin but can cause severe hepatic toxicity. Effective control of spasticity may require a combination of drugs in selected patients.[6]

Physical modalities that minimize tone include sustained stretching, vibration, cryotherapy, and the use of inhibiting postures. Splints are commonly used to maintain muscle length but to be most effective should be individually fabricated. Serial casting can dramatically increase muscle length and decrease spaticity. In addition, the circumferential pressure of the plaster may actually inhibit tone.

Peripheral nerve or motor point blocks can be effective in reducing spasticity localized to an extremity or muscle group, and should be considered as reasonable alternatives to systemic medications. Forty percent alcohol has been used, but 6% phenol has fewer side effects. Blocks should be performed using electrical stimulation to identify the myoneural junction or nerve sites for injection. Injections directly into mixed sensory-motor nerves may result in long-lasting dysesthesias. When spasticity is intense and cannot be adequately managed by the measures just mentioned, invasive orthopedic or neurosurgical measures may be indicated in the chronic phase. These might include tenotomies, muscle lengthening and releases, transposition, musculocutaneous and obturator neurectomies, and radio frequency rhizotomies.[7] Intrathecal phenol, simultaneous anterior and posterior rhizotomies or chordectomies are rarely indicated after brain injury.

CONTRACTURES

Increased tone and its attendant primitive flexor or extensor reactions lead to unbalanced motor activity and loss of muscle length. Bed rest and persistent immobility contribute dramatically to the development of contractures.[2] One major goal of early rehabilitation is mobilization and maintenance of functional muscle length.

Positioning the patient in bed requires avoidance of reflex patterns that may induce spasticity and ultimately contracture. Side lying with the hips flexed inhibits extensor tone of the lower extremities and should be used, if possible. Devices to prevent shoulder adduction and internal rotation, shoulder protraction, elbow flexion, wrist flexion and pronation, finger flexion and thumb adduction should be utilized prophylactically. Deforming forces of the lower extremity also should be avoided.[16]

Footboards should be avoided, since pressure over the metatarsal heads facilitates flexor spasticity with subsequent development of a plantar flexed contracture. The patient should not be allowed to maintain the hips and knees in constant flexion. Pillows, towel rolls, and foam wedges should be placed to abduct the shoulder, limit protraction, and in the lower extremities, partially abduct the hips. Trochanteric rolls can prevent excessive external rotation. Firm cones should be used to produce mild wrist dorsiflexion and functional positioning of the fingers. Careful attention must be directed toward maintaining the first interdigital web space. Soft rolls such as toweling may have limited utility, since their elastic effect may increase flexor tone. The use of air splints provides circumferential pressure and places the fingers in greater extension and may reduce tone most effectively.

In the presence of severe spasticity, contracture progression may be impossible to control, even in the most aggressive program.

SENSORY STIMULATION

The goals of sensory stimulation are to elicit first generalized then localized responses, to prevent "sensory deprivation" and increase environmental awareness, and, if possible, to mold responses into meaningful functions. It is an interdisciplinary effort, and should be incorporated into the routine daily nursing care plan.

Sensory stimulation should attempt not only to evoke normalized responses, but also should use appropriate environmental stimuli as well. When intracranial hypertension is a problem, a planned stimulation program should be delayed. Noxious stimuli should be avoided to reduce facilitation of abnormal primitive reflexes or reinforcement of spasticity. Stimuli should be introduced singly to allow for adequate evaluation of responses and to accommodate for the significant processing delay that is inevitably present. Planned stimulation should be provided for brief periods of time at first and eventually be incorporated into the overall treatment program.

If radio and television are to be used for stimulation, then they should be used for brief intervals so that habituation to the stimulus does not occur. Patients with severe neurologic deficits should be placed in rooms remote from the hospital paging system to control incidental auditory stimuli. When consistent responses appear, the program should try to obtain functional goals rather than provoke only response repetition.

The theoretical basis for sensory stimulation techniques as facilitators of recovery has not been established. Clearly, however, they require more discrete evaluation of the patient's functional responses than standard medical assessment allows. Such serial evaluations can frequently reveal subtle neurologic changes that are reflective of psychologic contact with the environment at an early phase. Also the potential negative aspects of sensory deprivation (all too common in intensive care units) are avoided.

FEEDING

It is imperative that the oral-bulbar structures be evaluated before instituting a safe oral feeding program. Methylene blue dye placed in a teaspoonful of food can help define when patients can safely tolerate oral feeding; blue or green dye in tracheal secretions confirm unsafe swallowing. Protective mechanisms such as the gag and cough reflexes should be at least weakly present before feeding is initiated. Videofluoroscopic analysis of swallowing can identify patients at risk for aspiration. The pharyngeal phase of swallowing cannot be identified by a bedside evaluation.[8]

Standard nasogastric tubes in addition to producing discomfort can cause pressure ulceration, granuloma formation, stenosis, chronic blood loss, reflux, esophagitis, and aspiration. If oral feeding does not progress at all after 2 weeks of an oral bulbar training program, the physician should consider placing a gastrostomy, jejunostomy, or esophagostomy tube. Endoscopic percutaneous gastrostomy can largely eliminate the problem of reflux, particularly if the feeding tube is placed in the jejunum and it eliminates the need to suture the stomach to the anterior abdominal wall to prevent leakage.[12]

Permanent gastrostomies generally are unnecessary, since many patients will resume oral feeding with continued training while feeding tubes are in place. Gastrostomy tubes should be located to allow full involvement in the physical rehabilitation program. Esophagostomies should be avoided if a strong asymmetric tonic neck reflex or torticollis is present.

COMMUNICATION

Language comprehension usually precedes expressive language in recovery from brain injury. Thus, evaluations of linguistic parameters may be more productive than evaluation of speech in determining deficits and appropriate remediation programs. During the period of post-traumatic amnesia, a substantial number of brain-injured patients will remain mute but still have useful language comprehension.

Dysarthria is the most common speech problem occurring after diffuse head injury; aphasia is far less frequent. The most commonly occurring deficits are linguistic, such as anomia and impaired comprehension for complex material. Attentional deficits also are characteristic of this group, and limit the patient's functional language abilities.

The initial steps in management hinge on the early development of functional communication. Since communication impairment often causes agitation, establishing communication will make the patient more cooperative and allow a more productive effort. Any motor act that can be repeated volitionally should be used to develop a communication system, be it control of finger movement or eye blink. Consistency in response to question or command is crucial. Therefore the entire treatment team, physician, nurse therapists, and family should be aware of and promote the development of this consistent response with a previously determined motor act.

Nonoral communication systems should be simple enough to be functional. Since the patient will improve as he proceeds through rehabilitation, purchase of expensive equipment should be deferred until such time as the patient's progress has stabilized and a long-term definitive solution is needed.

HETEROTOPIC OSSIFICATION

For many patients with central nervous system injury, ectopic calcifications and ossification of soft tissue remote from sites of trauma produces major functional problems. The commonly involved joints are the hips, elbows, and shoulders, occurring with greatest frequency in the most severely brain-damaged patients. Their incidence increases with prolonged coma, extremity fracture, traumatic calcification, and paralysis. Ectopic calcification may also occur secondary to direct trauma. Neurogenic heterotopic ossification (HO) may progress to total ankylosis of major joints, or cause compression of nerve or vascular structures. In patients at high risk, it may be advisable to consider prophylactic diphosphonate therapy.

Early presentation signs are the sudden onset of swelling, erythema, and pain in an extremity. Clinically, the ossification may be indistinguishable from deep vein thrombosis, but venography is negative. Bone scan studies clearly define the process. Serum alkaline phosphatase elevates early, but after the process has begun. This elevation usually precedes x-ray evidence of calcification.

Management includes routine, regular, full range of motion exercises: previously held concepts that therapy initiated the process have been discarded. Surgical removal of the anklylosing bony mass should be deferred until maturity of bone has occurred, usually about 1½ years post injury. In some cases with returning motor function, forceful manipulation of the mass under anesthesia has resulted in improved extremity use.[5]

AGITATION

Patients are often disoriented and confused as a result of amnesia and deficiencies of perception. This results in impaired self-control, uncooperativeness, and potential danger to patients and others. Management includes behavioral-environmental approaches, the use of restraints and pharmacologic interventions.[4]

Patients should be reassured both verbally and physically as often as possible and noxious stimuli removed whenever possible. Staffing should be consistent, since confused patients have little tolerance for change. Daily nursing and therapy routines should be brief to prevent cognitive overload, and on a consistent schedule that varies little from day to day. Activities that cause agitation should be minimized and other procedures substituted if possible. Automatic overlearned activities such as self-care should be incorporated whenever possible [15]

Vest restraints are reasonably well tolerated, and if necessary may be combined with soft extremity restraints. Four point restraints should be avoided if possible unless essential for patient safety. Even with the most agitated patient, planned periods of unrestrained extremity activities should be provided, since the restraints may contribute to increased confusion.

Drug therapy for agitated, disruptive behavior is indicated for safety and to allow the patient to participate in rehabilitation without impairing his ability to learn. Sedation to compensate for inadequate staffing ratios slows rehabilitation. Many of the commonly used medications, however, do impair learning and memory, may potentiate seizures, cause secondary neurologic syndromes, and theoretically may lead to state dependent learning. Thus, the potential benefits of medication must be balanced against their risks. Drugs such as propranolol and carbamazepine have less effect on cognition and attention and are therefore preferable to traditional psychotropic agents.[10]

FRACTURE MANAGEMENT

Intracranial injury and altered consciousness may obscure other injuries. As many as 10% of associated hip fractures have been undiagnosed at the time of admission to rehabilitation.

The patient's insensitivity to pain and impaired level of consciousness obscure some of the usual physical signs of fracture, and abnormal postures may be ascribed to spasticity. Persistent deformities may significantly limit the ultimate functional outcome, so that fractures and dislocations must be recognized and corrected early during acute care.

Trauma care should be given assuming that good neurologic recovery will occur. Given that spasticity, confusion, and agitation occur as coma resolves, uncontrolled limb movement should be anticipated. Therefore stable internal fixation of displaced fractures should be considered, preferrably soon after injury. Joint immobilization in flexed postures and prolonged traction (skeletal and skin) should be avoided.[3]

VISUAL SYSTEM

Injury to cranial nerves II, III, IV, and VI results in impaired acquisition of sensory information and perceptual processing. Diplopia also adds to patient confusion. An eye patch for the uninvolved eye can improve orientation and force maximal use of the involved eye. Alternative eye patching to prevent disuse amblyopia is unnecessary in the adolescent or adult. When a patient cortically supresses the second image, the eye patch should be discontinued. Many extraocular motor palsies resolve spontaneously; pleoptic strengthening exercises may speed recovery. Once the condition has stabilized, residual dysconjugate gaze can sometimes be improved by the use of prisms. If surgical correction is indicated (generally 9 to 12 months after injury) then the adjustable suture technique is preferred.

If visual field deficits are present, the patient may present with an abnormal head turn. Since this is a functional compensation strategy, no attempt to correct it should be made. Compensatory scanning techniques should be taught to the patient. For the patient with good cognitive function, fresnal lenses may increase functional scanning of the periphery.

Persistent convergence deficits are common after brain injury. Antiseizure drugs may also make it difficult for the patients to fuse an image for near vision. In some patients, eye convergence exercises may be beneficial.[6]

NEUROPSYCHOLOGIC RECOVERY

Physical recovery proceeds more rapidly than cognitive recovery, but the latter can continue to improve for a much longer time.

Post-traumatic amnesia is characterized by confusion and disorientation as well as an inability to learn new information and leads to a variety of aberrant behaviors. Most significant cognitive gains occur after the resolution of post-traumatic amnesia.

Language deficits are more common than speech problems, and characteristically consist of decreased verbal fluency, dysnomias, dysgraphia, and impairment of comprehension of complex material. Improving recovery of language usually also improves behavior and cognitive ability.[13]

NEUROPSYCHOLOGICAL TESTING

Neuropsychological testing that relies solely on IQ scores is inadequate in assessing the consequences of traumatic brain injury. Mental status evaluations fail to identify the functional deficits of higher order thought processing. An adequate evaluation should determine residual areas of function, the extent and nature of the deficits, how these deficits interact with functional abilities, what and how the patient can learn, and the efficiency of memory. The patient's capacity to learn new material including ability to access, store, and recall information should be established. It is only then that serial evaluations may contribute to the selection of appropriate intervention strategies.

A variety of medications including tranquilizers, antiseizure drugs, antihistamines, anticholinergics, may adversely affect patient performance in cognitive testing and rehabilitation. Drugs that interfere with cognitive performance should be used judiciously, if at all. Test batteries that determine the extent of impairment based on a single numerical value are of questionable value in diffuse brain injuries. Testing should emphasize linguistic functions rather than aphasia. Selection of specific tests based on identified deficits contribute more effectively to an understanding of the patient's deficits. Full neuropsychological testing is rarely profitable until well after post-traumatic amnesia has resolved.[14]

INTERVENTIONS DURING POST-TRAUMATIC AMNESIA

The neurotrauma unit should use environmental tools to reorient the patient. These include calendars, clocks, signs with the facility name and city in the patient's room and at the nursing station. Staff should be familiar with the patient's history, names of significant others and of pets to use in ordinary conversation. Pictures of familiar people and events should be in the room. The amount of visual information should not be overwhelming, in order to prevent a decay in information acquisition. Initial therapy is directed toward establishing a consistent motor act (such as finger movement, eye blinking) that can be developed into a simple communication system. It is important that physicians, nurses, other staff, and the family consistently use the same agreed on system. Prompt attention to linguistic potential may have a positive effect on patient cooperation as well as motoric recovery.

COGNITIVE REHABILITATION

Cognitive ability improves as a result of increased attention. Training the patient to attend to a task, to select the appropriate material for the task, and to process information from multiple sensory stimuli forms the basis of cognitive rehabilitation. Techniques that have long been successfully used in rehabilitation now are sometimes called "cognitive rehabilitation" and include orientation training, behavioral modification, compensation training, and perceptual motor training.[9] Cognitive rehabilitation now receives great emphasis in rehabilitation after brain injury. Despite this, cognitive rehabilitation still needs better definition, more consistent application, and stronger proof of efficacy.

As patients improve after the rehabilitation period, many may benefit from a structured learning program. Basic academic skills are the foundation on which higher order cortical functions (frontal lobe skills) can be built. Microcomputers are a valuable tool in this process, but are not a replacement for the therapist. Improved computer skills do not necessarily translate into improved cognitive or functional performance.

To benefit from cognitive retraining, the patient must have some intact ability, the therapist must select appropriate strategies, and the patient must be able to apply the skills learned beyond the narrow confines of the therapy session.

LATER REHABILITATION

Brain injury can result in long-term deficits in physical, cognitive, behavioral, and psychosocial spheres. Long-term intervention is frequently needed to maximize the process of recovery. Cost-effective intervention must rely on a supportive environment requiring involvement of family, friends, and the community. Although physical recovery occurs rather rapidly, years of intervention are required to integrate effectively the severely brain-injured survivor into society.

Specialized programs for behavioral interventions and for cognitive and academic restructuring offer substantial potential for appropriate patients. The development of learning disability programs for brain-injured patients in educational institutions substantially lowers the long-term costs and does so among a patient's peers. Supportive employment also allows for ongoing vocational rehabilitation and a chance to advance in one's career ladder. Adaptive physical education and recreation can improve physical skills and reduce the social isolation so common to patients after severe brain injury.

If rehabilitation is to succeed, the patient's family must be involved. Accurate information and comprehensive training throughout the patient's care can equip the family for the arduous task of reintegration into the family and into society. We must accept the responsibility of providing and overseeing this aspect of medical service. Failure to do so results in patient failure to reintegrate into the world. The process of rehabilitation after severe brain injury is indeed lifelong. It requires appropriate medical management, prevention of complications, aid in helping the patient to develop optimal relationships with family and friends, and to achieve a productive meaningful life within the limits of his nervous system injury.

REFERENCES

1. Berrol S: The rehabilitation process. Semin Neurol 5:205–211, 1985.
2. Booth FW: Effect of limb immobilization on skeletal muscle. J Appl Physiol 52:1113–1118, 1982.
3. Botte MJ, Moore TJ: The orthopedic management of extremity injuries in head trauma. J Head Trauma Rehabil 2:13–17, 1987.
4. Cohadon F: The importance of rehabilitation programs in the prevention and alleviation of head injury sequelae. Prog Neurol Surg 10:344–384, 1981.
5. Garland DE, Hanscom DA, Keenan MA, Smith C, Moore T: Resection of heterotopic ossification in the adult with head trauma. J Bone Joint Surg 67(A):1261–1269, 1985.
6. Glenn MB, Rosenthal M: Rehabilitation following severe traumatic brain injury. Semin Neurol 5:233–246, 1985.
7. Kasdon DL, Lathi ES: A prospective study of radiofrequency rhizotomy in the treatment of posttraumatic spasticity. Neurosurgery 15:526–529, 1984.
8. Lazarus C, Logemann JA: Swallowing disorders in closed head trauma patients. Arch Phys Med Rehabil 68: 79–84, 1987.
9. Luria AR, Naydin VL, Tsvetkova LS, Vinarskaya EN: Restoration of higher cortical function following local brain damage. In PJ Vinken, GW Bruyn (eds): Handbook of Clinical Neurology. Amsterdam: North Holland Publishing, 1969, pp 368–432.
10. O'Shanick GJ: Clinical aspects of psychopharmacologic treatment in head-injured patients. J Head Trauma Rehabil 2:59–67, 1987.

11. Perry J: Rehabilitation of the neurologically disabled patient: Principles, practice, and scientific basis. J Neurosurg 58:799–816, 1983.
12. Ponsky JL, Gauderer MW, Stellato TA: Percutaneous endoscopic gastrostomy. Review of 150 cases. Arch Surg 118:913–914, 1983.
13. Prigatano GP: Neuropsychological Rehabilitation after Brain Injury. Baltimore: Johns Hopkins University Press, 1986, pp 1–28.
14. Walsh KW: Understanding Brain Damage. A Primer of Neuropsychological Evaluation. New York: Churchill Livingstone, 1985, pp 144–182.
15. Wood RL: Behavioral disorders following severe brain injury: Their presentation and psychological management. In Brooks N: Closed Head Injury. Psychological, Social, and Family Consequences. Oxford: Oxford University Press, 1984.
16. Yarkony GM, Sahgal V: Contractures. A major complication of craniocerebral trauma. Clin Orthop 219:93–96, 1987.

20

Neurotrauma and Emergency Medical Services Organization

LAWRENCE H. PITTS

More than 140,000 Americans die after trauma each year and at least 25,000 or more are chronically institutionalized. Trauma accounts for more years of potential life lost than cancer and cardiovascular disease combined[13] (Table 20–1) because of its preponderance in the young[8] (Table 20–2). About 350 to 500 people per one million are hospitalized each year after craniocerebral trauma.[19] Head injury accounts for half or more of trauma deaths in most reported series, and more than 80,000 people in the United States are permanently disabled with head or spinal cord injuries each year.[8] More people die from head injury than any other disorder treated by neurosurgeons, and trauma is second only to stroke as a cause of death from neurologic diseases. In the aggregate, neurosurgeons spend almost 20% of their time treating patients with head and spinal cord injury.[24]

Numerous investigators have reported that the absence of regional trauma planning has led to as many as 20 to 30% of trauma deaths that would otherwise be preventable.[12,33] Recently, reports have noted significant improvement in trauma care where trauma centers existed[32] or after they were established,[10,11] including declines in the rates of preventable (14 to 3%) and of suboptimal treatment (32 to 4%) before and after institution of a regional trauma system.[28] Such information has prompted many local, county, and state governments to begin design and enactment of trauma care systems. The necessary resources for optimal care of trauma patients have been specified by the American College of Surgeons Committee on Trauma (ACS-COT)[1] and a number of hospitals are becoming trauma centers.[17]

Although central nervous system (CNS) damage is a major portion of serious trauma, there are far fewer neurosurgeons than other medical and surgical specialists who treat injury patients. In 1984, there were about ten times as many board certified general surgeons and six times as many orthopedists as the nearly 3500 neurosurgeons estimated to practice in the United States. Although not all general surgeons or orthopedists treat trauma patients, neither do all neurosurgeons, making an even smaller group of surgeons treating CNS

246

Table 20–1   Potential Years of Life Lost Before Age 65 Years*

Trauma	41%
Cancer	18%
Heart disease	16%
All others	25%

*From Centers for Disease Control.[13]

Table 20–2   Percentage of Deaths from Various Causes

AGE (YR)	INJURY	CANCER	HEART DISEASE	OTHER
1–4	46	7	4	43
5–14	55	14	3	28
15–24	79	5	3	13
25–34	62	10	6	22
35–44	31	21	20	28
45–64	7	32	36	25
≥65	2	19	48	31

*Adapted from Baker et al.[8]

injuries. Since many hospitals are expanding their emergency medicine facilities as a source of new patients, and hospital staffs are asked to cover these emergency rooms, the relative scarcity of neurosurgeons is even more noticeable. In some European countries, neurologists manage head injury patients not requiring surgery and, at times, they direct the postoperative care of patients with operated traumatic lesions. However, in agreement with the ACS-COT, neurosurgeons in the United States believe that "trauma is a surgical disease"[1] and that neurotrauma is best treated by neurosurgeons.

Urgent or emergency treatment of traumatic injuries often disrupts the smooth pattern of routine medical care and elective surgery schedules during the day, or more commonly, preempts emergency medical and hospital resources and physician energies at night or on weekends,[34] occurring at "unsocial hours," as noted by Bryan Jennett. For all of these reasons—the enormous impact of trauma on the public health, particularly of the young, the prevalence of CNS injury in patients with severe trauma, the relatively small numbers of neurosurgeons available to treat trauma patients, and the strains placed on medical resources by the care of trauma and neurotrauma patients—it is imperative that trauma care planning in general and the neurosurgeons role in particular be well defined in each locale to assure delivery of the quality of care that now is possible and that the public demands and deserves. Neurosurgeons must become involved in this planning process if their patients and their own needs and interests are to be met. The following elements should be considered during the planning process.

PREHOSPITAL EMERGENCY MEDICAL SERVICES

Explosive advances in the quality, diversity, and sophistication in Emergency Medical Services (EMS) systems in the past decade have produced significant changes in a number of emergency medical problems.[15] Except in some rural areas, ambulance services no longer are staffed by firemen, policemen, or volunteers. The overwhelming majority of EMS are manned by highly trained professional paramedics or Emergency Medical Technicians (EMTs) whose training programs include extensive exposure to didactic classroom presentations, practical clinical instruction, and on the job training in delivery of emergency medical care. These EMTs all are under medical control, which has ultimate responsibility for training and quality assurance, and it is through this medical control structure that trauma-receiving facilities must coordinate EMT activities. There often is a fierce pride among paramedics and EMTs, and a careful balance must be struck between too lax and too tight a control on their management of patients. The former can lead to their making medical judgments too complex for their training, and the latter can preclude their exercising good judgment under difficult circumstances in the field.

A number of important EMS issues must be addressed and settled during trauma system planning. Population density and distances to trauma facilities will dictate the style of initial EMS care. In urban environments, with designated trauma facilities nearby, a "scoop and run" technique will allow the most rapid delivery of critically injured patients to definitive care.[21] In remote locations, more time probably should be spent "at the roadside" stabilizing the patient for a fairly long transport time by surface or air. An initial brief stop at a hospital not normally part of the trauma system may provide temporizing but lifesaving medical care, such as placement of chest or endotracheal tubes, fracture splinting, or blood transfusions, before transfer for definitive care. In suburban areas, careful guidelines must be established for EMS personnel, directing them to transport patients according to a defined local trauma plan, either to designated trauma hospitals or to nearby hospitals as determined best by the planning process.

An essential feature of an appropriate EMS response is patient evaluation and triage. Only some 8 to 10% of trauma patients require care at a Level I[1] hospital.[31] Inadequate triage either will send too many patients to Level I facilities with overutilization of costly resources when a lower level facility could deliver proper and more economical care, or will send too few patients to Level I facilities with some severely injured patients arriving at hospitals unable to manage them properly. Neurosurgeons, in their planning efforts, should define proper triage tools for neurologic injuries and instruct EMS personnel in their use. It has been proposed, for example, that patients with a Glasgow Coma Score[29] of less than 13 be taken to a Level I facility.[2] Triage tools for trauma outside the nervous system also have been developed and should be considered by other surgeons in the trauma planning process.[7,9,14] It is important for neurosurgeons to develop and review EMS protocols, particularly regarding neural trauma, and for training EMS personnel to evaluate neurologic injuries.

EMERGENCY ROOM ORGANIZATION

Emergency resuscitation after major trauma is exacting and complex, and the spectrum of traumatic injuries demands considerable diagnostic skill. In the absence of a surgeon trained in trauma management, properly trained emergency room personnel, including emergency physicians, are required for optimum delivery of trauma care.[30]

The ACS-COT Hospital Resources guidelines,[1] recognizing the prevalence and urgency of severe neurologic injury, requires that a neurosurgeon be "in house" in Level I and Level II facilities. Because it is impossible for fully trained neurosurgeons physically to be in all of the trauma facilities across the country, non-neurosurgeons can meet this requirement if approved by that hospital's Chief of Neurosurgery as being able to initiate immediate therapy and diagnostic procedures while the neurosurgeon is en route to the hospital after his presence is requested by emergency room personnel. In teaching hospitals, this function may be fulfilled by resident house staff or an in-house surgeon or physician who has been trained by the hospital's neurosurgeons to begin care of neurologic injury. The trauma facility's neurosurgical staff should either provide neurosurgical coverage or train in-house trauma physicians to begin the therapy and diagnostic procedures most appropriate for the patient.

Outcome after severe head injury correlates adversely with shock and hypoxia,[18,25] and these secondary insults must be addressed aggressively in prehospital and emergency room neurotrauma care. Life-threatening hemorrhage or respiratory problems must be corrected immediately regardless of the neurologic status. Sequential neurologic evaluations carefully documented can be used to ascertain improvement or worsening and will dictate subsequent patient management.

Depending on the degree of neurologic abnormality or evidence of external injury, a number of diagnostic or therapeutic pathways may be taken. In patients who are either comatose or have significant mental status alterations, CT scanning usually is done. If a patient rapidly deteriorates[27] or has signs of transtentorial herniation or brainstem compression with clear-cut evidence of trauma,[5] diagnostic burr holes can be done without computed tomography (CT) scanning and probably will reduce the time required to obtain brain decompression by craniotomy. Patients with altered mental status following a generalized seizure should improve within an hour of seizure, and patients who are intoxicated should improve over 2 to 3 hours of observation; their initial management may include serial observation. However, if they do not improve within these general time frames and there is evidence of head injury, CT scanning should be considered to rule out intracranial pathologic conditions requiring urgent attention. Specific protocols can be developed to determine those patients who routinely require admission and those who can be observed initially in the emergency room.[16,20] It is incumbent on neurosurgeons to help develop these protocols and, by instruction and monitoring of emergency room personnel, ensure that the protocols are followed. Since many patients with minor head injury can be treated appropriately without neurousurgery consultation, it is important that neurosurgeons help define who those patients are and to encourage trauma physicians and emergency room physicians to treat them without consultation. Proper instruction of physicians who first see patients in the emergency room setting will reduce the number of unnecessary calls that neurosurgeons receive and allow their time to be spent more appropriately on patients with significant head injuries.

Thus, the neurosurgeon's role in the emergency management of patients with head injury is to help define appropriate patient categories and establish protocols for their diagnostic and therapeutic management, to instruct emergency room personnel in the use of their protocols, and, finally, to monitor periodically the skill with which these protocols are carried out.

OPERATING ROOM ORGANIZATION

It is possible for the vast majority of American hospitals to acquire necessary operating room equipment to manage even the most severe traumatic injuries, including cardiac bypass capabilities. Proper neurosurgical equipment will be available in any operating room where a full spectrum of elective neurosurgery cases are treated. Most neurotrauma cases do not require a microscope or microsurgical instrument, although they should be available if needed. Intraoperative ultrasound is being used more frequently for intracerebral hematomas or foreign bodies and to ensure adequate spinal canal decompression, and it should be available if requested by the neurosurgeon. X-ray technicians and equipment should be available for intraoperative radiographs when requested.

Equipment generally is not a problem; operating room staffing certainly can be. For Level I and II trauma hospitals, an operating room must be available at all times for emergency thoracotomy, laparatomy, or craniotomy, and appropriate anesthesia and nursing personnel must be available and in house for such cases. It is unpopular, and expensive, to commit resources in such a stand-by mode unless they are used frequently. Surgeons, particularly those with no interest in trauma care, seeking daytime elective operating room time are unsympathetic when an operating room is standing idle "waiting for a trauma case," and they want to begin another elective or added case. Hospital administrators want to minimize salary costs for in-house anesthesia and nursing staff, but they cannot reduce available personnel too far without losing the ability to initiate immediate surgery when needed. At least some minimal annual number of trauma cases is necessary for proper operating room staffing to be cost effective and to perform efficiently when emergency surgery is required.

Neurosurgeons and their trauma colleagues must assure themselves of proper and timely hospital support for operative cases, or refuse to support trauma designation at that institution. Differences in institution commitment in operating room, emergency room, and intensive care unit (ICU) staffing usually will dictate the most appropriate hospital for designation as a trauma-receiving facility, and neurosurgeons can best determine an institution's commitment to care of the neurotrauma patient.

NEUROTRAUMA INTENSIVE CARE

Intensive care management of trauma patients has changed dramatically in the past decade. Substantial numbers of ICU beds have been added in most acute care hospitals, improving intensive management of critically ill patients but usually lowering the acuity of care of patients on general medical or surgical wards. Substantial technological advancements in physiological monitoring and cardiopulmonary care have evolved in ICUs. Finally, with relatively large numbers of critically ill patients in ICUs, critical care specialists have arisen from a number of medical specialties, including neurosurgery, surgery, anesthesia, internal medicine, and pediatrics. In some institutions, neurological ICUs have remained under the direct control of neurologists and neurosurgeons, some of whom have had special fellowship training in intensive care. In other instances, local use of consultation from anesthesiologists, internists, and others has provided additional skills in appropriate cases. As in other areas of planning for the care of the neurotrauma patient, individual neurosurgeons must assess their own skills and availability in deriving a plan for the optimum management of patients with neurotrauma.[26]

No physician is better prepared than the neurosurgeon for the management of critically ill patients with nervous system injury.[26] Assessment of patient status, particularly including deterioration, should fall to his purview. Since the management of neurologic injury sometimes is at odds with the management of other problems and since neurologic injury so commonly dictates eventual patient outcome, the neurosurgeon must maintain an important influence in patient management as long as the nervous system is physiologically unstable. For instance, in many cases of general trauma, fluid management can be quite liberal and large fluid volumes commonly are used in resuscitation and in the acute phase of trauma management. However, when nervous system injury is present, overhydration in some patients can lead to increased cerebral swelling, particularly if serum sodium or osmolarity falls. The mild hypotension seen with many cervical spinal cord injuries is either best untreated or treated with low doses of vasopressor agents after possible internal hemorrhage has been excluded, instead of infusion of large fluid volumes so routinely used by trauma surgeons to treat hypotension. No other specialist will appreciate as well as the neurosurgeon these nuances of therapy, and thus, the neurosurgeon has an important role and obligation in the intensive management of patients with nervous system injuries.

The ACS-COT guidelines[1] require that a trauma service be an organizational unit of Level I and Level II trauma facilities. When such a service exists, multiple trauma patients often are managed by the trauma team[22] with essential input from other specialists, such as neurosurgeons, urologists, and orthopedic surgeons. Such an organization has been reported to reduce ICU mortality in severely injured patients.[6] In many instances, as the various injuries become less acute, the patient eventually is transferred to the care of the specialist with the greatest expertise in caring for the most problematic residual injury, for example, an orthopedist for the management of complex extremity fractures. Because of the prevalence in severity of injuries to the brain and spinal cord, often the patient is transferred to a neurosurgery service for management after the other organ injuries have become stable. This "trauma team" concept has been used successfully in a large number of trauma centers. However, for it to work satisfactorily, there has to be a strong commitment by the hospital's surgical staff. In these instances, the trauma team becomes an important resource for treating patients with complex injuries. The neurosurgeon is an important member of this team whenever CNS injuries are present and he or she can beneficially affect the management of the patient's neurologic injuries. If a well-developed trauma team does not exist in a given hospital, the neurosurgeon may need to become the trauma team leader and organize the efforts of various appropriate specialties. In patients with multiple complex injuries this is an arduous task that falls to a surgeon skilled in the management of trauma who, in some institutions, will be the neurosurgeon.

Since the neurosurgeon will rarely be in the ICU on a full-time basis, he or she has an important additional role in nursing and staff education. The neurosurgeon should help develop ICU charting and record-keeping so that adverse changes in patient status can be appreciated using routine neurologic status recording, such as the Glasgow Coma Score and standardized muscle strength testing. Once appropriate scales have been incorporated into patient observation charts, the nursing staff must be instructed in their use. ICU physicians and nursing staffs must be able to evaluate neurosurgical patients adequately so that they can accurately detect patient deterioration and notify the neurosurgeon promptly. After the neurosurgeon has instituted appropriate instruction of the nursing staff in the proper use of neurologic observation tools, he should help monitor their use to ensure appropriate and adequate use.

The neurosurgeon also needs to standardize management protocols insofar as possible. If intracranial pressure (ICP) monitoring is used in a given hospital, monitoring technique and ICP management protocols must be devised and the nursing staff become competent in their use. Careful instruction of nurses to increase their skills and allay their fears will produce valuable allies for the neurosurgeon and his patients in the ICU.

RELATIONSHIPS AMONG HOSPITALS

Not all hospitals are able or wish to participate in a region's trauma system. As already noted, there often will not be enough neurosurgeons in a given area to staff adequately all those hospitals that do seek trauma facility status. Finally, there will be instances when a trauma facility's neurosurgeon is unavoidably unavailable, such as with an on-going trauma case, and adequate neurosurgical back-up cannot be obtained. In all of these instances, it will be necessary to transfer patients with CNS trauma with or without other organ involvement to another facility inside or outside that region for definitive neurosurgical care. Appropriate plans must be made in advance for orderly transfer of such patients under medical control to other facilities where prompt neurosurgical attention is available.[4]

When a neurosurgeon who is responsible for trauma coverage at a given trauma-receiving facility is unavailable, he should notify the hospital and try to work with them to secure adequate coverage until he is again available.[3] In some cases for limited periods of time, one of the other neurosurgeons on the call schedule might be able to provide temporary coverage. If such coverage cannot be obtained, trauma cases involving the nervous system should be diverted to the nearest trauma-receiving facility that does have coverage at that time. As soon as neurosurgical coverage is available at the first hospital, the diversion can be canceled and trauma patients received in the usual fashion. EMS should be notified when diversion is temporarily in place so that they can most expeditiously take a trauma patient to the appropriate facility without the potentially disastrous delay of taking a patient to a first facility only to find that adequate care cannot be delivered.

This sort of structure and written transfer agreements must be designed and implemented in advance, including appropriate financial agreements if a local or regional government is financially responsible for a patient's emergency medical care. Prearrangement will avoid potentially life-threatening delays that can occur shortly after injury. These matters cannot be dealt with smoothly at night or on weekends when most trauma occurs, and adequate planning is necessary for smooth transfers or diversions to occur.

NEUROTRAUMA SYSTEM ORGANIZATION

In the early 1970s, regionalized trauma centers were strongly encouraged by federal legislation, but funding for that initiative waned by 1980. Recently, with urging from a number of groups because of the obvious economic and societal benefits of trauma systems,[15] trauma legislation has emerged again. Several states have mandated regional trauma organization and about one third of the states have trauma care guidelines that likely will become regulations in the next several years. Bills currently under discussion in both houses of Congress, if enacted, will require that virtually all states have trauma care plans.

Since neurotrauma is so prevalent in injured patients, and since "trauma is a surgical disease,"[1] neurosurgeons are central figures in trauma system design. The ACS optimal care guidelines[1] recognize neurotrauma's importance, and a neurosurgeon's presence or prompt availability is required at Level I and Level II trauma facilities. Since there are some 35,000 general surgeons and less than one tenth as many neurosurgeons, it is clear that a disproportionate trauma burden falls on individual neurosurgeons. This burden carries with it, however, the opportunity for neurosurgeons to claim their pivotal position in defining trauma care systems. It is imperative that neurosurgeons enter this planning process so that they can devise systems that work best for neurotrauma patients and also can be managed effectively by the nation's few neurosurgeons.

Many trauma system designs have been used in various areas around the United States. Generally speaking, smaller communities with only one hospital need little planning, since their one hospital is "the only show in town." Similarly, in well-organized urban centers, trauma centers have long been functioning, although there are some urban areas where trauma patients still are taken to the nearest hospital with little coordination among various institutions. In these latter urban areas and in many suburban areas, where multiple community hospitals often are in fierce competition, trauma plans frequently function poorly or do not exist.

Because legislated trauma organization is becoming the rule, it would be useful to consider several regional trauma care plans, devised with substantial neurosurgical input, which might be considered as models for new regional or local trauma systems. At least three states have mandated organization for trauma care. Virginia has established six Level I trauma centers geographically distributed throughout the state. Helicopter transport is frequently used for trauma patients to be taken to these centers. The Virginia trauma centers all contribute data to a centralized registry, which may, in the future, allow outcome assessment at and among trauma centers.

Pennsylvania has established a program for verifying trauma facility level designation throughout the state. Although there is no legislated distribution of trauma centers, this system allows uniform application of trauma standards to hospitals and allows them to qualify for participation in trauma systems.

California has established regulations for determining level designation among hospitals with emergency rooms. These regulations, like those in Virginia and Pennsylvania, closely parallel the ACS guidelines for level designation, with some modifications in each state. The California State Emergency Medical Services authority has delegated responsibility regionally, often on a county basis, to define a trauma care plan for any given region. Within the broad guidelines established by the state, at least five different systems have been adopted and, in each case, neurosurgeons played a central role in determining the specifics of the local plan. It would be instructive to review these plans as possible models for application in other parts of the United States.

San Francisco County has long been served by a single Level I trauma facility, which serves as the base station for the city ambulance service. All major specialties are represented by in-house resident house staff with in-house presence of attending surgeons and emergency physicians in the hospital most hours of the day. Occasionally, trauma cases are diverted to other hospitals in the city by prearrangement when the hospital cannot accept additional patients, usually because of unavailability of critical care beds. This model seems ideal for densely populated urban areas with the actual population dictating the number of such facilities required in a given city.

San Diego County adopted a carefully planned trauma care system in 1983, using six trauma-receiving facilities geographically distributed around the county. This system has a thorough quality assessment program and frequent meetings of system organizers to monitor closely the quality of trauma care. Neurosurgeons in San Diego County were instrumental in helping devise the plan and have supported it strongly. It is of interest that fewer trauma craniotomies have been required than was initially anticipated, and a current modification of the original plan is being investigated that would allow one group of neurosurgeons to designate an on-call member who will cover several hospitals simultaneously with a certain back-up system for the unusual need for a neurosurgeon in two hospitals simultaneously. This modification will be evaluated by the quality assessment process in San Diego County.

Orange County adopted a trauma care system using five Level I facilities within the county. This system was antedated by a system of neurotrauma-receiving centers that were established in the mid-1970s. Before that time, some 30 hospitals within Orange County received trauma patients by ambulance. An autopsy review[33] cited deficiencies in the adequacy of trauma care, and the neurotrauma receiving facilities were established to improve neurotrauma care. Orange County neurosurgeons assessed how many of themselves wished to treat trauma patients and which hospitals should be covered for trauma care. About 12 centers were initially designated, which number was subsequently reduced to nine. Major trauma is taken to the Level I trauma centers (now four in number) and isolated head or spinal cord injury patients are taken to one of the neurotrauma-receiving facilities (of which four also are Level I facilities). A recent review has indicated that the Orange County plan is working well and that field triage of multiple trauma patients has resulted in only rare multisystem trauma patients being taken to the neurotrauma-receiving facilities. The review raised some questions about the adequacy of coverage and the importance of establishing fail-safe call schedules and also raised questions about the adequacy of quality assessment. These issues will have to be monitored closely in the coming years as the Orange County model is evaluated.

Sonoma County had been served until 1987 by a single community hospital where that county's neurosurgeons practiced. Recently, a second hospital administered by the county sought permission to be a second trauma-receiving facility. This request initially was denied because of lack of neurosurgical coverage. However, the hospital upgraded their facilities to the point that the area's neurosurgeons were willing to provide neurotrauma care, and permission was granted for the second hospital to enter the trauma system. This, in essence, is a change from a single trauma facility, which follows the ACS guidelines more closely, to a two-hospital system with the second hospital having entered the process for a variety of economic, house staff training, and patient care reasons. This change from a one- to a two-hospital system should periodically be reevaluated to determine whether or not this will have a beneficial or adverse effect on neurotrauma care.

San Mateo County, covering a long, thin corridor of suburban population, considered various alternative systems for trauma care. Because of the distances and population densities involved, and against the recommendation of at least some well-known trauma surgeons, San Mateo County decided to have an eight hospital trauma system with the facilities distributed geographically throughout the region. The county's neurosurgeons supported this particular type of designation. This new process essentially has patients taken "to the nearest hospital." A careful quality assessment effort will be required to assure that this relatively diffuse trauma care system does not adversely affect patient outcome.

SUMMARY

For optimal care of neurotrauma, the neurosurgeon has an obligation to develop and implement schemes for emergency and urgent neurosurgical care. This must be done in advance of the need of such systems and further requires that a region's neurosurgeons and other trauma surgeons monitor the system that they have planned to assure its efficacy.[23] The planning process requires that neurosurgeons assess their region's needs and their own ability to meet those needs. They must determine how many hospitals are required to provide appropriate trauma care availability and how they will staff those hospitals. This may exclude some facilities from providing trauma care for lack of adequate neurosurgical coverage. A designation of trauma facilities is a political process[23] and neurosurgeons should learn how to have their recommendations accepted and acted on by regional and state trauma system directors. This obviously will be done best when neurosurgeons speak with a unified voice. It is in their and their patient's interest for neurosurgeons to agree to a single plan and then strive to have it accepted by other parts of the trauma care system.

The five particular areas that require neurosurgeons' involvement in planning include:

1. Development and implementation of EMS protocols regarding neurotrauma.
2. Emergency room management, including resuscitation and initiation of diagnostic procedures
3. Appropriate operating room organization, which will allow immediate surgical care of appropriate patients;
4. Trauma service and ICU organizational design to ensure appropriate neurosurgical input in the care of the trauma patient
5. Development of diversion and transfer plans when usual neurosurgical coverage at a trauma facility is unavoidably unavailable.

Trauma is a surgical disease and neurotrauma should be treated preponderantly by neurosurgeons. Their involvement in neurotrauma care planning will best ensure their appropriate dominance in this area and assure optimum care for their injured patients.

REFERENCES

1. American College of Surgeons Committee on Trauma: Hospital and Prehospital Resources for Optimal Care of the Injured Patient. Chicago: American College of Surgeons, 1988.
2. American College of Surgeons Committee on Trauma: Hospital and Prehospital Resources for Optimal Care of the Injured Patient. Chicago: American College of Surgeons, 1988, pp 37–41.
3. American College of Surgeons Committee on Trauma: Hospital and Prehospital Resources for Optimal Care of the Injured Patient. Chicago: American College of Surgeons, 1988, pp 51–52.
4. American College of Surgeons Committee on Trauma: Hospital and Prehospital Resources for Optimal Care of the Injured Patient Chicago: American College of Surgeons, 1988, pp 19–22.
5. Andrews BT, Pitts LH, Lovely MP, Bartkowski HM: Is computed tomographic scanning necessary in patients with tentorial herniation? Results of immediate surgical exploration without computed tomography in 100 patients. Neurosurgery 19:408–414, 1986.
6. Baker CC. Degutes LD, DeSantis J, Baue AE: Impact of a trauma service on trauma care in a university hospital. Am J Surg 149:453–458, 1985.
7. Baker SP, O'Neill B: The injury severity score: An update. J Trauma 16:882, 1976.
8. Baker SP, O'Neill B, Karpf R: The Injury Fact Book. Lexington, MA: Lexington Books, 1984.
9. Boyd CR, Tolson MA, Copes WS: Evaluating trauma care: the TRISS method. J Trauma 27:370–378, 1987.
10. Cales RH: Trauma mortality in Orange County: The effect of implementation of a regional trauma system. Ann Emerg Med 13:1–10, 1984.
11. Cales RH, Anderson PG, Heilig RW: Utilization of medical care in Orange County: The effect of implementation of a regional trauma system. Ann Emerg Med 14:853–858, 1985.
12. Cales RH. Trunkey DD: Preventable trauma deaths: A review of trauma care systems development. JAMA 254:1059–1063, 1985.

13. Centers for Disease Control. Morbid Mortal Weekly Rep 31:599, 1982.
14. Champion HR, Sacco WJ, Hannan DS, et al.: Assessment of injury severity: The Triage Index. Crit Care Med 8:201–208, 1980.
15. Craren EJ, Ornato JP, Nelson NM: The investment. jems 5:35–38, 1985.
16. Dacy RG, Alves WM: Neurological complications after apparently minor head injury. J Neurosurg 65:203–210, 1986
17. Dunn EL, Berry PH, Cross RE: Community hospital to trauma center. J Trauma 26:733–737, 1986.
18. Eisenberg HM: Outcome after head injury: General considerations. In Becker DP, Povlishock JT (eds): Central Nervous System Trauma Status Report. Bethesda, MD: National Institutes of Health, 1985, pp 271–280.
19. Frankowski RF, Annegers JF, Whitman S: Epidemiological and descriptive studies: The descriptive epidemiology of head trauma in the United States. In Becker DP, Povlishock JT (eds): Central Nervous System Trauma Status Report. Bethesda, MD: National Institutes of Health, 1985, pp 33–43.
20. Feuerman T, Wackym PA, Gade GF, Becker DP: Value of skull radiography, head computed tomographic scanning and admission for observation in cases of minor head injury. Neurosurgery 22:449–453, 1988.
21. Lewis FR: Prehospital intravenous fluid therapy: Physiologic computer modelling. J Trauma 26:804–811, 1986.
22. Maull KI, Haynes BW: The integrated trauma service concept. JACEP 6:497–499, 1977.
23. Maull KI, Schwab CW, McHenry SD, Leavy P, Carl L, Woo P, Overholt S, Sinclair T, Aprahamian C: Trauma center verification. J Trauma 26:521–524, 1986.
24. Mendenhall RC, Watts C, Radecki SE, Girard RA: Neurosurgery in the United States: Log-diary study. Neurosurgery 8:267–276, 1981.
25. Miller JD, Sweet RC, Narayan R, Becker DP: Early insults to the injured brain. JAMA 240:439–442, 1978.
26. Pitts LH: The neurointensive care unit—who's in charge? Clin Neurosurg 35:55–67, 1988.
27. Rockswold GL: Management of closed head injury patients who "talked and deteriorated." Neurosurgery 22:614, 1988.
28. Shackford SR, Hollingworth-Fridlund P, Cooper GF, Eastman AB: The effect of regionalization upon the quality of trauma care as assessed by concurrent audit before and after institution of a trauma system: A preliminary report. J Trauma 26:812–820, 1986.
29. Teasdale G, Jennett B: Assessment of coma and impaired consciousness: A practical scale. Lancet 2:81–84, 1974.
30. Thompson CT: The emergency physician, the trauma surgeon, and the trauma center. Ann Emerg Med 12:235–237, 1983.
31. Thompson CT: Trauma care: Commitment to excellence. Ann Emerg Med 9:538, 1980.
32. West JG, Cales RH, Gazzaniga AB: Impact of regionalization: The Orange County experience. Arch Surg 118:740–744, 1983.
33. West JG, Trunkey DD, Lim RC: Systems of trauma care—a study of two counties. Arch Surg 114:455, 1979.
34. Young JS, Burns PE, Bowen AM, McCutchen R: Spinal cord injury statistics. Good Samaritan Medical Center, Phoenix, Arizona, 1982.

Index

4